Clinical Focus on
ART

Clinical Focus on ART

Series Editors

Narendra Malhotra
MD FIAJAGO FICMU FICOG FICMCH FRCOG FICS FMAS FIAPM FICRM
Managing Director
Global Rainbow Health Care and MNMH (P) Ltd and
Ujala Cygnus Rainbow Hospital
Agra, Uttar Pradesh, India

Jaideep Malhotra
MD FICOG FICS FIUMB FICMCH FMAS FRCPI FRCOG FICRM FIAPM
Managing Director
ART Rainbow IVF Infertility
Agra, Uttar Pradesh, India

Neharika Malhotra
MD (Gold Medalist) DRM (Germany) DMIS FICMCH FMAS FICOG
ICOG Fellowship in Reproductive Medicine DGC
Consultant
Department of Obstetrics and Gynecology
Ujala Cygnus Rainbow Hospital
Agra, Uttar Pradesh, India

Neha Priyadarshini
MD FRM FICOG FICMCH
Medical Director
Department of IVF
Satvik IVF
Dhanbad, Jharkhand, India

Foreword

Jatin Shah

JAYPEE

JAYPEE BROTHERS MEDICAL PUBLISHERS

The Health Sciences Publisher

New Delhi | London

JAYPEE **Jaypee Brothers Medical Publishers (P) Ltd**

Headquarters
EMCA House, 23/23-B
Ansari Road, Daryaganj
New Delhi 110 002, India
Landline: +91-11-23272143, +91-11-23272703
+91-11-23282021, +91-11-23245672
e-mail: jaypee@jaypeebrothers.com

Corporate Office
4838/24, Ansari Road, Daryaganj
New Delhi 110 002, India
Phone: +91-11-43574357
Fax: +91-11-43574314
e-mail: jaypee@jaypeebrothers.com

Overseas Office
JP Medical Ltd.
83, Victoria Street, London
SW1H 0HW (UK)
Phone: +44-20 3170 8910
e-mail: info@jpmedpub.com

EU GPSR Authorised Representative
Logos Europe, 9 rue Nicolas Poussin
17000, La Rochelle, France
Phone: +33 (0) 6 67 93 73 78
e-mail: contact@logoseurope.eu

Website: www.jaypeebrothers.com
Website: www.jaypeedigital.com

Clinical Focus on ART

First Edition: **2026**

ISBN: 978-93-7545-433-5

Printed in India at Sterling Graphics Pvt. Ltd.

Dedication

We dedicate this work to our families,
who stand behind every commitment,
and to our patients, who remind us that ART is as much
about compassion as it is about science.

Contributors

Aakanksha Tiwari MBBS DNB (1st Year)
DNB Resident
Department of Obstetrics and Gynecology
Kamla Nagar Hospital
Jodhpur, Rajasthan, India

Aditi Nadkarni MBBS DGO FRM FICOG
Medical Director and Fertility Consultant
Department of Reproductive Medicine
Nadkarni IVF and 21st Century
Group of Hospitals
Vapi, Gujarat, India

Akansha Mishra MSc (Clinical Embryology)
Embryologist
Department of IVF
Yatharth Super Specialty Hospital
Noida, Uttar Pradesh, India

Akash More MSc Fellowship PhD in Infertility
Chief Embryologist
Department of IVF
Mayuri IVF and Fertility Center
Nagpur, Maharashtra, India

Amreen Singh MBBS MD
Senior Consultant
Department of IVF
Yatharth Super Specialty Hospital
Noida, Uttar Pradesh, India

Anindita Singh MBBS DGO
Fertility Consultant
Department of IVF
NOVA IVF Fertility
Kolkata, West Bengal, India

Ankita Kaushal MS (Obs & Gyne) DNB FRM
Consultant and Scientific Director
Department of Obstetrics and Gynecology
Dr Ankita's Fertility Centre
Mumbai, Maharashtra, India

Antara Mukherjee MSc (Microbiology)
Chief Embryologist
Department of IVF Lab
Urvaraa IVF
Kolkata, West Bengal, India

Apurba Kumar Dutta
MBBS MS (Gold Medalist) FIAOG FICOG PGDHHM PGDMLS
Assistant Professor
IQ City Medical College and Hospital, Durgapur
Consultant
Shree Durga Clinic and Fertility Centre
Dhanbad, Jharkhand, India
Chairperson, Sexual Health and STI Committee, FOGSI

Archana Kumari MBBS MS (Obs & Gyne) FICOG
Professor and Unit In-charge
Department of Obstetrics and Gynecology
Rajendra Institute of Medical Sciences
Ranchi, Jharkhand, India

Astha Ubeja
MD (Obs & Gyne) DRM (Keil University) FMAS FICOG
Consultant
Department of Obstetrics and Gynecology
Prakash Test Tube Baby Centre
Khandwa, Madhya Pradesh, India

Divya MB MBBS MS (Obs & Gyne) DNB (Obs & Gyne) MNAMS Postdoctoral Fellowship in Obstetric Medicine
Assistant Professor
Department of Obstetrics and Gynecology
All India Institute of Medical Sciences
Deoghar, Jharkhand, India

Gayatri Satpathy MS, DNB (Obs & Gyne) FNB (Reproductive Medicine)
Fertility Consultant
Department of Fertility
NOVA IVF Fertility
Bhubaneswar, Odisha, India

Gunupuru Gayatri Swetha MBBS MD DNB
Senior Resident (DM Resident in Reproductive Medicine and Surgery)
Department of Obstetrics and Gynecology
All India Institute of Medical Sciences
New Delhi, India

Himani Agarwal MBBS DNB
Medical Director and Fertility Consultant
Department of Obstetrics and Gynecology
Meerut IVF Test Tube Baby Centre
Vardhman Hospital
Meerut, Uttar Pradesh, India

Himanshu Roy MD FICOG
Chief Consultant
Department of Obstetrics and Gynecology
Srijan Fertility Clinic Pvt Ltd
Patna, Bihar, India

Indira Prasad MS DNB MNAMS
Additional Professor
Department of Obstetrics and Gynecology
All India Institute of Medical Sciences
Patna, Bihar, India

Indrani Lodh MS (Obs & Gyne)
Medical Director
Department of IVF
Urvaraa IVF
Kolkata, West Bengal, India

Jaideep Malhotra MD FICOG FICS FIUMB FICMCH FMAS FRCPI FRCOG FICRM FIAPM
Managing Director
ART Rainbow IVF Infertility
Agra, Uttar Pradesh, India

Jyoti Budi DGO MRM
Medical Director
Department of Reproductive Medicine
Ferty9 Fertility Center
Hyderabad, Telangana, India

Maitri Modh MBBS DGO
DNB 3rd year Resident
Department of Obstetrics and Gynecology
Kamla Nagar Hospital
Jodhpur, Rajasthan, India

Mayuri Assudani MBBS DGO
Gynecologist and Infertility Specialist
Department of IVF
Mayuri IVF and Fertility Center
Nagpur, Maharashtra, India

Monisha Singh MBBS MD
Consultant
Department of Obstetrics and Gynecology
Sarojini and Parul Hospital
Varanasi, Uttar Pradesh, India

Narendra Malhotra
MD FIAJAGO FICMU FICOG FICMCH FRCOG FICS FMAS FIAPM FICRM
Managing Director
Global Rainbow Health Care and MNMH (P) Ltd
and
Ujala Cygnus Rainbow Hospital
Agra, Uttar Pradesh, India

Neha Agrawal MBBS DGO
2nd year DNB Resident
Department of Obstetrics and Gynecology
Kamla Nagar Hospital
Jodhpur, Rajasthan, India

Neha Priyadarshini MD FRM FICOG FICMCH
Medical Director
Department of IVF
Satvik IVF
Dhanbad, Jharkhand, India

Neharika Malhotra
MD (Gold Medalist) DRM (Germany) DMIS FICMCH FMAS FICOG ICOG Fellowship in Reproductive Medicine DGC
Consultant
Department of Obstetrics and Gynecology
Ujala Cygnus Rainbow Hospital
Agra, Uttar Pradesh, India

Prachi Singh
MBBS (Hons) DGO DNB (HFH) FICOG Dip IVF (Munich)
Consultant
Department of IVF
Ayushman Hospital and Ashirwad IVF Centre
Muzaffarpur, Bihar, India

Pratibha Singh
Consultant, Laparoscopic Gynecologist and IVF Specialist
Director
Healing Touch Hospital
Bhagalpur, Bihar, India

Priyanka Rai MBBS MS
Additional Professor and Head
Department of Obstetrics and Gynecology
All India Institute of Medical Sciences
Deoghar, Jharkhand, India

Rajarshi Bir MBBS
Clinician
Department of IVF
Urvaraa IVF
Kolkata, West Bengal, India

Rajeev Agarwal MD (Obs & Gyne)
Director
Department of Obstetrics and Gynecology
Renew Healthcare
Kolkata, West Bengal, India

Rekha Rajendra Kumar MBBS MD DNB FICOG PGDMLE (law) FIRM FKCOG
Medical Director
Department of Reproductive Medicine
Chandana Hospital and Miracle IVF
Bengaluru, Karnataka, India

Rekha Ramappa MBBS MS FICOG
Senior Resident (DM Fellow in Reproductive Medicine and Surgery)
Department of Obstetrics and Gynecology
All India Institute of Medical Sciences
New Delhi, India

Rohit Gutgutia MBBS DGO
Medical Director
Department of IVF
NOVA IVF Fertility
Kolkata, West Bengal, India

Rutuja R Athawale
MBBS MD DGO FMAS FRM FAG CCGDM
Medical Director
Parency IVF Hospital
Unit of Parenthood Healthcare Pvt Ltd
Bengaluru, Karnataka, India

Shivani Jha DGO
Medical Director
Department of Obstetrics and Gynecology
Sri Krishna Matri Sadan
Dhanbad, Jharkhand, India

Shivani Sachdev Gour MD DNB MRCOG
Infertility Specialist
Department of Obstetrics and Gynecology
Founder and Director
SCI Healthcare and SCI IVF Hospital
New Delhi, India

Shruti P Shirodkar MBBS (Hon) MD (Obs & Gyne)
Senior Resident
Department of Obstetrics and Gynecology
All India Institute of Medical Sciences
Deoghar, Jharkhand, India

Shubhda Gupta MS FRM
Consultant Gynecologist and Fertility Specialist
Department of Obstetrics and Gynecology
SCI Healthcare and SCI IVF Hospital
New Delhi, India

Snigdha Soni MD DNB MRCOG DM
Senior Resident
Department of Obstetrics and Gynecology
All India Institute of Medical Sciences
New Delhi, India

Sudhanshu Dakre PhD Scholar
Senior Embryologist
Department of IVF
Oasis Fertility
Ranchi, Jharkhand, India

Sugandha Goel
MBBS MS FICOG PGDHHM PGDMLS
Director and Consultant, DNB Professor
Department of Obstetrics and Gynecology
Kamla Nagar Hospital
Jodhpur, Rajasthan, India

Sumavarsha MS DNB FRM
Senior Consultant
Department of Reproductive Medicine
Ferty9 Hospital
Vijayawada, Andhra Pradesh, India

Tanu Sharma MBBS MD (Obs & Gyne)
Fellow National Board in Reproductive medicine
Chief Infertility and IVF Specialist
Department of Obstetrics and Gynecology
Indira IVF Fertility Centre
Lucknow, Uttar Pradesh, India

Varsha Agrawal
MBBS MD (Obs & Gyne) MRCOG (UK)
Consultant
Department of Obstetrics and Gynecology
Life Care Nursing Home and Stone Center
Muzaffarpur, Bihar, India

Veneela Nallani MS (Obs & Gyne) FRM
Junior Consultant
Department of Reproductive Medicine
Ferty9 Fertility Center
Vijayawada, Andhra Pradesh, India

Message from the Series Editors

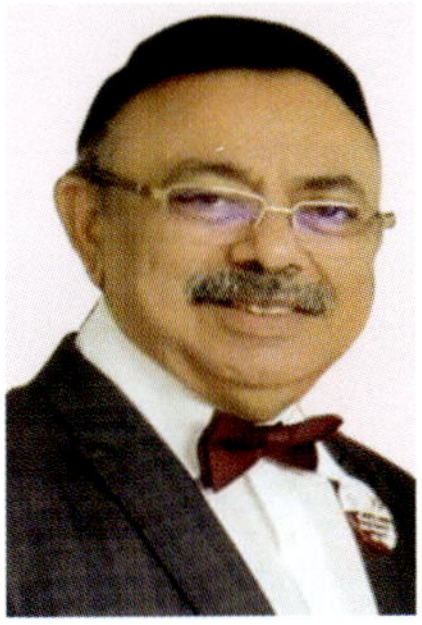

Narendra Malhotra

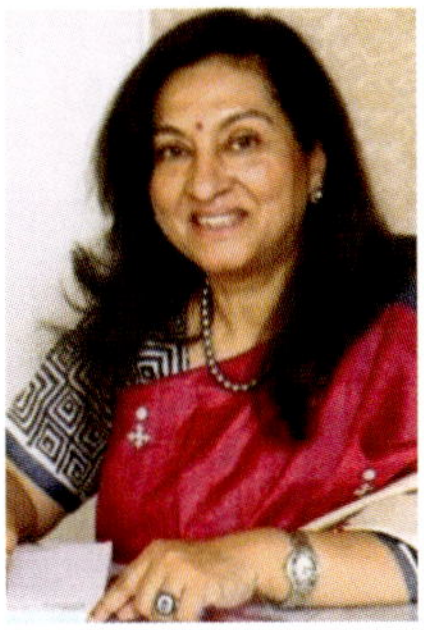

Jaideep Malhotra

It gives us immense pleasure to present *Clinical Focus on ART*, a comprehensive and contemporary series designed to serve as a reliable, practical, and evidence-based resource for clinicians, embryologists, postgraduate students, and all professionals engaged in the field of assisted reproduction.

As assisted reproductive technology (ART) touches millions of lives across the world, the responsibility of ensuring safe, ethical, and effective treatment becomes even more important. This compilation reflects our commitment to improving reproductive health outcomes and empowering practitioners with the knowledge needed to deliver the highest standards of care.

Assisted reproductive technology has evolved rapidly over the past few decades—transforming from hope to science and now to precision-driven, personalized care. With this series, our aim is to bridge the gap between cutting-edge research and daily clinical practice. Each chapter in this volume addresses a key pillar of ART, written by leading experts who bring their deep experience, scientific insight, and clinical wisdom to the table.

We extend our heartfelt gratitude to all contributing authors for their dedication, expertise, and timely efforts. Their contributions form the backbone of this project. We also thank the entire editorial and production teams at M/s Jaypee Brothers Medical Publishers (P) Ltd, New Delhi, India, for their constant support.

We hope this series becomes a valuable companion for every ART professional—enhancing understanding, improving decision-making, and ultimately contributing to better patient care and healthier families.

With warm regards,

Narendra Malhotra

Jaideep Malhotra

Editorial

It gives us immense pleasure to present the *Clinical Focus on ART*, a collective effort shaped by the expertise, commitment, and scholarly contributions of distinguished authors from across the country. As co-editors, we extend our heartfelt gratitude to each contributing author for their time, diligence, and dedication in creating chapters that are both clinically relevant and academically enriching.

The topics selected for this series reflect real-world challenges encountered daily in infertility practice. Each chapter focuses on practical, common clinical scenarios encountered by ART specialists—ranging from evaluation and diagnostics to advanced technologies, ethical dilemmas, and long-term reproductive outcomes. Our goal has been to curate content that not only deepens understanding but also empowers clinicians to make rational, informed decisions grounded in the principles of evidence-based medicine.

Every chapter in this series blends scientific rigor with clinical applicability, offering readers clarity on evolving concepts, updated guidelines, and decision-making pathways. We believe that this compilation will serve as a valuable resource for practitioners, fellows, and students striving to enhance patient care in reproductive medicine.

We once again thank all our authors for their exemplary contributions and shared vision. Their collective wisdom has transformed this series into a comprehensive, impactful, and practical guide for the ART community.

Neharika Malhotra
Neha Priyadarshini
(Co-Editors)

Foreword

Assisted reproductive technologies (ART) have witnessed remarkable scientific and technological advances over the past few decades. From refined ovarian stimulation strategies and laboratory innovations to improved embryo selection and cryopreservation, the field of in vitro fertilization (IVF) continues to evolve at a rapid pace. Amidst this progress, it has become increasingly clear that technological sophistication alone does not guarantee better outcomes—clinical judgment, individualization, and patient-centered decision-making remain the cornerstones of successful practice.

This textbook, *Clinical Focus on ART*, edited by Dr Neharika Malhotra and Dr Neha Priyadarshini under the guidance of Senior Editors Dr Narendra Malhotra and Dr Jaideep Malhotra, is both timely and relevant. It addresses a crucial need in contemporary ART practice: Translating evidence and experience into pragmatic, clinically applicable guidance. The emphasis on real-world scenarios, decision-making pathways, and problem-solving reflects the realities faced daily by clinicians working in IVF units.

One of the foremost priorities in modern IVF is the move away from a "one-size-fits-all" approach toward truly patient-centered and individualized care. Factors such as age, ovarian reserve, previous response, and patient preferences must guide protocols and interventions. Equally important is the judicious use of investigations and treatments. In an era where multiple add-ons are readily available, this book rightly underscores the importance of tailor-made approaches that are evidence-based, ethical, and cost-conscious—avoiding unnecessary interventions that may add complexity without improving outcomes.

By highlighting rational protocol selection, personalized treatment planning, and thoughtful restraint in the use of add-ons, this book reinforces a philosophy that places the patient—not the technology—at the center of care. It will serve as a valuable resource for postgraduate students, clinicians, and seasoned practitioners alike, helping them refine their clinical acumen while staying aligned with the fundamental principles of good medical practice.

I am confident that this textbook will contribute meaningfully to improving standards of care in ART and will inspire clinicians to combine scientific rigor with compassionate, individualized patient management.

Jatin Shah
Director
Mumbai Fertility Clinic and IVF Center
Mumbai, Maharashtra, India

Preface

Assisted reproductive technology (ART) has evolved rapidly over the past two decades, transforming infertility from a largely unexplained condition into a discipline guided by sophisticated diagnostics, advanced laboratory techniques, and expanding therapeutic options. While these advances have improved outcomes, they have also increased the complexity of clinical decision-making in everyday practice.

The book *Clinical Focus on ART* was conceived to address this very challenge. This book aims to provide a structured, evidence-based, and practical approach to the evaluation and management of infertility, with a special focus on clinical scenarios commonly encountered in India and South Asia.

Beginning with the epidemiology, psychosocial impact, and lifestyle influences on infertility, the book progresses through comprehensive clinical evaluation, imaging innovations, ovarian reserve assessment, male and female infertility, and unexplained infertility. Emerging areas such as genetic testing, AI-assisted embryo selection, fertility preservation, regenerative therapies, and long-term health outcomes of ART-conceived children are thoughtfully integrated. Ethical, legal, cultural, and access-related considerations—particularly relevant to resource-variable settings—form an essential part of this volume.

Each chapter has been authored by experienced clinicians and academicians who bring clarity to complex topics while maintaining a strong grounding in evidence-based medicine. The content is designed to support practicing clinicians in making informed decisions at the bedside while also serving as a valuable learning resource for fellows, postgraduate students, and young practitioners entering the field of reproductive medicine.

We hope this book serves not only as a reference, but also as a clinical companion—helping readers navigate the evolving landscape of ART with confidence, responsibility, and compassion.

Neharika Malhotra
Neha Priyadarshini

Preface

Acknowledgments

Bringing this book to completion has been a deeply fulfilling journey, made possible by the blessings of Almighty with guidance and support of many inspiring individuals. We are profoundly grateful to our mentors Dr Jaideep Malhotra and Dr Narendra Malhotra whose wisdom and clinical insight laid the foundation for this work and continues to influence our professional growth.

Our heartfelt gratitude goes to Dr Jatin Shah for agreeing to write foreword for this book, providing us with his invaluable insights and perspectives. We extend our sincere thanks to all contributors for sharing their expertise and experience and to the editorial and publishing team for their invaluable assistance in shaping this book.

Our heartfelt appreciation goes to Shri Jitendar P Vij (Group Chairman), Mr Ankit Vij (Managing Director), and Mr Sabyasachi Hazra (Director—PG and PNR Content) of M/s Jaypee Brothers Medical Publishers (P) Ltd, New Delhi, India, for their efforts in ensuring the timely publication of this book. Special thanks go to Ms Aarti Kushwah (Development Editor) for her expertise in streamlining the book and managing the final stages of editing.

We owe our deepest gratitude to our family for their unconditional love, patience, and encouragement. Their belief in us has been our greatest strength.

This book is dedicated to all learners and clinicians who strive every day to combine science with compassion.

Neharika Malhotra
Neha Priyadarshini

Acknowledgements

Contents

SECTION 1: Foundations and Epidemiology

1. **History and Epidemiology of Infertility** 3
   Archana Kumari, Tanu Sharma
2. **Psychosocial Impact on Individuals and Couples** 9
   Anindita Singh
3. **Environmental and Lifestyle Contributors to Infertility** 16
   Antara Mukherjee, Rajarshi Bir, Indrani Lodh

SECTION 2: Diagnostic Workup

4. **Comprehensive Clinical Evaluation and Basic Investigations** 25
   Mayuri Assudani, Akash More, Sudhanshu Dakre
5. **Advances in Semen Analysis and Sperm Deoxyribonucleic Acid (DNA) Fragmentation** 31
   Mayuri Assudani, Akash More, Sudhanshu Dakre
6. **Ovarian Reserve Assessment and Anti-Müllerian Hormone** 42
   Himani Agarwal
7. **Imaging Innovations: Hysterosalpingography, Three-dimensional Ultrasound, and Sonohysterography** 47
   Sugandha Goel, Maitri Modh, Neha Agrawal, Aakanksha Tiwari

SECTION 3: Emerging Biological Insights

8. **Unexplained Infertility: Folate Pathway Variants, Epigenetic Mechanisms, Immune Dysregulation** 57
   Himanshu Roy, Indira Prasad

SECTION 4: Artificial Reproductive

9. **Fertility Preservation Technologies** 67
   Amreen Singh, Akansha Mishra
10. **Embryo Selection: Artificial Intelligence-driven Multimodal Grading and Explainability** 78
    Snigdha Soni, Gunupuru Gayatri Swetha

11. Noninvasive and Minimally Invasive Preimplantation Genetic Testing and Advances in Next-generation Sequencing 89
Priyanka Rai, Shruti P Shirodkar, Divya MB

12. Ethical and Clinical Debates: Preimplantation Genetic Screening, Blastocyst Transfer, and BMI Limits 100
Rohit Gutgutia, Gayatri Satpathy

SECTION 5: Special Causes and Populations

13. Endometriosis-associated Infertility: Mechanisms and Clinical Pathways 109
Apurba Kumar Dutta

14. Polycystic Ovary Syndrome and Anovulation 113
Rajeev Agarwal, Ankita Kaushal

15. Age-related Ovarian Decline and Poor Ovarian Response 121
Neha Priyadarshini, Shivani Jha

16. Male Infertility: Emerging Diagnostics and Microsurgical Approaches 129
Gunupuru Gayatri Swetha, Snigdha Soni, Rekha Ramappa

17. Impact of Cancer Treatment on Fertility and Preservation Strategies 138
Prachi Singh, Varsha Agrawal

SECTION 6: Therapeutics and Adjuncts

18. Ovulation Induction Protocols and Assisted Reproductive Technology Medications 149
Astha Ubeja

19. Role of Antioxidants and Supplements in Infertility 156
Sumavarsha, Veneela Nallani, Jyoti Budi

20. Growth Factors and Regenerative Medicine: Platelet-rich Plasma in Uterine and Ovarian Applications 164
Monisha Singh, Neharika Malhotra

21. Lifestyle Modifications and Stress Management for Infertility Patients 170
Neharika Malhotra, Jaideep Malhotra

SECTION 7: Clinical Challenges and Controversies

22. Managing Unexplained and Idiopathic Infertility 181
Aditi Nadkarni

23. In Vitro Fertilization in Low-resource Settings: Challenges, Innovations, and Global Lessons 188
Rutuja R Athawale

SECTION 8: Support, Ethics, and Broader Outcomes

24. Counseling Strategies and Supporting Diverse Family Structures 197
Shivani Sachdev Gour, Shubhda Gupta

25. Ethical, Religious, and Legal Considerations in Assisted Reproductive Technology 209
Pratibha Singh

26. Long-term Health of ART: Conceived Children and Reproductive Outcomes 215
Rekha Ramappa, Gunupuru Gayatri Swetha

27. Endometriosis and Assisted Reproductive Technology 220
Rekha Rajendra Kumar

Index 233

SECTION 1

Foundations and Epidemiology

1. **History and Epidemiology of Infertility**
   Archana Kumari, Tanu Sharma
2. **Psychosocial Impact on Individuals and Couples**
   Anindita Singh
3. **Environmental and Lifestyle Contributors to Infertility**
   Antara Mukherjee, Rajarshi Bir, Indrani Lodh

CHAPTER 1

History and Epidemiology of Infertility

Archana Kumari, Tanu Sharma

INTRODUCTION

Infertility is a disorder defined by the inability to achieve a clinical pregnancy after 12 months of regular, unprotected sexual intercourse or by an impairment of a person's ability to reproduce, either alone or with their partner. It causes impairment, hence access to healthcare for those experiencing infertility must be given in accordance with the rules of the Convention on the Rights of Persons with Disabilities. It impacts millions of people, as well as their families and communities. According to estimates, one out of every six persons of reproductive age in the globe experiences infertility at some point in their lives.[1] It can be primary or secondary infertility. Fertility care includes the prevention, diagnosis, and treatment of infertility. Most poor and middle-income nations still struggle to provide equal and fair access to fertility treatment, and fertility care is not emphasized in national universal health coverage benefit packages.

The global sexual and reproductive health and rights (SRHR) agenda has not focused on addressing infertility, despite the fact that it is a significant determinant of SRHR. Given the severity of infertility, enhanced efforts are urgently needed to monitor, evaluate, and improve equitable access to high-quality fertility care services.[2]

PREVALENCE

A significant health concern, infertility affects 8–10% of couples globally.[3] Of the 60–80 million couples that experience infertility each year worldwide, 15–20 million (or 25%) most likely reside in India alone.[4,5] Infertility affects one in four couples in underdeveloped nations, according to a WHO survey. The exact number of couples affected by infertility remains uncertain. A comprehensive global analysis found that about 1.9% of women at risk of pregnancy faced primary infertility, while 10.5% experienced secondary infertility.[6] This study drew on data from 277 reproductive health surveys and applied Bayesian hierarchical modeling to generate age-standardized estimates across 190 countries and territories. A separate review of 25 population-based surveys, published in 2007, reported that infertility rates ranged between 3.5% and 16.7% in high-income nations and between 6.9 and 9.3% in lower-income regions.[7] A mean incidence of 10% worldwide was observed by another comprehensive evaluation of 52 research.[8] The Western Pacific had the highest incidence (23.4%), followed by America (20.5%), Europe (16.8%), Africa (13%), and the Eastern Mediterranean (10.8%), according to a different comprehensive assessment that included 133 research from 1991 to 2021. Both high-income and low-middle-income nations have comparable patterns of infertility.[2]

According to a National Survey of Family Growth research that surveyed 12,000 American women, the prevalence of infertility rose as women's ages climbed.[9] A woman's chances of becoming infertile rise with age and infertility rates among women aged 15–34 years varied from 7.3 to 9.1%. The rates rose to 25% among women aged 35 to 39 years, and the likelihood of infertility was 30% among women aged 40 to 44 years.[9] Globally, the Middle East, North Africa, and eastern Europe have greater rates of infertility.[6]

According to studies from 1997, around 5% of heterosexual couples worldwide struggle with infertility. About 17.5% of couples have infertility, according to a 2023 World Health Organization (WHO) report,[10] and that number has been rising. Depending on the criteria, infertility prevalence varies. Since the 1980s, infertility rates have risen by 4%, primarily as a result of fecundity issues brought on by aging.[11] In the UK, one in seven couples has fertility issues.[12] Both men and women make equal contributions to the incidence of in vitro fertilization (IVF) adoption in the UK.[13]

Of infertile couples in Britain, 25% have male factor infertility, while another 25% have no known cause. Anovulation accounts for 25% and tubal issues for 25% of the 50% contribution from females.[14] About 10% of couples in Sweden that wish to have children are infertile.[15] Due to stigmatization and a lack of knowledge, assessing infertility is challenging in many low-income nations. There are not many historical records on infertility because research and monitoring on the topic did not start until the early 1900s.

The lack of population-based studies, particularly in Asian nations, is one of the primary obstacles to determining the true cost of infertility. The WHO estimates that between 8 and 12% of couples in these areas who are of reproductive age have infertility.[3,16] Due to varying environmental, cultural, and socioeconomic factors as well as access to the healthcare system, there are notable regional variations in the prevalence.[7] India is a very diverse country with a wide range of customs, traditions, quality of life, healthcare system accessibility, and climate. The prevalence varied among states and tribes, but there are not many studies, so it is hard to compare the prevalence in different parts of India. An investigation of Central Indian urban populations revealed an 8.9% prevalence of primary infertility. Using the "age but no birth" criteria, the WHO study found that the prevalence of primary infertility in India was 3.9% (age standardized to 25–49 years) and 16.8% (age standardized to 15–49 years).[17] The frequency was 12.6% in another research from South India,[18] while a study from the Kashmir area[19] reported a similar prevalence. The incidence in southern states and union territories was found to be between 10 and 12%, according to DLHS-3. It ranges from 10 to 14% in northern states including UP, Bihar, West Bengal, and Haryana.[6]

SOCIODEMOGRAPHIC FACTORS

Research has identified several demographic and lifestyle factors associated with primary infertility. These include higher educational attainment, employment outside the home, living in nuclear family structures, delayed marriage and childbearing, increased body mass index (BMI), irregular menstrual cycles, and elevated socioeconomic status.[6,20,21] Some investigations have also observed a higher prevalence of infertility among women engaged in semi-skilled or skilled occupations compared to homemakers.[16] A family history of infertility, particularly among first-degree relatives, has been recognized as another important risk factor.[21,22] Moreover, poor menstrual hygiene practices may contribute to lower reproductive tract infections, menstrual irregularities, and eventually infertility.[23] Certain medical conditions, such as uterine fibroids and hypothyroidism, have also shown significant associations with infertility in some studies.[17,24] Additionally, psychological factors including anxiety, panic disorders, and other mental health challenges have been demonstrated to negatively influence fertility outcomes in couples.[25-27]

Fertility is a crucial milestone for a happy marriage in a traditional nation like India. Negative social outcomes for infertile women include maltreatment, stigmatization, and unstable marriages. Women's social and psychological well-being may suffer significantly as a result.[27,28] To ascertain the prevalence of infertility in India, its contributing variables, and its effects, more community-based research should be conducted.

CAUSES

- Female infertility is related to increasing age at conception, anatomical or functional abnormalities of genital organ, endocrine disorders and reproductive hormones imbalance or a combination of these factors.
- Male infertility can be brought on by hormonal imbalances, abnormal semen analysis, genital tract injuries, infections, or congenital problems.
- Fertility can be impacted by lifestyle choices such as smoking, using drugs recreationally, drinking too much alcohol, and being obese. Gametes may be directly poisoned by exposure to environmental contaminants and chemicals, which might make conception challenging.

The most common causes of female infertility are hormonal in nature like PCOS, and aging, which generally manifests as oligo- or hypomenorrhea. Ovarian follicles and oocytes decrease with age in women, resulting in a decreased ovarian reserve. Some women have infertility as a result of primary ovarian insufficiency. 10–15% of infertile couples have an unknown reason, whereas 85–90% have a known cause.[29] Male infertility, which is a gauge of male fecundity, is most frequently caused by abnormalities in the quantity and quality of semen. Retrograde ejaculation, functional azoospermia, and obstructive azoospermia can also be causes of male infertility.[29]

Every person is entitled to the best possible level of bodily and mental well-being. The decision on the number, timing, and spacing of children belongs to the individual or couple. The fulfillment of these fundamental human rights may be undermined by infertility.

- *Causes and the prevalence among couples:*[30]
  - *Male problems:* 35%
  - *Tubal and pelvic pathology:* 35%
  - *Ovulatory dysfunction:* 15%
  - *Unexplained infertility:* 10%
  - *Unusual problems:* 5%
- *Causes and its prevalence among women:*[30]
  - *Ovulatory dysfunction:* 40%
  - *Tubal and pelvic pathology:* 40%
  - *Unexplained infertility:* 10%
  - *Unusual problems:* 10%

The WHO subdivided ovulatory disorders into four classes:[31]

1. Hypogonadotropic hypogonadal anovulation
2. Normogonadotropic normoestrogenic anovulation [polycystic ovary syndrome (PCOS)]

3. Hypergonadotropic hypoestrogenic anovulation like premature ovarian failure
4. Hyperprolactinemic anovulation like pituitary adenoma

When to start evaluation?

An infertility evaluation is recommended for women who do not conceive after at least 12 months of regular, unprotected intercourse.

For women aged 35 years or older, diagnostic assessment should begin earlier after 6 months of unsuccessful attempts to achieve pregnancy.

From 40 years of age, start evaluating right away.

Many individuals may need fertility care services, including heterosexual couples, homosexuals, elderly couples with health issues, HIV-positive couples, and cancer survivors following fertility-sparing treatment. Unfair access to these services has a negative impact on disadvantaged groups such as the poor, unmarried, illiterate, and jobless. Reducing infertility can also help to lessen gender disparity. Infertility affects both men and women, however whether or not they are infertile, women frequently endure greater hardship. Infertile couples, and especially women, who often face violence, divorce, social stigma, emotional stress, despair, anxiety, and poor self-esteem, are significantly impacted socially and psychologically.

Because reproduction is highly valued in society, women and men may be discouraged from taking contraception due to fear of infertility if they feel compelled to demonstrate their fertility early in life. Interventions aimed at increasing knowledge of the prevalence and contributing factors of infertility and fertility are crucial in these circumstances.

CHALLENGES

The quality, accessibility, and availability of infertility therapies continue to be issues in the majority of nations. Public health funding seldom covers development programs and reproductive health measures, and the diagnosis and treatment of infertility are frequently not given priority in national population surveys. Significant obstacles, even for nations that are actively addressing the needs of individuals with infertility, include the high cost of treatment medications, a shortage of skilled workers, and thc infrastructure required. Assisted reproductive technology (ART) has been around for >30 years, and millions of children have been born all over the world, thanks to ART procedures like IVF. However, in low- and middle-income nations, these technologies are still mostly unavailable, inaccessible, and prohibitively expensive.[32]

The disparities in access to quality fertility treatment might be lessened by government initiatives. To provide universal access without discrimination and to safeguard the human rights of all parties concerned, enabling legislation and regulations that govern ART and third-party reproduction are crucial. WHO acknowledges that one of the fundamental components of reproductive health is the delivery of high-quality family planning services, including fertility care services.

There are several ethical issues associated with its implication like high-cost treatment, health insurance companies should cover infertility treatment, opposition to discarding the embryo not transferred, IVF increases the rates of multiple pregnancy, premature births, multiple health problems, and ethical issues related to surrogacy. Many countries have special frameworks for dealing with the ethical and social issues around fertility treatment.

CONCLUSION

In many nations, national data is either insufficient or indirect. Furthermore, it is important to carefully assess published research because the majority of them contain methodological issues. Researching the incidence of primary and secondary infertility presents challenges in particular. From a public health perspective, as well as when it comes to the planning, procurement, and delivery of medical services, this information is beneficial to the country. However, it is evident that infertility, which can occur for a variety of causes, is a widespread issue that affects a significant percentage of otherwise healthy people, typically in their 20s and 30s. The increasing prevalence is due to advanced age marriage and childbearing, lifestyle, and hormonal issues. It creates a stigma of childlessness specially in developing countries like India and mostly impact on social and psychological health of female in a community.

REFERENCES

1. European Society of Human Reproduction and Embryology. (2024). Factsheet on infertility- prevalence, treatment and fertility decline in Europe. [online] Available from https://www.eshre.eu/-/media/sitecore-files/ESHRE-internal/EU-Affairs/ESHRE_InfertilityFactsheet_April2024Final.pdf [Last accessed December, 2025].
2. Cox CM, Thoma ME, Tchangalova N, Mburu G, Bornstein MJ, Johnson CL, et al. Infertility prevalence and the methods of estimation from 1990 to 2021: a systematic review and meta-analysis. Hum Reprod Open. 2022;2022(4):hoac051.
3. World Health Organization. Infertility: a tabulation of available data on prevalence of primary and secondary infertility. Geneva: World Health Organization; 1991.
4. Poongothai JE, Gopenath TS, Manonayaki SW. Genetics of human male infertility. Singapore Med J. 2009;50:336-47.
5. Chander PP, Indira H, Kusum Z. Need and feasibility of providing assisted technologies for infertility management in resource poor settings. ICMR Bull. 2000;30:55-62.
6. Mascarenhas MN, Flaxman SR, Boerma T, Vanderpoel S, Stevens GA. National, regional, and global trends in infertility prevalence since 1990: a systematic analysis of 277 health surveys. PLoS Med. 2012;9:e 1001356.
7. Boivin J, Bunting L, Collins JA, Nygren KG. International estimates of infertility prevalence and treatment-seeking: potential need and demand for infertility medical care. Hum Reprod. 2007;22:1506-12.
8. Moghaddam AD, Delpisheh A, Sayehmiri K. An investigation of the worldwide prevalence of infertility as a systematic review. Qom Univ Med Sci J. 2016;10:76-87.
9. Chandra A, Copen CE, Stephen EH. Infertility and impaired fecundity in the United States, 1982-2010: data from the National Survey of Family Growth. Natl Health Stat Report. 2013;(67):1-18, 1 p following 19.
10. World Health Organization. (2023). "1 in 6 people globally affected by infertility: WHO". [online] Available from https://www.who.int/news/item/04-04-2023-1-in-6-people-globally-affected-by-infertility [Last accessed December, 2025].
11. Maheshwari A, Hamilton M, Bhattacharya S. Effect of female age on the diagnostic categories of infertility. Hum Reprod. 2008;23(3):538-42.
12. Taylor A. ABC of subfertility: extent of the problem. BMJ. 2003;327(7412):434-6.
13. "HFEA chart on reasons for infertility" Archieved from the original on 30 May 2008. Retrieved 15 September 2025.
14. Gupta J, Mires G, Khan K. Core clinical cases in obstetrics and gynaecology: a problem-solving approach. London: CRC Press; 2011.
15. "Till Spermadonator" [To Sperm donators] (PDF). Sahlgrenska University Hospital (in Swedish). Archieved from the original (PDF) on 26 June 2008. Retrieved on 15 September 2025.

16. World Health Organization. Reproductive health indicators for global monitoring: report of the second interagency meeting, WHO Geneva, 17-19 July 2000. Geneva: WHO; Geneva; 2001.
17. Padubidri VG, Daftary SN. Howkins and Bourne Shaw's Textbook of Gynaecology, 14th edition. Noida: Elsevier, A division of Reed Elsevier India Private Limited; 2008. pp. 251-60.
18. Adamson PC, Krupp K, Freeman AH, Klausner JD, Reingold AL, Madhivanan P. Prevalence & correlates of primary infertility among young women in Mysore, India. Indian J Med Res. 2011;134:440-6.
19. Zargar AH, Wani AI, Masoodi SR, Laway BA, Salahuddin M. Epidemiologic and etiologic aspects of primary infertility in the Kashmir region of India. Fertility and sterility. 1997;68:637-43.
20. Sundby J, Mboge R, Sonko S. Infertility in the Gambia: frequency and health care seeking. Soc Sci Med. 1998;46:891-9.
21. Katole A, Saoji AV. Prevalence of primary infertility and its associated risk factors in urban population of central India: A community-based cross-sectional study. Indian J Community Med. 2019;44:337-41.
22. Shamila S, Sasikala SL. Primary report on the risk factors affecting female infertility in South Indian districts of Tamil Nadu and Kerala. Indian J Community Med. 2011;36:59-61.
23. Das P, Baker KK, Dutta A, Swain T, Sahoo S, Das BS, et al. Menstrual hygiene practices, WASH access and the risk of urogenital infection in women from Odisha, India. PloS One. 2015;10:e0130777.
24. World Health Organization. Reproductive health indicators: guidelines for their generation, interpretation and analysis for global monitoring. Geneva: World Health Organization; 2006. pp. 1-63.
25. Rajashekar L, Krishna D, Patil M. Polycystic ovaries and infertility: our experience. J Hum Reprod Sci. 2008;1(2):65-72.
26. Ozkan M, Baysal B. Emotional distress of infertile women in Turkey. Clin Exp Obstet Gynecol. 2006;33:44-6.
27. Soltani M, Shairi MR, Roshan R, Rahimi CR. The impact of emotionally focused therapy on emotional distress in infertile couples. Int J Fertil Steril. 2013;7(4):337.
28. Musa R, Ramli R, Yazmie AW, Khadijah MB, Hayati MY, Midin M, et al. A preliminary study of the psychological differences in infertile couples and their relation to the coping styles. Compr Psychiatry. 2014;55: S65-9.
29. Carson SA, Kallen AN. Diagnosis and management of infertility: a review. JAMA. 2021;326:65-76.
30. Taylor HS, Pal L, Sell E. Speroff's Clinical Gynecologic Endocrinology and Infertility. Philadelphia: Lippincott Williams & Wilkins; 2019.
31. Walker MH, Tobler KJ. Female Infertility. StatPearls [Internet]. Treasure Island (FL): StatPearls Publishing. 2023.
32. Singh HD. "The World's Back Womb?": Commercial Surrogacy and Infertility Inequalities in India. Am. Anthropol. 2014;116(4):824-8.

CHAPTER 2

Psychosocial Impact on Individuals and Couples

Anindita Singh

INTRODUCTION

Infertility, defined clinically as the inability to achieve conception after 12 months of regular, unprotected intercourse, affects approximately 48 million couples and 186 million individuals worldwide.[1] The World Health Organization recognizes infertility as a disease of the reproductive system with major public health implications.[2] Beyond its biomedical dimensions, infertility constitutes a psychosocial life crisis with far-reaching effects on self-identity, relationships, and social participation.[3] For several couples, infertility is not only a medical condition but also a profound emotional experience resembling grief. Unlike bereavement for a visible loss, this grief is often unacknowledged or minimized by society, leading to what has been termed "disenfranchised grief." The concept highlights the unique challenges of infertility, where individuals mourn the loss of anticipated parenthood, face ongoing ambiguity about outcomes, and struggle with feelings of invisibility and isolation. This framework has been pivotal in validating the emotional reality of infertility and in shaping supportive interventions that acknowledge the depth of this hidden loss.[4] Subsequent work integrated models from health psychology and psychotherapy to describe infertility as a chronic stressor requiring ongoing coping and adaptation rather than a single clinical event.[5] Contemporary studies show consistent elevations in anxiety and depressive symptoms among people experiencing infertility and document meaningful decrements in quality of life across emotional, relational, and social domains.[6] Crucially, the relationship between stress and infertility is bidirectional: psychological distress can influence neuroendocrine pathways relevant to reproduction, while infertility and its treatments generate and sustain distress over time.[7] This chapter integrates global literature to examine the psychosocial impact of infertility, highlighting stress pathways, gender differences, relational effects, sociocultural contexts, coping strategies, and long-term consequences. Our aim is to provide in vitro fertilization (IVF) specialists with a concise, clinically actionable synthesis to complement biological care.

INFERTILITY AS A PSYCHOSOCIAL STRESSOR

The lived experience of infertility is punctuated by cyclical hope and disappointment, serial diagnostic testing, and invasive treatments—dynamics that resemble chronic illness and, for many, elements of bereavement.[3] Neuroendocrine and psychobiological models offer plausibility for the impact of stress on fecundability.

Dysregulation of the hypothalamic–pituitary–adrenal (HPA) axis leads to prolonged elevations of cortisol, which can disrupt the delicate balance of reproductive hormones. Excess cortisol suppresses the release of gonadotropin-releasing hormone (GnRH) from the hypothalamus, thereby impairing luteinizing hormone (LH) and follicle-stimulating hormone (FSH) secretion. Over time, this hormonal imbalance negatively affects ovarian and testicular function, leading to irregular ovulation, impaired spermatogenesis, and reduced fertility.[7] Prospective studies also link stress biomarkers (e.g., salivary α-amylase) with reduced fecundability and lower assisted reproductive technology (ART) success, though causality remains debated.[8] Qualitative and quantitative studies converge on a picture of substantial emotional burden—including sadness, guilt, shame, anger, and loss of control—that may persist beyond treatment and, for some, long after the fertility journey concludes.[9] Standardized instruments help clinicians to identify and monitor psychosocial need: the Fertility Problem Inventory (FPI) assesses infertility-related stress across domains such as social concerns, sexual concerns, and relationship strain,[10] while the Fertility Quality of Life (FertiQoL) tool quantifies QoL impacts and has been validated internationally.[11] The FertiQoL tool is a standardized questionnaire developed to assess the impact of infertility and measures emotional, relational, social, and physical dimensions of quality of life, providing valuable insights for both clinicians and researchers.

GENDERED PERSPECTIVES

Gender norms shape the psychosocial impact of infertility in powerful ways. In many settings, womanhood is tightly linked to motherhood; as a result, women often bear stigma and blame regardless of medical etiology.[12] Empirical studies consistently show that women undergoing fertility care experience significantly higher rates of anxiety and depression compared to their male partners. This disparity is partly due to the biological treatment burden women face, such as invasive procedures, hormonal therapies, and physical side effects. Additionally, sociocultural expectations that place greater responsibility for reproduction on women amplify psychological stress, leading to a more profound emotional impact.[6] Gender-role conformity further moderates outcomes: women adhering to traditional norms report greater decrements in quality of life following an infertility diagnosis.[13] Clinically, the ART pathway adds gender-specific stressors—hormonal stimulation, oocyte retrieval, side effects (e.g., mood change and sleep disruption), and embodied reminders of treatment—that amplify emotional vulnerability.

Male infertility remains comparatively under-recognized despite contributing to approximately half of infertility presentations. Men often experience infertility as a threat to their masculinity, leading to feelings of diminished self-esteem and personal inadequacy. Cultural taboos and societal expectations further contribute to their reluctance to openly disclose or discuss infertility.[14] Quantitative and qualitative studies describe shame, secrecy, and a tendency toward protective silence intended to shield partners from distress;[15] yet reviews underscore that men also experience clinically significant anxiety, depression, and relationship strain.[16] Cross-cultural ethnography highlights how ideals of virility shape help-seeking and disclosure patterns, with implications for adherence and engagement in care.[17]

RELATIONAL DIMENSIONS OF INFERTILITY

Infertility affects couple functioning through multiple pathways. Marital satisfaction can decline as partners navigate uncertainty, differing coping styles, and altered sexual intimacy. Empirical research highlights that marital satisfaction and the psychosocial impact of infertility influence each other in a bidirectional manner. Couples with stronger marital bonds tend to cope better with infertility, whereas strained relationships often intensify emotional distress. Gender differences in anxiety levels further shape these outcomes, with women generally reporting greater psychological vulnerability than men.[18] Structured psychosocial interventions have been shown to strengthen marital satisfaction among couples facing infertility. When delivered in group settings, these programs allow couples to share experiences and strategies, fostering a sense of mutual support. Peer learning and social comparison help to normalize their struggles, reducing feelings of isolation and stigma.[19] At the dyadic level, perceived social support within the couple buffers distress and predicts better adjustment.[20] Dyadic coping frameworks suggest that viewing infertility as a shared stressor fosters unity between partners. Collaborative problem solving in this context helps preserve and even strengthen relationship quality.[21] Communication skills such as empathic listening and shared meaning-making play a crucial role in helping couples navigate the stress of infertility. These skills can be taught effectively through brief training programs incorporated into routine clinical care. Evidence shows that couples who develop these abilities report better emotional adjustment, stronger relationships, and improved treatment experiences.[22]

Sexual intimacy is frequently medicalized—shifted from spontaneous pleasure to scheduled, goal-directed intercourse with attendant performance pressure. This change can reduce desire, increase avoidance, and undermine sexual satisfaction. Stigma and rigid social expectations often intensify the emotional strain of infertility across many cultural contexts. Women are more frequently blamed for childlessness, facing judgment and pressure from families and communities. At the same time, men are socially encouraged to suppress their emotions, limiting their willingness to disclose or seek support.[23] Psychosexual counseling provides couples with tools to reframe intimacy and separate it from reproductive pressure. Such interventions can ease performance anxiety and restore confidence in sexual expression. When combined with treatment planning, they help to rebuild erotic connection and strengthen relational closeness.

SOCIOCULTURAL AND ETHICAL CONSIDERATIONS

Sociocultural context strongly determines how infertility is experienced and expressed. In multiple African settings, infertility is associated with social exclusion and, in severe cases, vulnerability to intimate partner violence or marital instability.[23] Stigma measurement tools are valuable for capturing the hidden psychosocial impact of infertility and tailoring care to patient needs. Instruments such as the Infertility Stigma Scale (ISS), the Female Infertility Stigma Instrument (ISI-F), and infertility perception scales provide culturally sensitive ways to assess how stigma is experienced. These measures are useful both for screening and needs assessment in clinical practice, as well as for evaluating the outcomes of psychosocial or medical interventions. Incorporating them into fertility care helps normalize experiences, guide targeted support, and track progress in reducing stigma over time.[24-26] A short-form stigma instrument has recently been validated to facilitate brief screening in busy clinics.[27]

Assisted reproductive technologies bring with them a range of ethical and practical challenges that extend beyond medical care. Choices regarding embryo disposition can raise difficult moral and legal questions for couples. Third-party reproduction, including donor gametes or surrogacy, may conflict with deeply held personal, religious, or cultural beliefs. Similarly, decisions around genetic testing often force couples to navigate sensitive value systems while balancing medical guidance.[12] Financial inequity continues to be one of the most significant stressors for individuals and couples pursuing fertility treatment. Even in settings where insurance coverage exists, the combined burden of out-of-pocket expenses, repeated medical appointments, travel, and time away from work often leads to treatment discontinuation. These pressures not only create economic strain but also compound emotional distress, contributing to feelings of hopelessness and inequity in access to care. Such realities highlight the importance of transparent counseling that sets realistic expectations regarding success probabilities, timelines, and potential setbacks. Moreover, integrating discussions about alternatives—such as adoption, donor options, or embracing a child-free life—ensures that care is patient-centered and aligned with individual values, preferences, and long-term well-being.

COPING STRATEGIES AND INTERVENTIONS

Patients adopt diverse coping strategies. Adaptive responses—seeking social support, problem-solving, cognitive reappraisal—are associated with better emotional outcomes, whereas avoidance, denial, and overinvestment in treatment correlate with greater distress. Routine measurement using FPI and FertiQoL can flag maladaptive trajectories early and prompt timely referral.[10,11]

Randomized trials and systematic reviews support multiple psychosocial interventions. Mindfulness-based programs have been shown to significantly reduce anxiety and emotional distress in women undergoing IVF. By fostering relaxation, emotional regulation, and present-moment awareness, these interventions enhance overall quality of life during treatment. Some studies even suggest an association with higher pregnancy rates, highlighting their potential therapeutic value.[28,29] A brief and skills-based psychological intervention delivered during IVF has been shown to reduce patient distress. Exploratory analyses further suggest that it may contribute to lower treatment discontinuation rates.[30] Online psychoeducational support demonstrates benefits in emotional well-being and offers scalable access to care.[31] A self-administered coping protocol specifically targeting the 2-week wait improved emotional outcomes and reduced negative affect.[32] Professional societies now recommend that routine fertility care incorporate psychosocial screening and support, with clear referral pathways to specialized mental health providers.[33]

Complementary therapies—yoga, acupuncture, and relaxation training—are commonly used adjuncts. A systematic review found moderate evidence for reductions in distress and improved emotional well-being among women undergoing IVF, although effects on live birth remain uncertain.[34] From a practical perspective, shared decision-making allows patients to actively participate in choices about their fertility care. Aligning complementary approaches with medical evidence and patient preferences helps to restore a sense of control while maintaining high-quality treatment.

LONG-TERM PSYCHOSOCIAL OUTCOMES

Psychosocial effects can persist regardless of reproductive outcome. Couples who conceive via ART sometimes report residual anxiety, grief for lost years, and fear of future infertility or pregnancy loss—responses that mirror trajectories observed after other chronic stressors.[9] For those who remain involuntarily childless, long-term adjustment involves identity reconstruction, meaning-making, and the development of alternative life goals and roles within families and communities. Some evidence suggests that even when medical issues are addressed (e.g., after surgical management), psychosocial sequelae may endure, emphasizing the importance of continued support and follow-up.[35] Clinicians should normalize these experiences, set expectations about the emotional course of treatment, and offer ongoing support options beyond the last clinical encounter.

CONCLUSION

Infertility is both a medical and psychosocial condition. It destabilizes identity, strains partnerships, invites stigma, and raises ethical dilemmas. Evidence-based psychological care—including routine distress screening, brief skills-based interventions, and timely referral—should be regarded as core to high-quality fertility practice, not an optional extra. Multidisciplinary models that integrate counselors, psychologists, and nursing staff improve patient experience and may reduce treatment discontinuation. Finally, culturally sensitive counseling that acknowledges diverse values, religious frameworks, and resource constraints is essential to equitable and person-centered reproductive care.

REFERENCES

1. Feng J, Wu Q, Liang Y, Liang Y, Bin Q. Epidemiological characteristics of infertility, 1990–2021, and 15-year forecasts: an analysis based on the global burden of disease study 2021. Reprod Health. 2025;22:26.
2. World Health Organization. Infertility: a public health issue and disease of the reproductive system. Geneva: WHO; 2020.
3. Menning BE. The psychosocial impact of infertility. Nurs Clin North Am. 1982;17(1): 155-63.
4. Doka KJ. Disenfranchised grief and infertility. Omega (Westport). 1989;20(1):81-90.
5. Cousineau TM, Domar AD. Psychological impact of infertility. Best Pract Res Clin Obstet Gynaecol. 2007;21(2):293-308.
6. Braverman AM, Davoudian T, Levin IK, Bocage A, Wodoslawsky S. Depression, anxiety, quality of life, and infertility: a global lens on the last decade of research. Fertil Steril. 2024;121(3):379-83.
7. Rooney KL, Domar AD. The relationship between stress and infertility. Dialogues Clin Neurosci. 2018;20(1):41-7.
8. Zhou FJ, Liu JH, Dai SJ, Kun K, Cai YN, Dong YZ. [The level of the stress biomarker salivary alpha amylase is correlated with semen quality in infertile young men]. Zhonghua Nan Ke Xue. 2021;27(11):1001-5.
9. Greil AL, Slauson-Blevins K, McQuillan J. The experience of infertility: a review of recent literature. Sociol Health Illn. 2010;32(1):140-62.
10. Newton CR, Sherrard W, Glavac I. The Fertility Problem Inventory: measuring perceived infertility-related stress. Fertil Steril. 1999;72(1):54-62.
11. Boivin J, Takefman J, Braverman A. The Fertility Quality of Life (FertiQoL) tool: development and general psychometric properties. Hum Reprod. 2011;26(8):2084-91.
12. Leyser-Whalen O, Temple JR, Phelps JY. Ethical and psychosocial impact of female

infertility. Curr Obstet Gynecol Rep. 2012; 1(4):153-8.

13. Bueno-Sánchez L, Alhambra-Borrás T, Gallego-Valadés A, Garcés-Ferrer J. Psychosocial impact of infertility diagnosis and conformity to gender norms on the quality of life of infertile Spanish couples. Int J Environ Res Public Health. 2024; 21(2):158.
14. de Vries CEJ, Veerman-Verweij EM, van den Hoogen A, de Man-van Ginkel JM, Ockhuijsen HDL. The psychosocial impact of male infertility on men undergoing ICSI treatment: a qualitative study. Reprod Health. 2024;21(1):26.
15. Dooley M, Dineen T, Sarma K, Nolan A. The psychological impact of infertility and fertility treatment on the male partner. Hum Fertil (Camb). 2014;17(3):203-9.
16. Fisher JR, Hammarberg K. Psychological and social aspects of infertility in men: an overview of the evidence and implications for psychologically informed clinical care and future research. Asian J Androl. 2012;14(1):121-9.
17. Inhorn MC, Patrizio P. Infertility around the globe: new thinking on gender, reproductive technologies and global movements in the 21st century. Hum Reprod Update. 2015;21(4):411-26.
18. Chamorro PP, Herruzo J, Pino MJ. Study on the interdependent relationship between marital satisfaction and the psychosocial impact of infertility and anxiety disposition, according to gender. J Sex Marital Ther. 2022;48(5):461-74.
19. Chamorro PP, Pino MJ, Casas-Rosal JC, Herruzo J. A longitudinal comparative study of a multicouple group and single-couple psychosocial intervention while experiencing infertility. Fam Process. 2023;62(2): 557-75.
20. Martins MV, Peterson BD, Almeida VM, Costa ME. Dyadic dynamics of perceived social support in couples facing infertility. Hum Reprod. 2014;29(1):83-9.
21. Chaves C, Canavarro MC, Moura-Ramos M. The role of dyadic coping on the marital and emotional adjustment of couples with infertility. Fam Process. 2019;58(2):509-23.
22. Schmidt L, Holstein B, Christensen U, Boivin J. Does infertility cause marital benefit? An epidemiological study of 2250 women and men in fertility treatment. Patient Educ Couns. 2005;59(3):244-51.
23. Roomaney R, Salie M, Jenkins D, Eder C, Mutumba-Nakalembe MJ, Volks C, et al. A scoping review of the psychosocial aspects of infertility in African countries. Reprod Health. 2024;21(1):123.
24. Fu B, Qin N, Cheng L, Tang G, Cao Y, Yan C, et al. Development and validation of an infertility stigma scale for Chinese women. J Psychosom Res. 2015;79(1):69-75.
25. Taebi M, Kariman N, Montazeri A, Majd HA. Development and psychometric evaluation of the female infertility stigma instrument (ISI-F): protocol for a mixed method study. Reprod Health. 2020;17(1):70.
26. Kim M, Ban M. Development of an infertility perception scale for women (IPS-W). BMC Womens Health. 2024;24:513.
27. Li R, Luo L, Qin N, Guan M, Peng E, Qu J, et al. Development and validation of the infertility stigma scale short form (ISS-SF): a cross-sectional study. J Psychosom Res. 2025;194:112160.
28. Li J, Long L, Liu Y, He W, Li M. Effects of a mindfulness-based intervention on fertility quality of life and pregnancy rates among women subjected to first in vitro fertilization treatment. Behav Res Ther. 2016;77:96-104.
29. Wang G, Liu X, Lei J. Effects of mindfulness-based intervention for women with infertility: a systematic review and meta-analysis. Arch Womens Ment Health. 2023;26(2):245-58.
30. Domar AD, Gross J, Rooney K, Boivin J. Exploratory randomized trial on the effect of a brief psychological intervention on emotions, quality of life, discontinuation, and pregnancy rates in in vitro fertilization patients. Fertil Steril. 2015;104(2):440-51.e7.
31. Cousineau TM, Green TC, Corsini EA, Barnard T, Seibring AR, Domar AD. Online psychoeducational support for infertile

women: a randomized controlled trial. Fertil Steril. 2008;89(3):537-46.

32. Ockhuijsen H, van den Hoogen A, Eijkemans M, Macklon N, Boivin J. The impact of a self-administered coping intervention on emotional well-being in women awaiting the outcome of IVF: a randomized controlled trial. Hum Reprod. 2014;29(7):1459-67.
33. Gameiro S, Boivin J, Dancet E, de Klerk C, Emery M, Lewis-Jones C, et al. ESHRE guideline: routine psychosocial care in infertility and medically assisted reproduction—a guide for fertility staff. Hum Reprod. 2015;30(11):2476-85.
34. LoGiudice JA, Massaro J. The impact of complementary therapies on psychosocial factors in women undergoing in vitro fertilization: a systematic literature review. Appl Nurs Res. 2018;39:220-8.
35. Lalos A, Lalos O, Jacobsson L, von Schoultz B. The psychosocial impact of infertility two years after completed surgical treatment. Acta Obstet Gynecol Scand. 1985;64(7):599-604.

CHAPTER 3

Environmental and Lifestyle Contributors to Infertility

Antara Mukherjee, Rajarshi Bir, Indrani Lodh

INTRODUCTION

Infertility is now recognized as a major global health concern, affecting nearly one in six couples worldwide and presenting a profound clinical and psychosocial challenge.[1] While anatomical and genetic factors remain important, contemporary evidence highlights that environmental exposures and lifestyle behaviors play a critical role in shaping reproductive health outcomes.[2]

This recognition has led to the emergence of the *exposome*—the cumulative measure of environmental and lifestyle exposures across the lifespan—as a valuable framework for understanding how nongenetic factors influence fertility.[3] The exposome approach goes beyond identifying isolated risk factors, instead acknowledging the complex interplay between pollutants, diet, stress, and personal habits.

This chapter explores the impact of environmental and lifestyle contributors on male and female fertility. The discussion is structured in two parts: (1) environmental exposures, including endocrine-disrupting chemicals, heavy metals, air pollution, and pesticides, and (2) lifestyle factors such as nutrition, body mass index (BMI), substance use, and psychological stress. Clinical implications are considered throughout, with emphasis on prevention, counseling, and patient-centered care.

ENVIRONMENTAL EXPOSOME: THREATS TO REPRODUCTION (TABLE 1)

Endocrine-disrupting Chemicals

Endocrine-disrupting chemicals (EDCs) are exogenous substances that interfere with endogenous hormone function by mimicking, blocking, or altering hormonal signaling.[4] These chemicals are pervasive, found in plastics [e.g., bisphenol A (BPA) and phthalates], pesticides, cosmetics, and industrial by-products.

Effects in females: Exposure to EDCs has been associated with earlier puberty, reduced ovarian reserve, impaired oocyte quality, and higher risk of endometriosis and polycystic ovary syndrome (PCOS).[5,6] Perfluoroalkyl substances (PFAS) and BPA have been linked to reduced anti-Müllerian hormone (AMH) levels and implantation failure.

Effects in males: Global declines in sperm counts over recent decades have been partly attributed to EDCs.[7] Phthalates and BPA impair spermatogenesis, reduce motility, and increase sperm DNA fragmentation. Prenatal exposure to some pesticides is linked to testicular dysgenesis syndrome (TDS), manifesting later as infertility.[8]

Mechanisms of action include receptor binding (agonist/antagonist), altered steroid

TABLE 1: Environmental contributors to infertility.

Factor	*Common sources*	*Mechanisms*	*Reproductive effects*
Endocrine disruptors	Plastics, pesticides, and cosmetics	Hormone mimicry/blocking, altered biosynthesis, and epigenetic changes	↓ Sperm quality, ovarian dysfunction, and implantation failure
Heavy metals	Industrial waste, fish (mercury), and tobacco (cadmium)	Oxidative stress, mineral competition, and endocrine disruption	Ovarian aging, miscarriage, ↓ sperm count, and DNA damage
Air pollution	Vehicle emissions, $PM_{2.5}$, and industrial activity	Inflammation, oxidative stress, and genetic/epigenetic damage	↓ Ovarian reserve, miscarriage, and poor semen parameters
Pesticides	Agricultural chemicals and food residues	Hormonal disruption, oxidative stress, and DNA damage	↓ Sperm quality, miscarriage, and ovulatory dysfunction

biosynthesis, and epigenetic modifications that may be transmitted across generations.[9]

Heavy Metals

Heavy metals such as lead, mercury, cadmium, and arsenic accumulate through industrial emissions, contaminated water, food, and tobacco smoke.

- *Oxidative stress:* Metals generate reactive oxygen species (ROS), overwhelming antioxidant defenses and damaging DNA, lipids, and proteins[10] inside the body.
- *Endocrine disruption:* Heavy metals compete with essential minerals, disrupt steroid hormone synthesis, and impair gonadal function.[11]

Effects in females: Associated with accelerated ovarian aging, diminished ovarian reserve, spontaneous abortion, and adverse pregnancy outcomes.[12]

Effects in males: Linked to reduced sperm count and motility, testicular degeneration, and increased DNA fragmentation.[13]

Cadmium exposure, often from smoking, is particularly detrimental, underscoring the overlap between environmental and lifestyle risks.

Air Pollution

Air pollution—particularly fine particulate matter ($PM_{2.5}$), nitrogen dioxide (NO_2), sulfur dioxide (SO_2), and carbon monoxide (CO)—is a pervasive hazard. Pollutants enter the bloodstream via the lungs, triggering systemic inflammation and oxidative stress.[14]

Effects on female fertility: Linked to reduced ovarian reserve, poorer oocyte and embryo quality, implantation failure, and miscarriage.[15]

Effects on male fertility: Associated with decreased sperm concentration, motility, and morphology.[16] Adverse effects are especially evident during spermatogenesis (70–90 days pre-ejaculation).

Epidemiological studies report significantly lower live birth rates among women undergoing assisted reproductive technologies (ARTs) in areas with high air pollution.[17]

Pesticides

Agricultural pesticides, particularly organochlorines and organophosphates, persist in the environment and bioaccumulate in human tissues.

Effect in females: Hormonal disruption, ovarian dysfunction, accelerated ovarian aging, and higher risks of miscarriage and preterm birth.[18]

Effects in males: Reduced sperm count and altered morphology, motility, and high DNA fragmentation.[19]

Occupational exposures in farming communities are strongly correlated with impaired fertility in both men and women.[20]

LIFESTYLE EXPOSOME: MODIFIABLE FACTORS (TABLE 2)

Epigenetics

Epigenetics refers to heritable changes in gene function without any alteration in the nucleotide sequence of the DNA molecule. These changes can impact a person's ability to conceive by regulating genes that are important for reproduction. Studies have shown lifestyle choices, environmental factors such as diet, stress, and exposure to toxins can induce epigenetic changes that affect reproductive health.

Nutrition and Body Mass Index

Body mass index (BMI) is a critical determinant of fertility. Both underweight (<18.5 kg/m^2) and obesity (>30 kg/m^2) are associated with reproductive dysfunction.[21]

- *Women:* Obesity contributes to insulin resistance and anovulation, while underweight status disrupts gonadotropin release and ovulation.[22]
- *Men:* Extremes of BMI impair testosterone production and reduce semen quality.[23]

Dietary patterns play a major role. The "Western diet" (high in trans fats, refined sugars, and red meat) is linked with lower fertility, whereas a Mediterranean-style diet rich in fruits, vegetables, whole grains, and omega-3 fatty acids improves gamete quality and ART success rates.[24] Supplementation with folic acid and antioxidants further enhances reproductive outcomes.[25]

Substance Use

Tobacco: Smoking accelerates follicular depletion, lowers ovarian reserve, and

TABLE 2: Lifestyle contributors to infertility.

Factor	*Mechanisms*	*Male effects*	*Female effects*
BMI	Hormonal dysregulation, insulin resistance, and HPG axis suppression	↓ Testosterone and poor semen quality	Anovulation, irregular cycles, and ↓ endometrial receptivity
Diet	Oxidative stress, altered microbiota, and nutrient deficiencies	↓ Motility and sperm quality	Poor oocyte quality and implantation failure
Smoking	Oxidative stress, DNA damage, and tubal injury	↓ Sperm count/motility and DNA fragmentation	↓ Ovarian reserve, ectopic pregnancy, and premature menopause
Alcohol	Hormonal disruption and testicular toxicity	↓ Testosterone and impaired spermatogenesis	Menstrual irregularities and implantation failure
Stress	HPA–HPG axis suppression and oxidative stress	Impaired spermatogenesis	Anovulation, ↓ IVF success, and menstrual dysfunction

(BMI: body mass index; HPA: hypothalamic–pituitary–adrenal; HPG: hypothalamic–pituitary–gonadal; IVF: in vitro fertilization)

advances menopause by 1–4 years.[26] In men, it increases oxidative stress, sperm DNA damage, and erectile dysfunction.[27]

Alcohol: Excessive alcohol disrupts ovulation, menstrual regularity, and implantation in women. In men, it reduces testosterone and impairs spermatogenesis.[28] Moderate-to-heavy drinking consistently prolongs time to conception.[29]

Caffeine: High intake (>300–400 mg/day) is associated with irregular cycles, miscarriage, and reduced semen quality.[30]

Stress and Psychological Health

Infertility itself is a stressor, creating a bidirectional cycle where stress worsens reproductive outcomes.

- *Mechanism:* Stress activates the hypothalamic–pituitary–adrenal (HPA) axis, increasing cortisol, which suppresses the hypothalamic–pituitary–gonadal (HPG) axis.[31] This reduces secretion of gonadotropin-releasing hormone (GnRH), luteinizing hormone (LH), and follicle-stimulating hormone (FSH), impairing ovulation and spermatogenesis.[32]
- *Effects:* Stress is associated with lower in vitro fertilization (IVF) success, menstrual irregularities, and abnormal semen characteristics.[33]

Interventions such as cognitive-behavioral therapy, mindfulness, and acupuncture may improve outcomes by mitigating stress.[34]

CLINICAL IMPLICATIONS AND PATIENT COUNSELING

Recognizing the role of environmental and lifestyle factors in infertility has important implications for practice. Clinicians should incorporate proactive counseling that emphasizes prevention alongside treatment.

- *Weight management:* Maintaining a healthy BMI improves ovulatory function and semen quality.[21]
- *Substance avoidance:* Patients should be strongly advised to abstain from smoking and limit alcohol and caffeine.[26,28]
- *Dietary interventions:* Adopting a Mediterranean-style diet rich in antioxidants improves fertility outcomes.[24]
- *Environmental avoidance:* Patients can reduce exposure to toxins by limiting plastic use (especially when heated), consuming organic produce, and avoiding occupational hazards.[6,12]
- *Stress reduction:* Incorporating stress-management strategies into infertility care enhances both emotional well-being and clinical outcomes.[33]

Although biomarkers of exposure (e.g., urinary phthalate metabolites and blood lead levels) are under investigation, their clinical utility remains limited.[35]

CONCLUSION

Infertility or subfertility is a multifactorial condition shaped not only by biological and genetic determinants but also by the lifelong accumulation of environmental exposures and lifestyle choices. Across diverse risk factors—ranging from endocrine disruptors and heavy metals to smoking, poor diet, and stress—a consistent theme emerges: oxidative stress and hormonal dysregulation as central pathways.

The exposome framework provides a valuable perspective for integrating these risks into prevention, clinical counseling, and policy. Future research should prioritize longitudinal studies, transgenerational impacts of epigenetic changes, and the development of reliable biomarkers.

By embracing a holistic approach, clinicians can move beyond treatment alone, contributing to prevention, patient empowerment, and improved reproductive health outcomes for future generations.

REFERENCES

1. World Health Organization. Infertility prevalence estimates, 1990–2021. Geneva: WHO; 2023.
2. Vander Borght M, Wyns C. Fertility and infertility: Definition and epidemiology. Clin Biochem. 2018;62:2-10.
3. Wild CP. The exposome: from concept to utility. Int J Epidemiol. 2012;41(1): 24-32.
4. Endocrine Society. Endocrine-disrupting chemicals. [online] Available from https://www.endocrine.org/topics/edc [Last accessed December, 2025].
5. Seli E, Taylor H. The impact of endocrine disruptors on reproduction. J Clin Endocrinol Metab. 2022;107(3):e4876-88.
6. Lauria G, Trombino S, D'Alessandro D. Environmental factors affecting female fertility. Resgate. 2024;381:1-8.
7. Levine H, Jørgensen N, Martino-Andrade A, Mendiola J, Weksler-Derri D, Mindlis I, et al. Temporal trends in sperm count: A systematic review and meta-regression. Hum Reprod Update. 2017;23(6):646-59.
8. Skakkebaek NE, Rajpert-De Meyts E, Main KM. Testicular dysgenesis syndrome: An increasingly common developmental disorder. Hum Reprod. 2001;16(5):972-8.
9. Miller GW, Jones DP. The nature of nurture: refining the definition of the exposome. Toxicol Sci. 2014;137(1):1-2.
10. Akinloye O, Arowojolu AO, Shittu OB, Adejuwon CA. Cadmium toxicity: A possible cause of male infertility in Nigeria. Reprod Biol. 2006;6(1):17-30.
11. Borujeni H, Hemmati M, Zandi S. The effects of lead and mercury on male fertility. Andrologia. 2020;52(2):e13880.
12. Bloom MS, Parsons PJ, Steuerwald AJ, Schisterman EF, Browne RW, Kim K, et al. Toxic trace metals and human oocytes during in vitro fertilization (IVF). Reprod Toxicol. 2010;29(3):298-305.
13. Jurasovic J, Cvitkovic P, Pizent A, Colak B, Telisman S. Semen quality and reproductive endocrine function with regard to blood cadmium in Croatian men. Reprod Toxicol. 2004;18(6):743-51.
14. Schraufnagel DE, Balmes JR, Cowl CT, To T, Vanker A, Wuebbles DJ, et al. Air pollution and noncommunicable diseases: A review by the Forum of International Respiratory Societies' Environmental Committee, Part 1: The Damaging Effects of Air Pollution. Chest. 2019;155(2):409-16.
15. Legro RS, Sauer MV, Mottla GL, Richter KS, Li X, Dodson WC, et al. Effect of air quality on assisted human reproduction. Hum Reprod. 2010;25(5):1317-24.
16. Lao XQ, Zhang Z, Lau AKH, Chan TC, Chuang YC, Chan J, et al. Exposure to ambient fine particulate matter and semen quality in Taiwan. Occup Environ Med. 2018;75(2):148-54.
17. Conforti A, Mascia M, Cioffi G, De Angelis C, Coppola G, De Rosa P, et al. Air pollution and assisted reproduction: A systematic review. Reprod Biol Endocrinol. 2018;16(1):117.
18. Arbuckle TE, Sever LE. Pesticide exposure and reproductive outcomes. Am J Epidemiol. 1998;148(11):1052-76.
19. Fuortes L, Clark MK, Kirchner HL, Smith EM. Association between female infertility and agricultural work history. Am J Ind Med., 1997;31(4):445-51.
20. Larsen SB, Spanò M, Giwercman A, Bonde JP. ASCLEPIOS Study Group. Semen quality and sex hormones among organic and traditional farmers. Occup Environ Med. 1999;56(2):139-44.
21. Silvestris E, de Pergola G, Rosania R, Loverro G. Obesity as disruptor of the female fertility. Reprod Biol Endocrinol. 2018;16:22.
22. Pasquali R, Gambineri A. Impact of obesity on reproduction in women with PCOS. Hum Reprod Update. 2006;12(6):573-84.
23. Sermondade N, Faure C, Fezeu L, Shayeb AG, Bonde JP, Jensen TK, et al. BMI and male infertility: A systematic review and meta-analysis. Hum Reprod Update. 2013;19(3):221-31.

24. Karayiannis D, Kontogianni MD, Mendorou C, Mastrominas M, Yiannakouris N. Adherence to the Mediterranean diet and IVF success rate among non-obese women attempting fertility. Hum Reprod. 2018;33(3):494-502.
25. Gaskins AJ, Chavarro JE. Diet and fertility: A review. Am J Obstet Gynecol. 2018;218(4):379-89.
26. ASRM Practice Committee. Tobacco or marijuana use and infertility: a committee opinion. Fertil Steril. 2023;120(4):783-92.
27. Sharma R, Harlev A, Agarwal A, Esteves SC. Cigarette smoking and semen quality: a new meta-analysis. Reprod Biomed Online. 2016;32(2):147-59.
28. Ricci E, Al Beitawi S, Cipriani S, Candiani M, Chiaffarino F, Viganò P, et al. Alcohol intake and infertility in women: A systematic review and meta-analysis. Reprod Biomed Online. 2017;34(1):38-47.
29. Muthusami KR, Chinnaswamy P. Effect of chronic alcoholism on male fertility hormones and semen quality. Fertil Steril. 2005;84(4):919-24.
30. Lyngsø J, Ramlau-Hansen CH, Bay B, Ingerslev HJ, Hulman A, Kesmodel US. Association between coffee or caffeine consumption and fecundity and fertility: a systematic review and dose-response meta-analysis. Clin Epidemiol. 2017;9:699-719.
31. Liang J, Kumar P, et al. The relationship between psychological stress and ovulatory disorders: a review of the molecular mechanisms. J Psychosom Obstet Gynaecol. 2024;45(1):2418110.
32. Csemiczky G, Landgren BM, Collins A. The influence of stress and state anxiety on IVF outcome. Hum Reprod. 2000;15(10):2152-7.
33. Rooney KL, Domar AD. The relationship between stress and infertility. Dialogues Clin Neurosci. 2018;20(1):41-7.
34. Frederiksen Y, Farver-Vestergaard I, Skovgård NG, Ingerslev HJ, Zachariae R. Efficacy of psychosocial interventions for infertility: A meta-analysis. Hum Reprod Update. 2015;21(6):807-20.
35. Vrijheid M, Slama R, Robinson O, Chatzi L, Coen M, van den Hazel P, et al. The human early-life exposome (HELIX): project rationale and design. Environ Health Perspect. 2014;122(6):535-44.

SECTION 2

Diagnostic Workup

4. **Comprehensive Clinical Evaluation and Basic Investigations**
   Mayuri Assudani, Akash More, Sudhanshu Dakre

5. **Advances in Semen Analysis and Sperm Deoxyribonucleic Acid (DNA) Fragmentation**
   Mayuri Assudani, Akash More, Sudhanshu Dakre

6. **Ovarian Reserve Assessment and Anti-Müllerian Hormone**
   Himani Agarwal

7. **Imaging Innovations: Hysterosalpingography, Three-dimensional Ultrasound, and Sonohysterography**
   Sugandha Goel, Maitri Modh, Neha Agrawal, Aakanksha Tiwari

CHAPTER 4

Comprehensive Clinical Evaluation and Basic Investigations

Mayuri Assudani, Akash More, Sudhanshu Dakre

INTRODUCTION

Infertility is defined as the inability to conceive after 12 months or more of uninterrupted, regular sexual intercourse. It represents a worldwide health concern that is steadily on the rise, impacting approximately one in six couples of childbearing age.[1] It is generally classified as either primary infertility (if never conceived) or secondary infertility (if conceived but cannot conceive again).[2] Infertility affects couples on several levels, well beyond physical health, as it can impact social and psychological health as well.[3]

In several cultures, the stigma and emotional burden of childlessness are so significant that they can affect the individual or couple's emotional well-being and quality of life. The consequences are dire, underscoring the necessity of timely, comprehensive, and accurate assessments that can inform prompt treatment and/or care for the affected couple.[4]

A systematic and methodical technique is ultimately important for a thorough diagnostic workup in managing infertility. The evaluation aims to (1) determine any treatable etiologic factors, (2) present clear options for treatment based on the couple's needs, and (3) avoid unnecessary evaluation.[5] Because infertility is often multifactorial, both partners should be evaluated and treated simultaneously to minimize delay in diagnosis and treatment with the patient.[6] This chapter will outline the key features of clinical evaluation and baseline evaluations/factors assessments that can represent the basic framework of infertility evaluation according to the declaration and position statements of professional organizations, including the World Health Organization (WHO), American Society for Reproductive Medicine (ASRM), and European Society of Human Reproduction and Embryology (ESHRE)[7] **(Flowchart 1)**.

GENERAL PRINCIPLES OF INFERTILITY WORKUP

The evaluation of infertility should be an organized and evidence-based process. For couples in whom the female is <35 years old,

Flowchart 1: Basic diagnostic workup of infertility.

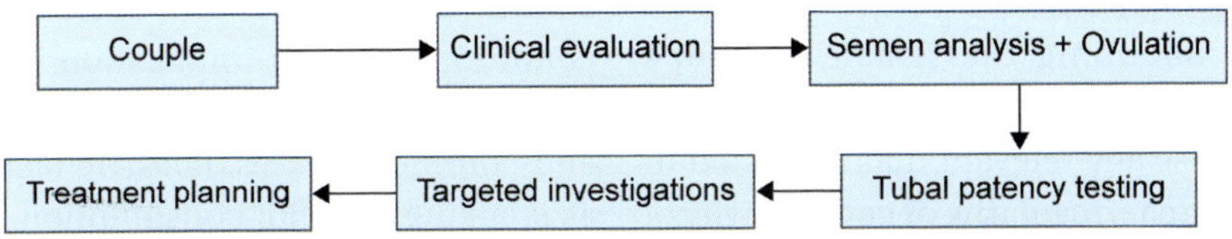

the evaluation usually begins after 12 months of regular and unprotected intercourse. For couples in which the female is over 35 years, the evaluation should begin after 6 months due to the more rapid decline of ovarian reserve with advancing age. In certain circumstances (such as in the presence of amenorrhea, pelvic inflammatory disease, prior pelvic surgery, or a known male factor), the evaluation can begin earlier.[8]

Assessment of infertility should be undertaken in a careful and A couple-centered evaluation approach is at the core of the assessment of infertility. The cause of infertility can be due to female factors, male factors, a combination, or, in rare cases, could be unexplained despite the complete evaluation. The assessment should follow the steps of a diagnostic plan that is organized in a stepwise approach beginning with basic, noninvasive tests, and proceeding to more invasive tests only if warranted. The importance of cost-effectiveness emerges as it is common to practice in the clinical medicine world to carry out unnecessary investigations or repeat them, which could further add to the stress and harm to the emotional health of the couple seeking help. In addition to the medical assessment, counseling and psychological support are needed as infertility is an emotional stress that could further jeopardize reproductive success.[8]

CLINICAL EVALUATION

History Taking

A thorough and empathetic history-taking is the first and often most informative step in evaluating infertility.

When obtaining the female partner's history, menstrual history is critical and should assess any relevant details related to age at menarche, regularity or compulsivity of cycle, flow, dysmenorrhea (which may suggest endometriosis). It is important to recognize that irregular cycles, oligomenorrhea, and amenorrhea are suggestive of anovulation or an endocrine abnormality of some kind, including polycystic ovary syndrome (PCOS) or thyroid issues. It is also very helpful to obtain obstetric history, including any prior conceptions/pregnancy losses and problems with any prior pregnancies, which may affect reproductive potential. Any history of gynecological problems should be evaluated in detail [i.e., sexually transmitted infections (STIs), pelvic inflammatory disease, and surgery related to the uterus, ovaries, or fallopian tubes]. Similarly, any history of systemic disease (including diabetes, thyroid Disease, or autoimmune diseases) would be considered and recollected for details when it comes to potential effect on fertility. Lifestyle is also an important consideration, including body mass index (BMI), smoking, alcohol use, and exercise, which can all directly and considerably influence reproductive health. The sexual history should also be evaluated in detail, including detailing frequency and timing of coitus, whether there is dyspareunia, and noting any vaginal lubricants used for penetration, as certain lubricants may compromise sperm function.[9]

In the male partner, the history should focus on pubertal development and past testicular conditions, as well as sexual functions (libido, erectile function, and ejaculatory pattern). Childhood infections (notably mumps orchitis) are pertinent because they can cause long-term reproductive harm. The medical history should discuss past and current systemic conditions with an implication for fertility, previous pelvic or urogenital/other surgeries, and chronic illnesses. Lifestyle factors, such as smoking, alcohol consumption, anabolic

TABLE 1: Key points in history and examination.

Aspect	*Female partner*	*Male partner*
History	Menstrual and obstetric details; past pelvic disease/surgery; lifestyle	Pubertal/sexual history; systemic illness; lifestyle
Examination	Body mass index (BMI), hirsutism, thyroid, and pelvic exam	Testicular size, varicocele, and genital anomalies

steroid use, and occupational issues relating to excessive heat exposure or environmental toxins, are particularly relevant to men, given their potential detrimental effects on spermatogenesis. Although this could already be obvious, it is usually the reproductive and sexual history that contributes to the most relevant clinical information before noninvasive or potentially invasive procedures.[10]

Physical Examination

Clinical examination is an essential complement to history-taking, as it helps identify underlying conditions that may require more specific evaluation. In the female partner, a general examination may include measurement of height, weight, and body mass index, given that extremes of body composition are often associated with anovulatory disorders. There may be physical signs of hyperandrogenism, such as acne, hirsutism, and alopecia, that are consistent with PCOS. Careful investigation for any thyroid enlargement, galactorrhea, or other evidence of systemic disease is also warranted. The pelvic examination is especially important as it provides information (uterine size and contour; adnexal masses, tenderness, perhaps endometriosis; cervical or vaginal abnormalities impeding fertility), which would be helpful later in fertility assessment.[11] Some general examination and history of the female Partner is provided in **Table 1**.

In the male partner, general physical examination should evaluate body habitus, secondary sexual characteristics, and signs supporting the chance of endocrine disorders.[12] Genital examination should be performed with care, looking specifically for testis size and consistency, and evidence of epididymal thickening. The presence of varicoceles, common and potentially correctable causes of male infertility, should be specifically evaluated.[13] Some history and examination of the male Partner is summarized in **Table 1**.

BASIC INVESTIGATION

Female Partner

The evaluation of female infertility primarily focuses on ovulation, ovarian reserve, tubal patency, and uterine anatomy.

Hormonal assessment is usually performed during the early follicular phase. Measurement of follicle-stimulating hormone (FSH) and luteinizing hormone (LH) provides insight into pituitary and ovarian function.[14] Elevated estradiol levels at this stage may suggest diminished ovarian reserve. Anti-Müllerian hormone (AMH) has become one of the most reliable indicators of ovarian reserve, as it reflects the pool of antral follicles and offers the advantage of being independent of the menstrual cycle. Thyroid function testing and serum prolactin evaluation are essential, since disturbances in either can contribute to an ovulation. In women with suspected PCOS, assessment of androgen levels, including testosterone and dehydroepiandrosterone sulfate (DHEAS), is particularly informative.[15]

Confirmation of ovulation is a critical step in infertility assessment. Midluteal serum progesterone measurement remains a widely accepted method, with values exceeding 3 ng/mL providing evidence of ovulation.[16] Ultrasound folliculometry offers direct visualization of follicular growth and rupture, while urinary LH detection kits are useful for identifying the preovulatory surge and optimizing the timing of intercourse or assisted reproductive procedures.[17]

Evaluation of tubal patency is an essential step, as tubal pathology accounts for nearly one-third of female infertility. Hysterosalpingography (HSG) remains a common first-line test, allowing visualization of both the uterine cavity and fallopian tubes. Alternatives such as saline infusion sonohysterography (SIS) or hysterosalpingo contrast sonography (HyCoSy) provide less invasive assessments. Laparoscopy with chromopertubation is considered the gold standard but is reserved for cases where high suspicion of tubal disease exists or when other pelvic pathology, such as endometriosis, is suspected.[18]

Evaluation of the uterus is equally important. Transvaginal ultrasound provides information on fibroids, endometrial thickness, and polyps, while hysteroscopy allows direct visualization and treatment of intrauterine pathology.[18]

Male Partner

Semen analysis forms the cornerstone of male infertility evaluation and remains the most informative initial test. According to the WHO 2021 guidelines, the lower reference limits for normal semen parameters include a volume of at least 1.4 mL, a sperm concentration of 16 million/mL, total motility of 42%, progressive motility of 30%, and normal morphology of 4% or more. Any abnormal finding should be confirmed with a repeat analysis, usually after an interval of two to three weeks, to account for natural variability.[19]

In cases where semen parameters are markedly abnormal, further evaluation with hormonal testing is indicated.[20] Measurement of serum FSH, LH, testosterone, and prolactin is particularly useful in men with azoospermia or severe oligozoospermia. Imaging studies may also be required: Scrotal ultrasonography can help detect varicocele, obstruction, or testicular pathology, while transrectal ultrasonography is valuable for identifying ejaculatory duct obstruction.[21]

Combined Investigation

Alongside partner-specific evaluations, certain general investigations are recommended for both individuals. Screening for infections such as HIV, hepatitis B, hepatitis C, and syphilis is essential, particularly before initiating assisted reproductive procedures. In selected cases, genetic testing may also be required. For example, karyotyping and Y-chromosome microdeletion analysis are indicated in men with azoospermia or severe oligozoospermia. While valuable, these tests extend beyond the scope of basic evaluation and are generally categorized as part of advanced diagnostic workups.[22]

■ SPECIAL CONSIDERATIONS

There are particular clinical circumstances that require a deviation from the usual diagnostic pathway. In women over the age of 35, it is important to move quickly if baseline investigations and ovulation concerns are fairly typical. Primarily, women in this age group need to consider that ovarian reserve will decline with age. If all baseline investigations are normal, the diagnosis of unexplained infertility can be accurately considered (accounting for approximately 10–20% of infertility cases).[23] Careful assessments of previous pregnancy outcomes and obstetric complications is also important for couples with secondary infertility, as fertility issues may contribute to key learning from previous pregnancies. Then, consider how a diagnosis of infertility and subsequent reproductive challenges often include psychological components to the experience. Emotional distress facing women and men could impact biological influences and fertility potential, leading to loss of sexual health or adherence to a treatment plan.[24]

PRACTICAL ASPECTS IN RESOURCE-LIMITED SETTINGS

Infertility investigation in low-resource settings should aim for a limited but essential number of diagnostic tests that are evidence-based, effective, and low-cost. Key investigations include semen analysis, an assessment of ovulation based on midluteal serum progesterone or ultrasound, and at least one test of tubal patency (such as HSG or HyCoSy). Secondary investigations should only be conducted when the indication for advanced investigations is convincing to save costs and limit stress for couples.[25]

CONCLUSION

Infertility is a multifactorial phenomenon that can best be approached in a systematic and structured way. A complete clinical history and careful physical examination are core to any evaluation, which should also include some important basic tests, including semen analysis, ovulation assessment, hormonal assessment, tubal patency testing, and uterine assessment. The objective of the evaluation is to find treatable causes, reduce unnecessary tests, and provide each couple with an individual evidence-based management plan. If clinicians can follow expected diagnostic pathways and respect a sense of balance between completeness and cost-effectiveness, we will increase the likelihood of positive conception outcomes for couples and lessen emotional distress and financial burden for couples.

REFERENCES

1. Vander Borght M, Wyns C. Fertility and infertility: Definition and epidemiology. Clin Biochem. 2018;62:2-10.
2. Jabeen F, Khadija S, Daud S. Prevalence of Primary and Secondary Infertility. Saudi J Med. 2022;7(1):22-8.
3. Sharma A, Shrivastava D. Psychological Problems Related to Infertility. Cureus. 2022;14(10):e30320.
4. Xie Y, Ren Y, Niu C, Zheng Y, Yu P, Li L. The impact of stigma on mental health and quality of life of infertile women: A systematic review. Front Psychol. 2023;13:1093459.
5. In: Weeks GR, Fife ST (Eds). Couples in treatment, 3rd edition. New York: Routledge; 2014.
6. Carson SA, Kallen AN. Diagnosis and management of infertility: A Review. JAMA. 2021;326(1):65.
7. Gianaroli L, Racowsky C, Geraedts J, Cedars M, Makrigiannakis A, Lobo R. Best practices of ASRM and ESHRE: a journey through reproductive medicine. Hum Reprod. 2012; 27(12):3365-79.
8. Kamel RM. Management of the infertile couple: an evidence-based protocol. Reprod Biol Endocrinol. 2010;8(1):21.
9. Missmer SA, Hankinson SE, Spiegelman D, Barbieri RL, Malspeis S, Willett WC, et al. Reproductive History and Endometriosis Among Premenopausal Women. Obstet Gynecol. 2004;104(5 Pt 1):965-74.

10. Weinbauer GF, Luetjens CM, Simoni M, Nieschlag E. Physiology of Testicular Function. In: Nieschlag E, Behre HM, Nieschlag S (Eds). Andrology. Berlin, Heidelberg: Springer Berlin Heidelberg; 2010. pp. 11-59.
11. Darıcı E, Pais F, Leemans L, Strypstein L, Tournaye H, De Vos M, et al. From body mass index to body composition in female infertility. Reprod Biomed Online. 2025;51(3):104941.
12. Jarow JP, Sharlip ID, Belker AM, Lipshultz LI, Sigman M, Thomas AJ, et al. Best Practice Policies for Male Infertility. J Urol. 2002;167(5):2138-44.
13. Levine DA, Powers ME. The Evidence-Based Physical Examination of the Child and Adolescent Male. In: Heidelbaugh JJ (Ed). Men's Health in Primary Care. Cham: Springer International Publishing; 2016. pp. 57-87.
14. Targonskaya A, Maslowski K. Gonadotropin and Ovarian Hormone Monitoring: Lateral Flow Assays for Clinical Decision Making. Women. 2023;3(4):471-85.
15. Patrelli TS, Gizzo S, Sianesi N, Levati L, Pezzuto A, Ferrari B, et al. Anti-Müllerian Hormone Serum Values and Ovarian Reserve: Can It Predict a Decrease in Fertility after Ovarian Stimulation by ART Cycles? Zakar T, editor. PLoS ONE. 2012;7(9):e44571.
16. Su H, Yi Y, Wei T, Chang T, Cheng C. Detection of ovulation, a review of currently available methods. Bioeng Transl Med. 2017;2(3):238-46.
17. Mittal P, Ghuman NK. Detection of Ovulation and Aetiology of Anovulation. In: Ghumman S, editor. Principles and Practice of Controlled Ovarian Stimulation in ART. New Delhi: Springer India; 2015. pp. 3-12.
18. Okeke T, Agwuna K, Ezenyeaku C, Ikeako L. Application of ultrasonography in female infertility: a comprehensive review. Int J Reprod Contracept Obstet Gynecol. 2015; 1246-56.
19. Barbăroşie C, Agarwal A, Henkel R. Diagnostic value of advanced semen analysis in evaluation of male infertility. Andrologia. 2021;53(2):e13625.
20. Hofny ERM, Ali ME, Abdel-Hafez HZ, Kamal EED, Mohamed EE, Abd El-Azeem HG, et al. Semen parameters and hormonal profile in obese fertile and infertile males. Fertil Steril. 2010;94(2):581-4.
21. Ragheb D, Higgins JL. Ultrasonography of the Scrotum: Technique, Anatomy, and Pathologic Entities. J Ultrasound Med. 2002;21(2):171-85.
22. Alswaidi FM, O'brien SJ. Premarital screening programmes for haemoglobinopathies, HIV and hepatitis viruses: review and factors affecting their success. J Med Screen. 2009; 16(1):22-8.
23. Pearlstone AC, Fournet N, Gambone JC, Pang SC, Buyalos RP. Ovulation induction in women age 40 and older: the importance of basal follicle-stimulating hormone level and chronological age. Fertil Steril. 1992; 58(4):674-9.
24. Fisher JR, Hammarberg K. Psychological and social aspects of infertility in men: an overview of the evidence and implications for psychologically informed clinical care and future research. Asian J Androl. 2012;14(1):121-9.
25. De Sutter P. Rational diagnosis and treatment in infertility. Best Pract Res Clin Obstet Gynaecol. 2006;20(5):647-64.

CHAPTER 5

Advances in Semen Analysis and Sperm Deoxyribonucleic Acid (DNA) Fragmentation

Mayuri Assudani, Akash More, Sudhanshu Dakre

INTRODUCTION

Infertility is defined as the inability to conceive after 12 months of regular, unprotected sexual intercourse. Globally, the prevalence of infertility among reproductive-age couples is estimated to range from 12.6 to 17.5%, affecting approximately 48.5–72.4 million couples worldwide.[1] Male factors alone are responsible for nearly 50% of all infertility cases and directly account for approximately 20–30% of them.[2] Seminal plasma, commonly referred to as semen, consists of spermatozoa suspended in glandular secretions and is produced by the testes along with accessory sex glands. The testes, functioning as dual glands, have both exocrine and endocrine roles—they generate spermatozoa and testicular fluid (exocrine function) while also secreting hormones such as testosterone and inhibin (endocrine function).[3] Semen analysis is a laboratory test that evaluates a man's sperm and overall reproductive health. It is an essential tool in investigating male infertility and helps in understanding the possible causes of difficulty in conceiving. Semen analysis evaluates several parameters, including total semen volume, sperm count sperm concentration, and sperm characteristics such as motility, morphology, and viability, along with the composition of seminal secretions. Examining these factors provides valuable insight into the causes of male infertility. Besides, semen examination is an important test used in estimating the male reproductive health, monitoring the success of various procedures, like vasectomy, and guiding assisted reproductive technologies, including intrauterine insemination (IUI) and in vitro fertilization (IVF).[4]

METHOD OF SEMEN COLLECTION

Semen collection is an essential step in assessing male fertility and supporting assisted reproductive treatments. Depending on the individual's condition and the purpose of the test or procedure, various methods can be used to collect semen.

- *Masturbation:* The man ejaculates into a clean, wide mouthed container made of glass or plastic by self-stimulation. It is the most common and safest method. The sample should be collected in a clean container and taken to the lab quickly.
- *Collection during inter course (using a special condom):* A condom that does not contain spermicide is used during intercourse to collect semen. This method may be used when masturbation is not possible or acceptable.
- *Penile vibratory stimulation (PVS):* A device is placed on the penis to create vibrations that help induce ejaculation. It is used when masturbation is difficult or not possible.

- *Electro-ejaculation:* A medical device applies small electrical pulses to the nerves controlling ejaculation. It is performed under sedation or anesthesia and is used for men with spinal cord injuries or other conditions.
- *Microsurgical epididymal sperm aspiration (MESA):* A small incision is made to extract sperm from the epididymis under a microscope. Surgical sperm retrieval—percutaneous epididymal sperm aspiration (PESA)—sperm is retrieved from the epididymis using a needle.
- *Testicular sperm extraction (TESE):* Sperm is surgically removed from the testicle. These methods are used when sperm cannot be obtained through ejaculation.[5]

HANDLING OF SEMEN

A minimum duration of 2 days and maximum of 7 days of sexual abstinence is required prior to the collection of the sample. The sample must be gathered in a clean wide mouthed container either plastic or glass and then kept at ambient temperature at 37C°. The sample should preferably be collected in a separate room (semen collection room) adjacent to the laboratory to prevent temperature variation.[6] In exceptional situations such as failure to ejaculate (possibly by masturbation) in the clinic or under stress etc., a sample may be collected at home. In such case the patient should record the time of semen production and deliver the sample to the laboratory within 1 hour of collection with proper labelling on container.[4] Microscope stage should be cleaned with the help of 70% alcohol and distilled water. Right after the collection, sample should be kept on the heating block in the laminar for liquefaction. While performing semen analysis or processing gently pipetting should be done to avoid formation of bubbles. Do not use alcohol in between the procedure for cleaning or washing the hands.[7]

Safety measures for laboratory staff are:

- Hepatitis immunization of all laboratory personnel should be done.
- No one should apply cosmetics, smoke, eat, or drink in the andrology laboratory.
- Semen sample may contain infectious agents example HIV, hepatitis, herbs, etc. In such case use of safety gears such as sterile dress, powder free gloves, face mask, and hair cap should be used.
- Always wash your hands before entering and leaving the laboratory.

PARAMETERS ASSESSED IN SEMEN ANALYSIS

Semen analysis involves both microscopic and macroscopic evaluation of the ejaculate. These parameters provide critical information about the functional competence of spermatozoa and the secretory activity of accessory sex glands **(Table 1)**.

MACROSCOPIC EXAMINATION

Macroscopic examination refers to the visual and physical assessment of semen immediately after ejaculation and during liquefaction, without the use of a microscope which includes.

Specimen Liquefaction

Within the first 10 minutes after collection, semen is typically kept at room temperature or placed in an incubator at 37°C to allow liquefaction. This process makes the sample more uniform and fluid, though small areas of coagulation may remain.[8] During liquefaction, sperm trapped within the coagulum are released and gain motility. Normally, liquefaction is completed within 15 minutes; if it does not occur within

TABLE 1: Nomenclature of semen.

Parameter	*Term (nomenclature)*	*Definition/WHO criteria (2021)*	*Clinical notes*
Overall semen quality	Normozoospermia	All semen parameters (volume, concentration, motility, morphology, vitality) within WHO reference ranges	Indicates normal semen profile but does not guarantee fertility
Sperm concentration	Oligozoospermia	Sperm concentration <15 million/mL • *Mild:* 10–15 million/mL • *Moderate:* 5–10 million/mL • *Severe:* <5 million/mL	May result from testicular failure, varicocele, obstruction, hormonal or genetic causes
	Azoospermia	No spermatozoa seen in ejaculate (confirmed after centrifugation)	May be obstructive (ductal blockage) or non-obstructive (spermatogenic failure)
	Cryptozoospermia	No sperm in initial exam, but very few observed after centrifugation	Indicates severely impaired spermatogenesis
	Polyzoospermia	Very high sperm concentration (>250 million/mL)	Rare; may be linked with inflammation or hyperandrogenism
Ejaculate volume	Hypospermia	Volume <1.4 mL	Suggests ejaculatory duct obstruction, retrograde ejaculation, androgen deficiency, or incomplete collection
	Hyperspermia	Volume >6.0 mL	May be due to prolonged abstinence, infection, or seminal vesicle hypersecretion
	Aspermia	Complete absence of ejaculate	Seen in retrograde ejaculation, obstruction, or anejaculation (neurological/psychological)
Motility	Asthenozoospermia	*Reduced motility:* • Total motility <40% OR • Progressive motility <32%	May be due to tail defects, oxidative stress, infections, or varicocele
	Complete asthenozoospermia	100% immotile spermatozoa	Rare; sperm may still be alive (differentiated using vitality test)
Vitality	Necrozoospermia	Majority or all spermatozoa dead (<54% viable)	Indicates testicular damage, infections, or toxic exposures
	Mixed necrozoospermia	Some sperm alive but proportion below WHO lower reference (54%)	May coexist with asthenozoospermia
Morphology	Teratozoospermia	<4% normal morphology (strict Kruger criteria)	Often linked to genetic/chromosomal abnormalities, varicocele, toxins
	Monomorphic teratozoospermia	All spermatozoa show same abnormality (e.g., globozoospermia – round heads)	Strongly associated with genetic defects, fertilization failure

Contd...

Contd...

Parameter	*Term (nomenclature)*	*Definition/WHO criteria (2021)*	*Clinical notes*
Semen appearance	Hematospermia	Presence of blood in semen	Can result from infection, trauma, obstruction, or tumors
	Leukocytospermia (Pyospermia)	Leukocyte concentration >1 million/mL	Suggests genital tract infection or inflammation, linked with oxidative stress
Multiple defects	Oligoasthenozoospermia	• Low sperm concentration (<15 million/mL) + reduced motility (<32% progressive) • Total sperm number also typically <39 million/ejaculate (WHO limit)	Common cause of subfertility
	Asthenoteratozoospermia	• Reduced motility (<32%) + abnormal morphology (<4% normal forms) • Often associated with a low total sperm count (<39 million/ejaculate)	Indicates combined functional and structural defects
	Oligoteratozoospermia	• Low concentration (<15 million/mL) + abnormal morphology (<4% normal forms) • Total sperm number falls below WHO limit of 39 million	Severe reduction in natural fertility potential
	Oligoasthenoteratozoospermia (OAT syndrome)	*Combination of:* • Low concentration (<15 million/mL) • Reduced motility (<32%) • Abnormal morphology (<4%) • Always associated with total sperm number <39 million/ejaculate	Represents one of the most severe semen abnormalities; often requires ART (IVF/ICSI)

30–45 minutes, chemical agents may be applied to assist the process. However, the use of such reagents can alter seminal plasma composition and affect sperm motility and morphology, which should be documented.

Volume: The semen volume is determined by aspirating the sample from the collection container, using a syringe or a pipette. Normal reference value according to the WHO is ≥1.4 mL per ejaculate.[9]

Appearance: Appearance refers to the consistency and color of semen. Sample is examined as soon as the collected sample is received. Normal color of the semen is opaque gray and abnormalities is considered when the color is yellowish which indicates infection or prolonged abstinence, Reddish/brown (hematospermia) which indicates presence of blood, often from infection, trauma, or tumors,[10] Clear/watery which indicates low sperm concentration or incomplete collection. Normal semen has a characteristic odor due to polyamines, i.e., seminal. A foul odor may suggest infection.

Viscosity: It refers to the thickness and flow characteristics of semen after liquefaction. After liquefaction, a pipette is dipped into the sample and allowed to drop; normal semen should form droplets, not long threads. Increased viscosity often associated with infection, high leukocyte content, or prostatic/seminal vesicle dysfunction. High viscosity can impair sperm motility and sperm retrieval for ART.[11]

pH: pH measures the alkalinity or acidity of semen. The pH scale ranges from 0 to 14, with 7 being neutral. Values >7 are alkaline, and <7 are acidic. The normal semen pH range is 7.2–8.0. Abnormal pH can indicate issues such as:

- *Low pH (<7.2):* May suggest problems like blockage in seminal vesicles or infection.
- *High pH (>8.0):* May indicate inflammation, infection, or blockage in accessory glands like the prostate or seminal vesicles.

MICROSCOPIC EXAMINATION OF SEMEN

Microscopic examination of semen is an essential laboratory test performed to evaluate the physical and cellular characteristics of semen, particularly to assess male fertility potential. It involves observing the semen sample under a microscope to analyze sperm count, motility, morphology, and other parameters.

Procedure

- Semen is collected by masturbation into a sterile container after 2–7 days of abstinence.
- The sample is allowed to liquefy at room temperature (usually 15 minutes).
- A small drop is placed on a Makler chamber.
- It is observed under a microscope at different magnifications (commonly 20×).

PRIMARY MICROSCOPIC EXAMINATION

Cell Count/Concentration

It measures the number of cells (e.g., sperm, blood cells, microorganisms) in a given volume. Sperm concentration is determined by counting number of sperm in a row of 10 squares in Makler's chamber at 20× magnification as shown in **Figures 1A and B**. Average of 3 counting is recorded for precision. The lower reference limit for sperm concentration per ejaculation is 15 million/ml as mentioned in **Table 2.**[12]

Makler's Chamber

Makler's chamber is a specialized counting device used in semen analysis to assess sperm concentration, motility, and morphology under the microscope.

The chamber is composed of two parts:

- *Lower part:* The base is metallic with two side handles. At its center lies a flat disc made of optical-grade glass, which serves as the platform for placing the specimen.
- *Upper part:* The top component consists of a cover glass bordered by a metal ring. On the underside of this cover, at the center, is a grid measuring 1 mm^2, subdivided into 100 smaller squares, each with dimensions of 0.1 × 0.1 mm.

Motility/Movement

Sperm motility refers to the ability of sperm to move efficiently, which is a critical factor in male fertility. Motility is evaluated by observing how sperm swim under the microscope, with particular attention to the speed, direction, and type of movement. It is

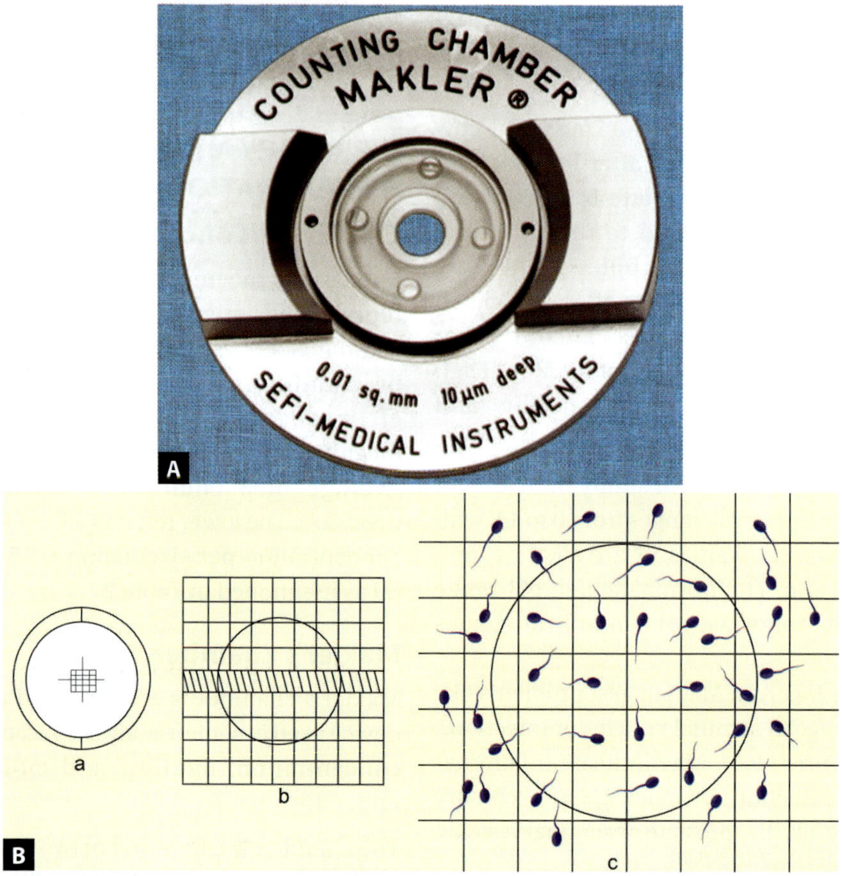

Figs. 1A and B: Makler chember and chamber grids for sperm concentration and motility evaluation.

TABLE 2: WHO semen analysis reference values (2010 vs. 2021).

Parameter	*WHO 2010*	*WHO 2021*
Semen volume (mL)	1.5 (1.4–1.7)	1.4 (1.3–1.5)
Total sperm number (10^6 per ejaculate)	39 (33–46)	39 (35–40)
Total motility (%)	40 (38–42)	42 (40–43)
Progressive motility (%)	32 (31–34)	30 (29–31)
Non-progressive motility (%)	1	1 (1–1)
Immotile sperm (%)	22	20 (19–20)
Vitality (%)	58 (55–63)	54 (50–56)
Normal forms (%)	4 (3–4)	4 (3.9–4)

classified into categories such as progressive motility (sperm moving actively and in a straight line), immotility (sperm showing no movement at all), non-progressive motility (sperm moving but in circles or without forward progression). The lower reference limit for total motility (PR + NP) is 40% and progressive motility (PR) is 32% as mentioned in **Table 2.**[13]

Agglutination

Agglutination refers to the abnormal clumping or sticking together of sperm cells, often caused by the presence of anti-sperm antibodies or other factors that interfere with sperm function. Unlike normal aggregation, which may be random and temporary, agglutination involves sperm binding head-to-tail, tail-to-tail, or head-to-head, forming clusters that restrict movement.[9] This condition can significantly affect motility and reduce the likelihood of fertilization.[14]

- *Grade 1 (isolated):* Fewer than 10 sperm/agglutinate, with many sperm remaining free.
- *Grade 2 (moderate):* Aggregates contain 10–50 spermatozoa, while free sperm are still present.
- *Grade 3 (large):* More than 50 spermatozoa per agglutinate, with only a small number of sperm remaining free.
- *Grade 4 (gross):* Complete agglutination, with virtually all spermatozoa clumped together.

Aggregation

Non-specific aggregation refers to the adherence of immotile spermatozoa to each other, or of motile spermatozoa to mucus strands, non-sperm cells, or cellular debris.[15]

Cellular Components and Contaminants in Semen

These are cells such as white blood cells, immature germ cells, epithelial cells, or pus cell found in semen besides sperm. Their presence may indicate infections, inflammation, contamination, or issues with sperm development, helping in diagnosing underlying reproductive problems.[16]

SECONDARY MICROSCOPIC EXAMINATION

Vitality/Life Status

Vitality refers to the assessment of the life status of cells by determining the proportion of living cells compared to dead ones. This parameter is particularly important in evaluating the functional health of cells, such as sperm in semen analysis. Specialized staining techniques are used to distinguish between dead and live cells, as non-viable cells absorb them while viable cells exclude certain dyes. For example, in semen examination, stains such as eosin-nigrosin are applied to the sample, allowing observers to count how many sperm are alive and capable of movement versus those that are dead or non-functional. A higher percentage of live cells is associated with better fertility potential, while a reduced vitality count may indicate underlying problems affecting cell integrity or health. Assessing vitality helps in diagnosing issues, guiding treatment options, and improving outcomes in reproductive and other medical contexts.

Morphology

Morphology refers to the detailed examination of the form, structure, and physical characteristics of cells or organisms under the microscope. This assessment helps in identifying both normal cells and those with structural abnormalities that may affect their function.[17] For example, in semen analysis, sperm morphology is evaluated to determine the proportion of sperm with a normal shape, including a well-formed head, midpiece, and tail. Defects such as coiled or bent tails, misshapen heads, or irregular midpieces can

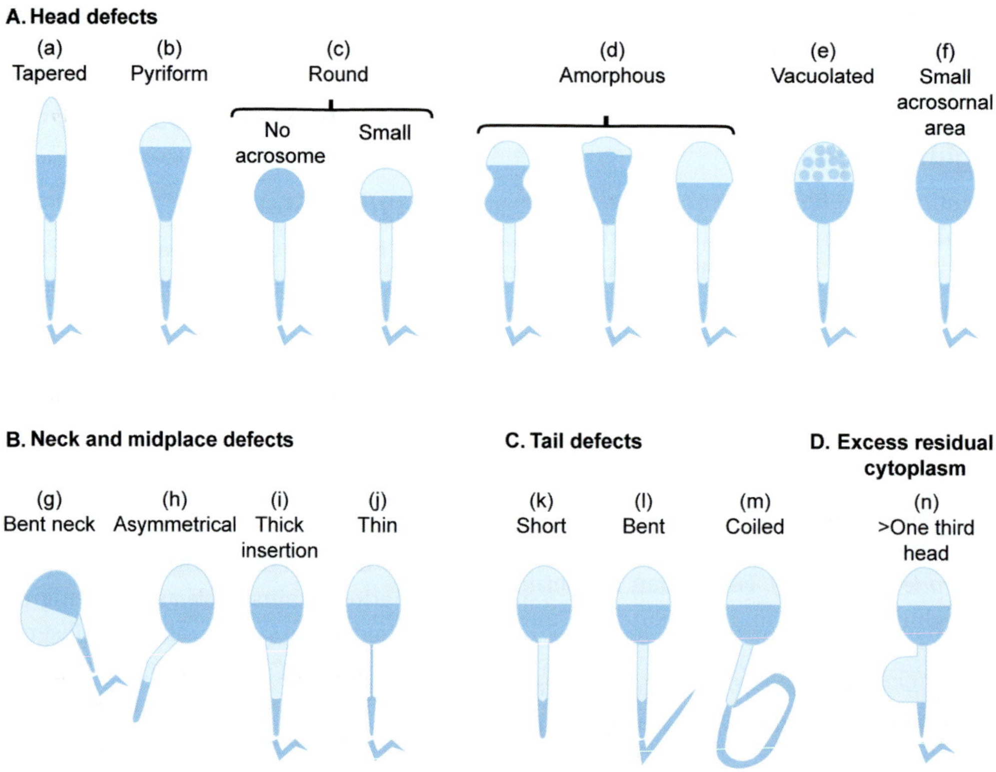

Figs. 2A to D: Defects in sperms.

impair the sperm's ability to swim properly and fertilize an egg, contributing to infertility **Figs. 2A to D)**.

The evaluation focuses on three main parts of the sperm—the head, neck (midpiece), and tail—and identifies structural defects in each that may impair fertility.

- *Head defects:* The head contains the genetic material necessary for fertilization. Abnormalities in the head can include being too large or too small, having an irregular shape, tapered or flattened forms, double heads, or amorphous structures. Such defects can interfere with the sperm's ability to penetrate the egg or carry the correct deoxyribonucleic acid (DNA).
- *Neck/midpiece defects:* The midpiece connects the head to the tail and houses mitochondria that provide energy for movement. Defects here include thickened or bent necks, irregular shapes, or disruptions that impair energy production, reducing the sperm's capacity to swim effectively.[18]
- *Tail defects:* The tail is responsible for propelling the sperm forward. Common abnormalities include coiled, bent, short, or absent tails. These defects can significantly decrease motility, preventing the sperm from reaching and fertilizing the egg.

LOWER REFERENCE VALUE

In semen analysis, the "lower reference value" according to WHO means the 5th percentile value of semen parameters obtained from a population of fertile men whose partners conceived within 12 months of unprotected intercourse.[19]

Lower reference limit for semen characteristics are:

DEOXYRIBONUCLEIC ACID FRAGMENTATION

Deoxyribonucleic acid fragmentation of sperm DNA as displayed in **Figure 3** (breakages or damages of the genetic material) is a leading cause of male infertility because it impairs the functional ability of the sperm. Generally, sperm DNA fragmentation index below 15% is normal, 15–30% is moderate and over 30% is correlated with poor potential fertility. Different assays are widely adopted in visualizing and quantifying sperm DNA fragmentation, e.g., the SCSA (sperm chromatin structure assay) as presented in **Figure 3**.[20]

Procedure

- Determine the concentration of the sperm sample and dilute it with culture media to produce a concentration of 5–10 million sperm cells per milliliter.
- Heat the agarose to 90°C using the sperm chroma warmer 1 and maintain it at this temperature for 5 minutes.
- Transfer the melted agarose to sperm chroma warmer 2, that is kept it at 37°C and allow it to stabilize for 5 minutes.
- Add 25 μL of the semen sample to the agarose and ensure thorough mixing.
- Immediately place the sperm cell suspension onto pre-treated slides and cover it with a glass cover slip carefully to avoid formation of bubbles.
- Let this slide sit at 4°C for 5 minutes.
- After 5 minutes, remove the slide. Gently slide off the cover glass with care.
- Ensure the slide remains horizontal throughout its immersion in solution A for 7 minutes.
- Keep the slide in the incubator horizontally for 7 minutes in solution A.
- After 7 minutes incubates the slide horizontally in Lysis solution for 25 minutes.
- Following the 7-minute incubation in solution A, soak the slides horizontally in Lysis solution (solution B) for 25 minutes. Submerge the slides in distilled water for 5 minutes.
- Submerge the slides for 2 minutes in 70% ethanol, secondly in 90% ethanol, and lastly in a solution of 100% ethanol.
- Leave them to air dry at room temperature.
- Mix solution C and solution D in a 1:1 ratio to make a staining solution. Apply a layer of stain and leave it to dry for 15–20 minutes.
- Carefully pour off the excess stain and gently wash the slides with distilled water. Let them dry it at the room temperature.
- Examine the slides under a bright field microscope using 20X or 40X objectives and assess the spermatozoa.

Cause:

- *Age:* Advanced paternal age has been associated with increased sperm DNA fragmentation.

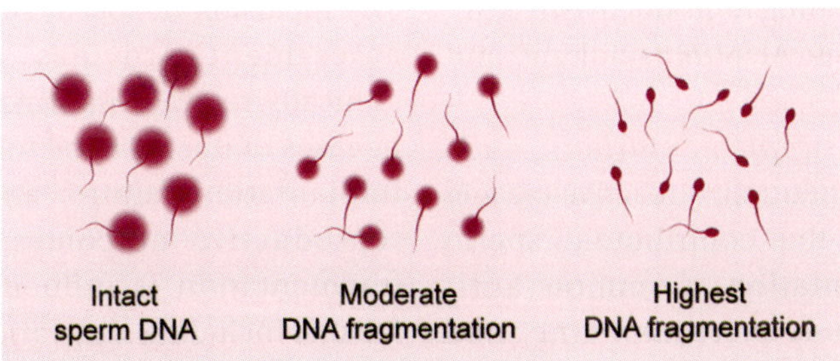

Fig. 3: Schematic representation of sperm deoxyribonucleic acid (DNA) fragmentation.

- *Varicocele:* A varicocele is a condition characterized by the enlargement of veins within the scrotum.
- *Infections:* Sexually transmitted infections (STIs) or other genital infections can cause inflammation and lead to sperm DNA damage.
- *Environmental factors:* Radiation, pollutants, and industrial chemicals can contribute to sperm DNA fragmentation.
- *Lifestyle factors:* Lack of exercise, poor diet, unhealthy lifestyle choices, obesity, and substance abuse (such as tobacco and recreational drugs), can negatively impact sperm quality and DNA integrity.
- *Genetic factors:* Genetic mutations or abnormalities can contribute to increased vulnerability to DNA damage.
- *Medications and treatments:* Certain medications and medical treatments, such as radiation therapy and chemotherapy, can affect sperm DNA integrity.
- *Poor semen quality:* Factors such as abnormal sperm morphology (shape), poor sperm motility, and low sperm count can be associated with increased DNA fragmentation.

Treatments:

- *Lifestyle modification:*
  - *Healthy diet:* Balanced and nutritious diet rich in antioxidants, vitamins, and minerals can positively impact sperm health.
  - *Regular Exercise:* Improve overall health including reproductive health.
  - *Avoid toxins*: Alcohol, smoking, and tobacco.
- *Antioxidant supplementation:* Antioxidants help neutralize reactive oxygen species (ROS) that contribute to sperm DNA fragmentation. Common antioxidants include selenium, zinc, and vitamins C and E.
- *Varicocele repair:* If a varicocele is identified as a contributing factor, surgical correction (varicocelectomy) may be considered to improve sperm parameters and reduce oxidative stress.
- *Sperm selection techniques:* Techniques such as intracytoplasmic sperm injection (ICSI) during IVF can be used to directly inject a single, healthy sperm into an egg. Bypassing potential DNA fragmentation issues.
- *Sperm cryopreservation (sperm freezing):* Freezing sperm samples before fertility treatments may be considered. This allows for the selection of healthier sperm during subsequent-assisted reproductive procedures.

CONCLUSION

Semen analysis remains a fundamental investigation in the evaluation of male infertility, offering critical insight into sperm concentration, motility, morphology, vitality, and seminal plasma characteristics. Standardized semen collection, handling, and microscopic assessment are essential to ensure reliable and clinically meaningful results. The adoption of updated World Health Organization reference values has further strengthened the diagnostic accuracy of routine semen analysis.

However, conventional semen parameters alone do not fully reflect the functional competence of spermatozoa. The inclusion of sperm DNA fragmentation assessment provides additional and clinically relevant information, particularly in cases of unexplained infertility, recurrent implantation failure, and poor assisted reproductive outcomes. Elevated DNA fragmentation is influenced by multiple factors, including age, varicocele, infections, environmental exposures, and lifestyle habits.

A comprehensive evaluation combining routine semen analysis with advanced sperm DNA integrity testing allows for improved diagnosis, targeted interventions, and optimized use of assisted reproductive technologies. This integrated approach enhances clinical decision-making and contributes to better reproductive outcomes in male factor infertility.

REFERENCES

1. Vander Borght M, Wyns C. Fertility and infertility: Definition and epidemiology. Clin Biochem. 2018;62:2-10.
2. Leslie SW, Soon-Sutton TL, Khan MA. Male Infertility. In: StatPearls. Treasure Island (FL): StatPearls Publishing; 2025.
3. Adelman MM. Semen Analysis Training Tool. Lab Med. 1999;30(10):687-8.
4. Mortimer D. Practical Laboratory Andrology. Oxford University Press: New York, NY; 1994.
5. Mendeluk G, Flecha FLG, Castello PR, Bregni C. Factors Involved in the Biochemical Etiology of Human Seminal Plasma Hyperviscosity. J Androl. 2000;21(2):262-7.
6. Lin MC, Tsai TC, Yang YS. Measurement of viscosity of human semen with a rotational viscometer. J Formos Med Assoc Taiwan Yi Zhi. 1992;91(4):419-23.
7. Stephen EH, Chandra A. Declining estimates of infertility in the United States: 1982–2002. Fertil Steril. 2006;86(3):516-23.
8. Carrell DT, De Jonge CJ. The troubling state of the semen analysis. Andrology. 2016;4(5):761-2.
9. Levine H, Jørgensen N, Martino-Andrade A, Mendiola J, Weksler-Derri D, Jolles M, et al. Temporal trends in sperm count: a systematic review and meta-regression analysis of samples collected globally in the 20th and 21st centuries. Hum Reprod Update. 2023;29(2):157-76.
10. Agarwal A, Henkel R, Huang CC, Lee MS. Automation of human semen analysis using a novel artificial intelligence optical microscopic technology. Andrologia. 2019;51(11):e13440.
11. Huang J, Chen L, Wan L, Yang JG, Wang H, Zhou XY, et al. [An analysis of donor semen quality in Chongqing Human Sperm Bank]. Zhonghua Nan Ke Xue Natl J Androl. 2018; 24(8):700-4.
12. Crissman JW. Postulated Human Sperm Count Decline May Involve Historic Elimination of Juvenile Iodine Deficiency: A New Hypothesis with Experimental Evidence in the Rat. Toxicol Sci. 2000;53(2):400-10.
13. Dhumal SS, Naik P, Dakshinamurthy S, Sullia K. Semen pH and its correlation with motility and count - A study in subfertile men. JBRA Assist Reprod. 2021;25(2):172-5.
14. Brown GJ, Nöthling JO, De Cramer KGM. Canine-specific tail-in, head-out sperm agglutination. Reprod Domest Anim Zuchthyg. 2021;56(10):1363-5.
15. Xie Y, Ren Y, Niu C, Zheng Y, Yu P, Li L. The impact of stigma on mental health and quality of life of infertile women: A systematic review. Front Psychol. 2023;13:1093459.
16. Moulik S, Gopalkrishnan K, Hinduja I, Shahani SK. Presence of sperm antibodies and association with viscosity of semen. Hum Reprod. 1989;4(3):290-1.
17. Viswambharan N, Manavalan M. Sperm Abnormalities: In the Male Partners of Infertile Couples from Kanyakumari District. Int J Infertil Fetal Med. 2021;11(1):16-9.
18. Eisenberg ML. The past, present, and future of the semen analysis. Fertil Steril. 2022;117(2):235-6.
19. Cooper TG, Noonan E, Von Eckardstein S, Auger J, Baker HWG, Behre HM, et al. World Health Organization reference values for human semen characteristics. Hum Reprod Update. 2010;16(3):231-45.
20. Stavros S, Potiris A, Molopodi E, Mavrogianni D, Zikopoulos A, Louis K, et al. Sperm DNA Fragmentation: Unraveling Its Imperative Impact on Male Infertility Based on Recent Evidence. Int J Mol Sci. 2024;25(18):10167.

CHAPTER 6

Ovarian Reserve Assessment and Anti-Müllerian Hormone

Himani Agarwal

INTRODUCTION

The endocrinology of ovarian function is very dynamic in nature. Traditionally, the aging process of the reproductive system is centered on the basic principle that during fetal life, oocytes peak in number; thereafter, they undergo ovulation or atresia and thence do not regenerate. However, some ovarian functions persist even after menopause.

The effect of ovaries is not only confined to the reproductive system. Estrogen affects mental health and skeletal and cardiovascular systems also. Thus, ovarian dysfunction can lead to disequilibrium related to various conditions.

Efficient ovarian reserve assessment can definitely give valuable clues regarding women's fertility potential, possible time to menopause, and postmenopausal symptoms that they face.

OVARIAN RESERVE

Ovarian reserve refers to the number of oocytes left in the ovary. It is different from oocyte quality which refers to the ability of a fertilized oocyte to result in a live-birth. Ovarian reserve is inversely proportional to the woman's age; however, it may vary among women of the same chronological age.[1]

OVARIAN RESPONSE

Ovarian response refers to the quantity and quality of follicular response and thereby the oocyte yield during controlled ovarian stimulation. It is usually assessed through transvaginal ultrasound scan and is considered as an important parameter to interpret the success of an ART procedure as the number of mature oocytes retrieved during ovum pickup strongly correlates with livebirth rate.[2]

OVARIAN RESERVE ASSESSMENT

Ovarian reserve assessment can primarily be done by both biochemical tests and ultrasound imaging of the ovaries.

Biochemical Tests

Biochemical tests directly or indirectly measure the follicular or oocyte pool. These tests can further be divided into early-follicular-phase measurement of follicle-stimulating hormone (FSH), E2, and inhibin B levels; measurement of cycle-day-independent anti-Müllerian hormone (AMH) levels; and provocative tests like clomiphene citrate challenge test (CCCT).

Basal Serum FSH Levels

Serum concentrations of FSH are usually elevated on the second or third day of menstrual cycle in females with diminished ovarian reserve (DOR). Though not sensitive, but it is a highly specific test for DOR.[3] Single FSH level measurement is not completely reliable as it has significant intercycle and intracycle variability.[3,4]

Basal Serum E2 Levels

Basal serum E2 levels seldom should be used to assess ovarian reserve. It can be used as an adjunct for interpretation of a normal basal FSH level. Early increased E2 levels are highly indicative of reproductive aging. This can cause misinterpretation by lowering an otherwise elevated basal FSH level into near-normal values. Additionally, if basal E2 levels are elevated (>60–80 pg/mL) and basal FSH levels are normal, this may point toward ovarian dysfunction due to DOR.[5]

Inhibin B

Inhibin B is a glycoprotein hormone secreted mainly by preantral follicles. With advancing age, both the number of ovarian follicles and early follicular phase inhibin B levels decline. This decrease leads to lowering the level of negative feedback which in turn results in increased pituitary FSH secretion. This leads to early onset of growth of new follicles and increased E2 levels, ultimately leading to shorter length of the follicular phase and the overall menstrual cycle. Overall measurement of inhibin B levels is not recommended as its clinical relevance is limited.

Anti-Müllerian Hormone

Anti-Müllerian hormone is one of the members of the transforming growth factor beta family. Its name is derived because of its pivotal role inducing regression of müllerian ducts during male sex differentiation. It is a glycoprotein hormone expressed by granulosa cells of growing follicles. It is secreted from the primary up to the small antral stage and is therefore a direct measurement of the follicular pool.

After FSH-dependent selection, the expression of AMH disappears. Its expression is also lost in corpus luteum and atretic follicles. This window of increased AMH expression is detected in follicles ≤8 mm and absent in follicles >8 mm **(Fig. 1A)**.[6]

The term functional ovarian reserve (FOR) has evolved to differentiate between the pool of growing follicles and the pool of resting primordial follicles. This pool of growing follicles is called AMH-producing follicles. Thus, AMH levels directly reflect FOR **(Fig. 1B)**.

Till date, AMH is considered as the best serum marker for ovarian function. Its levels can be assessed at both ends of the spectrum, i.e., polycystic ovarian syndrome and DOR.

Clomiphene Citrate Challenge Test

The CCCT is based on serum FSH level measurement before (day 3) and after (day 10) menstrual cycle treatment with clomiphene citrate (100 mg/day for 5 days, from day 5 to day 9). With growing ovarian follicles, inhibin B and E2 levels will rise which in turn will suppress FSH in females with responsive ovaries. However, smaller follicular cohorts recruited in females with DOR will produce less inhibin B and E2 levels, leading to decreased negative feedback inhibition of FSH secretion and hence higher stimulated serum FSH concentrations. This increased FSH concentration post clomiphene stimulation thus suggests DOR. Such provocative tests like CCCT may increase sensitivity for DOR[7] but are not superior in any way for predicting poor

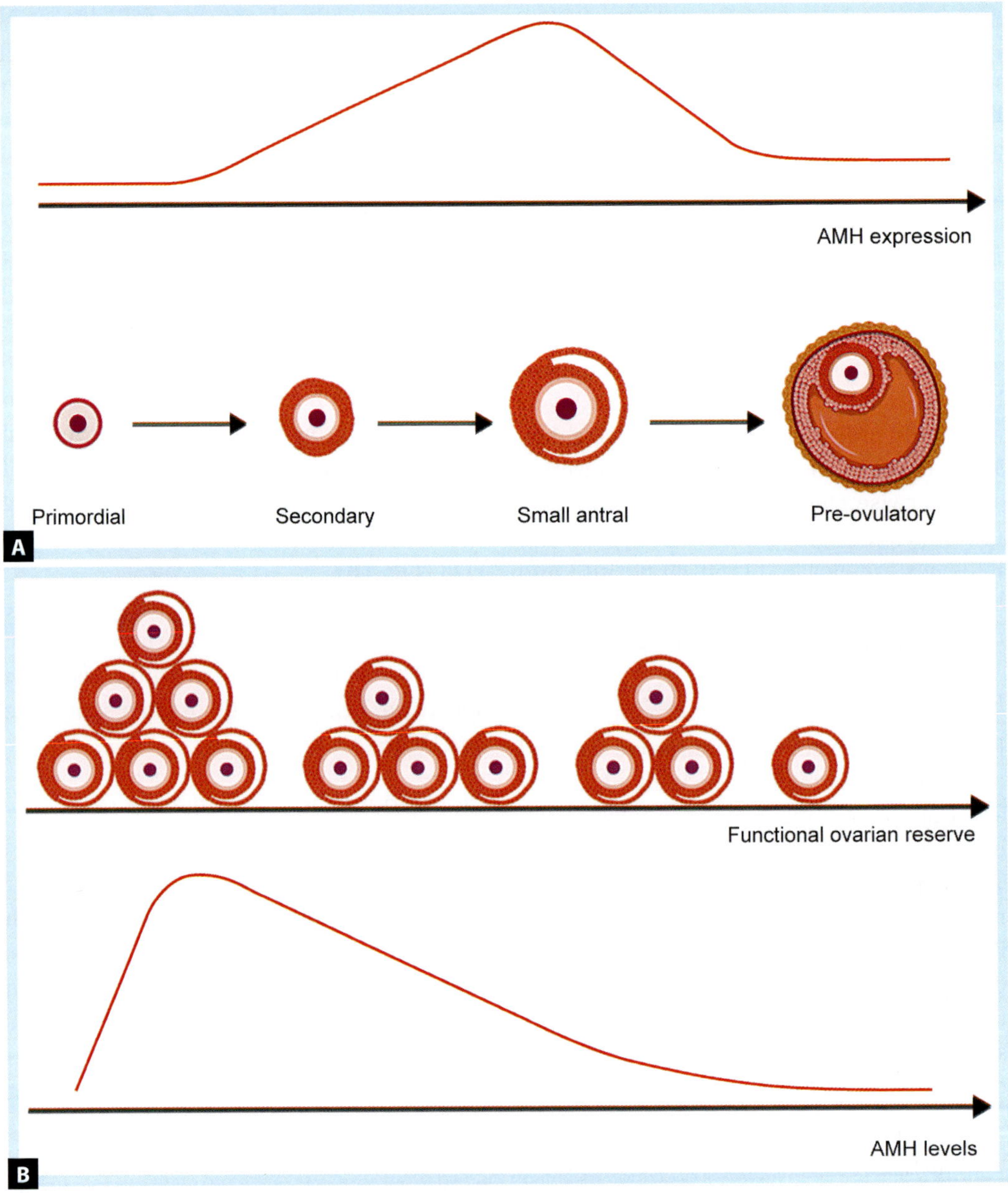

Figs. 1A and B: AMH expression in relation to FOR. (A) Increased AMH expression from secondary follicle till small antral follicle. In preovulatory stage, AMH is expressed only in cumulus granulosa cells which are surrounding the oocyte; and (B) With advancing age, primordial follicle pool gets exhausted leading to a decrease in the functional ovarian reserve. This decreases small AFC and consequently leads to a decrease in AMH levels, which reach undetectable levels nearing menopause. (AFC: antral follicle count; AMH: anti-Müllerian hormone)

ovarian response or pregnancy after IVF and hence should be abandoned.[7-9]

Ultrasound Imaging of the Ovaries

Antral Follicle Count and Ovarian Volume

- Ultrasound imaging of the ovaries as a measure of ovarian reserve involves assessment of AFC and ovarian volume.
- With increasing age, the ovarian volume decreases and thus ovarian reserve declines. However, because of significant intercycle and intracycle variability and also lack of sensitivity, it is less commonly used as a marker of ovarian reserve assessment.[3]
- Antral follicles are the follicles measuring 2–10 mm in diameter in the greatest two-dimensional plane across the ovary. AFC is the total number of antral follicles seen in both ovaries on transvaginal ultrasonography during the early follicular phase of the menstrual cycle. Besides having high interobserver reliability, AFC has very low intercycle variability.[10-14]

CONCLUSION

- Among various ovarian reserve assessment assays, serum AMH is probably most applicable in general practice. It is the most reliable indicator of female reproductive aging and declines in ovarian reserve. It is very closely related to AFC, which is also considered as one of the best predictors of ovarian reserve.
- Although no test is perfect, AMH and AFC promise more sensitive and specific results allowing continuum of ovarian function and are advantageous over other biochemical tests.
- In the quest to standardize a panel test for ovarian reserve assessment, FSH and AFC are advisable to be performed in low socioeconomic and poor resource settings. A combination of FSH, AMH, and AFC aids better in ovarian reserve determination in well-established tertiary centers.

REFERENCES

1. Hansen KR, Knowlton NS, Thyer AC, Charleston JS, Soules MR, Klein NA. A new model of reproductive aging: the decline in ovarian nongrowing follicle number from birth to menopause. Hum Reprod. 2008;23:699-708.
2. Sunkara SK, Rittenberg V, Raine-Fenning N, Bhattacharya S, Zamora J, Coomarasamy A. Association between the number of eggs and live birth in IVF treatment: an analysis of 400 135 treatment cycles. Hum Reprod Oxf Engl. 2011;26(7):1768-74.
3. Jayaprakasan K, Campbell B, Hopkisson J, Clewes J, Johnson I, Raine Fenning N. Establishing the intercycle variability of three-dimensional ultrasonographic predictors of ovarian reserve. Fertil Steril. 2008;90:2126-32.
4. Kwee J, Schats R, McDonnell J, Lambalk CB, Schoemaker J. Intercycle variability of ovarian reserve tests: results of a prospective randomized study. Hum Reprod. 2004;19:590-5.
5. Evers JL, Slaats P, Land JA, Dumoulin JC, Dunselman GA. Elevated levels of basal estradiol-17b predict poor response in patients with normal basal levels of follicle-stimulating hormone undergoing in vitro fertilization. Fertil Steril. 1998;69:1010-4.
6. Jeppesen JV, Anderson RA, Kelsey TW, Christiansen SL, Kristensen SG, Jayaprakasan K, et al. Which follicles make the most anti-mullerian hormone in humans? Evidence for an abrupt decline in AMH production at the time of follicle selection. Mol Hum Reprod. 2013;19(8):519-27.
7. Hendriks DJ, Mol BW, Bancsi LF, te Velde ER, Broekmans FJ. The clomiphene citrate challenge test for the prediction of poor ovarian response and non pregnancy in

patients undergoing in vitro fertilization: a systematic review. Fertil Steril. 2006;86: 807-18.
8. Hendriks DJ, Broekmans FJ, Bancsi LF, de Jong FH, Looman CW, te Velde ER. Repeated clomiphene citrate challenge testing in the prediction of outcome in IVF: a comparison with basal markers for ovarian reserve. Hum Reprod. 2005;20:163-9.
9. Yanushpolsky EH, Hurwitz S, Tikh E, Racowsky C. Predictive usefulness of cycle day 10 follicle-stimulating hormone level in a clomiphene citrate challenge test for in vitro fertilization outcome in women younger than 40 years of age. Fertil Steril. 2003;80: 111-5.
10. Eldar-Geva T, Ben-Chetrit A, Spitz IM, Rabinowitz R, Markowitz E, Mimoni T, et al. Dynamic assays of inhibin B, anti-Mullerian hormone and estradiol following FSH stimulation and ovarian ultrasonography as predictors of IVF outcome. Hum Reprod. 2005;20:3178-83.
11. Kwee J, Schats R, McDonnell J, Themmen A, de Jong F, Lambalk C. Evaluation of anti-Müllerian hormone as a test for the prediction of ovarian reserve. Fertil Steril. 2008;90:737-43.
12. Bancsi LF, Broekmans FJ, Looman CW, Habbema JD, te Velde ER. Impact of repeated antral follicle counts on the prediction of poor ovarian response in women undergoing in vitro fertilization. Fertil Steril. 2004;81: 35-41.
13. Frattarelli JL, Levi AJ, Miller BT, Segars JH. A prospective assessment of the predictive value of basal antral follicles in in vitro fertilization cycles. Fertil Steril. 2003;80:350-5.
14. Pache TD, Wladimiroff JW, de Jong FH, Hop WC, Fauser BC. Growth pat terns of nondominant ovarian follicles during the normal menstrual cycle. Fertil Steril. 1990;54:638-42.

CHAPTER 7

Imaging Innovations: Hysterosalpingography, Three-dimensional Ultrasound, and Sonohysterography

Sugandha Goel, Maitri Modh, Neha Agrawal, Aakanksha Tiwari

INTRODUCTION

Infertility affects an estimated 10–15% of couples worldwide, with female factors contributing to nearly half of all cases.[1] Among these, uterine and tubal abnormalities are particularly important, as they account for implantation failure, miscarriage, and difficulty in achieving natural conception. Accurate and timely evaluation of the uterine cavity and fallopian tubes is, therefore, a cornerstone of infertility workup.

Traditionally, laparoscopy and hysteroscopy were considered the reference standards for tubal and intrauterine assessment. While these techniques remain invaluable, they are invasive, require anesthesia, and are resource-intensive. The drive toward less invasive, more accessible diagnostics has accelerated innovation in reproductive imaging.

Hysterosalpingography (HSG), three-dimensional ultrasound (3D USG), and saline infusion sonohysterography (SIS) have emerged as pivotal tools in infertility assessment. Each modality offers unique benefits: HSG provides robust evaluation of tubal patency, 3D USG revolutionizes visualization of uterine anomalies, and SIS enhances detection of intrauterine pathology. The integration of these tools has redefined infertility evaluation by improving diagnostic accuracy, patient comfort, and cost-effectiveness. This chapter explores these imaging innovations in depth, covering their evolution, techniques, diagnostic accuracy, clinical roles, limitations, and future directions, with a focus on optimizing care in assisted reproduction.

HYSTEROSALPINGOGRAPHY

Historical Background and Evolution

Introduced in 1917 by Carette and Sicard, HSG was initially performed using oil-based contrast agents such as Lipiodol.[2] While effective for tubal visualization, these agents were associated with intravasation, embolization, and inflammatory reactions. The shift to water-soluble contrast media in the 1970s significantly improved safety.[3] Modern digital fluoroscopy has further enhanced resolution, reduced radiation exposure, and facilitated storage and review of images.[4]

Technique

The procedure is performed in the proliferative phase of the menstrual cycle. After cervical cleansing and placement of a cannula or balloon catheter, contrast medium is injected under fluoroscopic guidance. The uterine cavity, tubal outline, and peritoneal spill are visualized in real time.[5] Recent advances include:

- *Soft catheters and balloon-tipped devices:* Reduce leakage and patient discomfort.
- *Low-osmolar iodinated contrast agents:* Provide sharp imaging with lower risk of adverse reactions.
- *Digital subtraction HSG:* Improves contrast resolution by eliminating background structures[6] **(Figs. 1 and 2)**.

Indications

- Primary evaluation of tubal patency in infertility workup.
- Assessment of uterine cavity abnormalities such as synechiae or submucosal fibroids.
- Follow-up after tubal surgery (salpingostomy and tuboplasty).
- Evaluation after recurrent pregnancy loss or repeated implantation failure.[7]

Radiation Safety

While radiation exposure in HSG is relatively low (0.1–1.5 mSv), concern exists, especially in younger women and in repeated procedures. ALARA (As Low As Reasonably Achievable) principles are applied through pulsed fluoroscopy, collimation, and digital imaging.[8]

Diagnostic Accuracy

Hysterosalpingography remains a valuable test for tubal patency. A systematic review showed sensitivity of 65–85% and specificity of 80–90% compared with laparoscopy with chromopertubation.[9] However, it has limited utility for intrauterine pathology, with SIS or hysteroscopy providing superior accuracy.[10]

Patient Experience and Complications

Pain, cramping, and anxiety are frequently reported during HSG. Complications include:

- Pelvic infection (1–3%)
- Allergic reactions to contrast
- Uterine perforation (rare)[11]

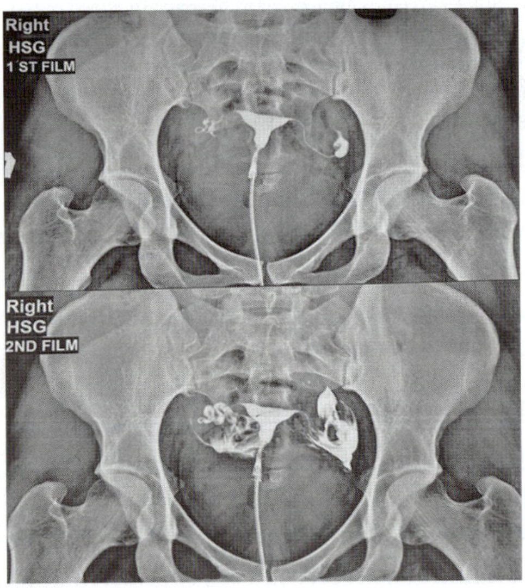

Fig. 1: Hysterosalpingography (HSG) images showing the uterine cavity and fallopian tubes. normal uterine cavity and bilateral tubal patency with contrast spillage into the peritoneal cavity.

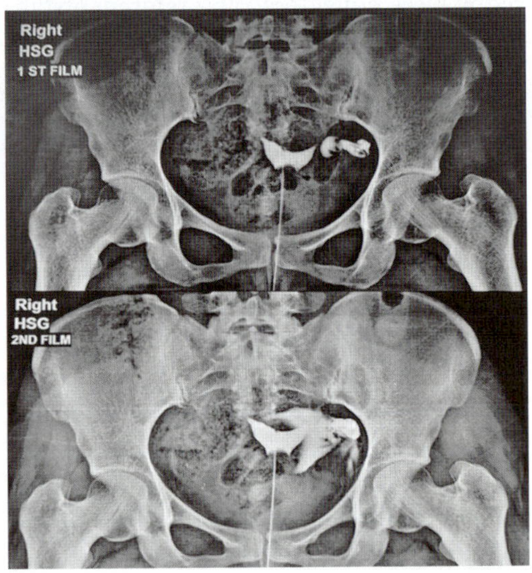

Fig. 2: Serial hysterosalpingogram (HSG). Hysterosalpingogram demonstrating right proximal tubal obstruction with left dilated tube (hydrosalpinx), suggestive of tubal factor infertility.

Strategies to improve tolerability include nonsteroidal anti-inflammatory drugs (NSAIDs), paracervical block, and preprocedure counseling.[12]

Unique Insights

Interestingly, oil-based contrast has been linked to increased pregnancy rates following HSG, possibly due to a "tubal flushing" effect, though its use remains controversial due to safety concerns.[13]

THREE-DIMENSIONAL ULTRASOUND

Technical Principles

3D ultrasound uses transvaginal probes with mechanical or electronic sweep capability to acquire volumetric datasets **(Fig. 3)**. These can be reconstructed into multiplanar or rendered images, enabling evaluation of coronal, sagittal, and transverse planes.[14]

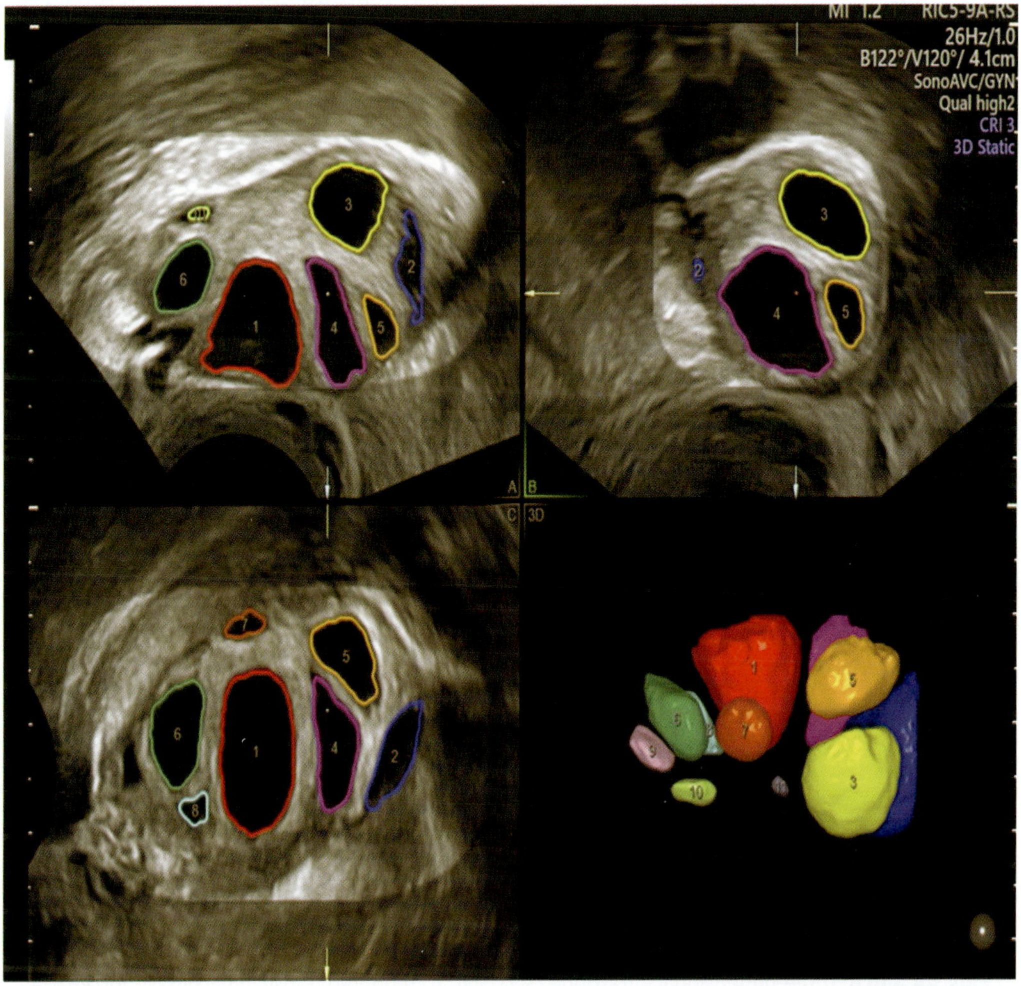

Fig. 3: Three-dimensional (3D) transvaginal ultrasound with follicular volume rendering.

Newer techniques include:

- *Volume contrast imaging (VCI):* Enhances border definition.
- *Omniview:* Allows customized plane reconstruction.
- *4D ultrasound:* Provides dynamic imaging in real time.[15]

Applications

- *Congenital uterine anomalies:*
  - Differentiating septate from bicornuate uteri is critical, as surgical correction is indicated only in septate cases. 3D USG demonstrates sensitivity of 98% and specificity of 100%, outperforming 2D USG.[16]
  - Useful in recurrent miscarriage evaluation.
- *Endometrial assessment:*
  - 3D power Doppler indices (vascularization index, flow index) correlate with endometrial receptivity and implantation success.[17]
  - Provides accurate endometrial volume measurement, aiding in assisted-reproductive technology (ART) planning **(Figs. 4A and B)**.
- *Myometrial and adnexal lesions:*
  - Detects fibroids, adenomyosis, and ovarian cysts with high precision.[18]
- *Guiding embryo transfer:*
  - Assessment of endometrial morphology and uterine anomalies optimizes embryo transfer strategy.[19]

Advantages

- Noninvasive and radiation-free.
- High reproducibility and interobserver agreement.
- Comparable to magnetic resonance imaging (MRI) for uterine anomalies, but more cost-effective.[20]

Limitations

- Operator dependency and learning curve
- Limited accessibility in resource-poor regions
- Requires advanced equipment and software[21]

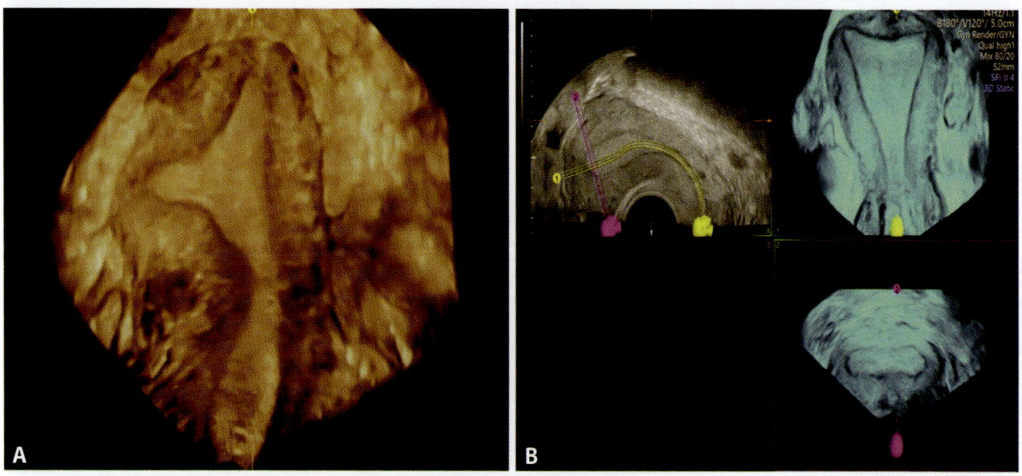

Figs. 4A and B: Three-dimensional ultrasound (3D USG). 3D rendered transvaginal ultrasound image demonstrating a normal, symmetrical, triangular uterine cavity with regular endometrial contour.

SALINE INFUSION SONOHYSTEROGRAPHY AND HYSTERO CONTRAST SONOGRAPHY/ HYSTEROSALPINGO-FOAM SONOGRAPHY

Principle and Technique

Sonohysterography involves instilling 5–10 mL of sterile saline into the uterine cavity, creating contrast that outlines intrauterine structures. HyCoSy (Hysterosalpingo-Contrast Sonography) and HyFoSy (Hysterosalpingo-Foam Sonography) extend this principle to tubal evaluation by using echogenic contrast media such as:

- Air–saline mixtures
- Galactose-based microbubbles (Echovist)
- SonoVue (sulfur hexafluoride microbubbles)
- Foam-based agents (ExEm foam)[22]

Applications

- *Intrauterine pathology:* Detection of polyps, submucous fibroids, adhesions, and hyperplasia with sensitivity and specificity >90%.[23]
- *Tubal patency:* HyFoSy has demonstrated comparable accuracy to HSG, with better patient tolerability.
- *Postsurgical evaluation:* Useful after adhesiolysis or myomectomy.

Patient Experience

Multiple randomized controlled trials (RCTs) confirm that HyFoSy is less painful than HSG and better accepted by patients. The absence of radiation and use of noniodinated agents make it particularly appealing.

Innovations

- *3D-SIS:* Combines volumetric reconstruction with saline contrast for detailed evaluation.
- *4D-HyCoSy:* Real-time dynamic visualization of tubal spill.
- *Contrast-enhanced ultrasound (CEUS):* Offers better visualization of tubal patency with microbubble agents.

Limitations

- Requires expertise for optimal interpretation.
- Inconclusive results in obese patients or in cases of suboptimal acoustic windows.
- Tubal spasm may mimic occlusion.

A cost-effectiveness analysis found HSG to be the cheapest but least tolerated, whereas SIS and HyFoSy, though slightly more expensive, offered superior diagnostic yield and patient experience. Combining modalities often yields the most comprehensive assessment **(Table 1)**.

TABLE 1: Comparative effectiveness and cost-efficiency.

Feature	*HSG*	*3D USG*	*SIS/HyFoSy*
Invasiveness	Minimally invasive, radiation	Non-invasive, no radiation	Minimally invasive, no radiation
Best for	Tubal patency	Uterine anomalies, endometrium	Intrauterine lesions, tubal patency
Patient comfort	Moderate pain	High comfort	Better tolerated than HSG
Availability	Widely available	Limited in low-resource areas	Increasing availability
Limitations	Radiation, discomfort	Operator-dependent	Visualization challenges

APPLICATIONS IN ASSISTED REPRODUCTIVE TECHNOLOGY

Pre-In Vitro Fertilization Screening

Sonohysterography and 3D USG are increasingly used to rule out intrauterine pathology before in vitro fertilization (IVF), reducing implantation failure.

Recurrent Implantation Failure

Three-dimensional USG identifies subtle anomalies such as small septa or arcuate uteri that may not be visible on 2D USG.

Unexplained Infertility

HyFoSy offers radiation-free tubal testing, especially appealing for women planning multiple ART cycles.

Embryo Transfer Guidance

Three-dimensional-derived endometrial volume and blood flow indices are predictive of implantation potential, guiding embryo transfer decisions.

GLOBAL PERSPECTIVE

In high-resource countries, advanced modalities such as 3D USG and HyFoSy are increasingly first-line, aligning with patient-centered and minimally invasive approaches. In contrast, HSG remains dominant in low- and middle-income countries due to its wide availability and lower cost. The challenge lies in improving access to advanced imaging while balancing affordability and sustainability.

FUTURE DIRECTIONS

- *Artificial intelligence (AI):* Automated interpretation of 3D datasets may reduce operator dependency and improve reproducibility.
- *Contrast-enhanced ultrasound (CEUS):* Microbubble contrast agents improve visualization of uterine and tubal structures and may offer therapeutic potential in the future.
- *Fusion imaging:* Integration of ultrasound and MRI datasets may provide a comprehensive anatomical and functional assessment.
- *Portable devices and telemedicine:* Handheld ultrasound combined with remote reporting may expand infertility care access in underserved regions.
- *Integration with omics and personalized medicine:* Linking imaging biomarkers with genetic and proteomic data may refine ART success prediction.

CONCLUSION

Imaging innovations have dramatically reshaped infertility evaluation. HSG, while traditional, remains vital for tubal assessment, particularly in resource-limited settings. 3D ultrasound has revolutionized the evaluation of uterine anomalies and endometrial receptivity, while SIS and HyFoSy provide accurate, patient-friendly alternatives for intrauterine and tubal pathology assessment.

The integration of these tools, guided by international recommendations, allows for a tailored, comprehensive, and patient-centered approach to infertility workup. Looking forward, advances in AI, contrast agents, and telemedicine will further enhance precision, accessibility, and efficiency in reproductive imaging.

REFERENCES

1. Mascarenhas MN, Flaxman SR, Boerma T, Vanderpoel S, Stevens GA. National, regional, and global trends in infertility prevalence since 1990: a systematic analysis of 277 health surveys. PLoS Med. 2012;9(12):e1001356.

2. Carette J, Sicard JA. Hysterosalpingography: early applications. Arch Med. 1917;12:85-92.
3. Kerin JF. Evolution of hysterosalpingography in infertility evaluation. Clin Radiol. 2021;76(9):711-20.
4. Jeans WD. The development and use of digital subtraction angiography. Br J Radiol. 1990;63:161-8.
5. Pellerito JS, McCarthy SM, Doyle MB, Glickman MG, DeCherney AH. Diagnosis of uterine anomalies: relative accuracy of MR imaging, endovaginal sonography, and hysterosalpingography. Radiology. 1992;183(3):795-800.
6. Toussant K, Khan T, Velez CK, Alicea C. Importance of collimation for image quality and radiation exposure. Radiol Technol. 2023;94:206-7.
7. Torre A, Pouly JL, Wainer B. [Anatomic evaluation of the female of the infertile couple]. J Gynecol Obstet Biol Reprod (Paris). 2010;39(8 Suppl 2):S34–44.
8. Tur-Kaspa I, Gal M, Hartman M, Hartman J, Hartman A. A prospective evaluation of uterine abnormalities by saline infusion sonohysterography in 1,009 women with infertility or abnormal uterine bleeding. Fert Steril. 2006;86:1731-5.
9. Nyambura E, Sonigra K, Mwangi O, Mutabari E, Omanwa K. A fatal outcome following uterine perforation and pelvic abscess after hysterosalpingography: A case report. JOGECA. 2025;37(3):99-102.
10. Hindocha A, Beere L, O'Flynn H, Watson A, Ahmad G. Pain relief in hysterosalpingography. Cochrane Database Syst Rev. 2015;2015(9):CD006106.
11. Mathews DM, Peart JM, Sim RG, Johnson NP, O'Sullivan S, Derraik JGB, et al. Iodine and other factors associated with fertility outcome following oil-soluble contrast medium hysterosalpingography: a prospective cohort study. Front Endocrinol (Lausanne). 2024;15:1257888.
12. Smith WL, Fenster A. Optimum scan spacing for three-dimensional ultrasound by Speckle statistics. Ultrasound Med. Biol. 2000;26:551-62.
13. Jurkovic D, Geipel A, Gruboeck K, Jauniaux E, Natucci M, Campbell S. Three-dimensional ultrasound for the assessment of uterine anatomy and detection of congenital anomalies: a comparison with hysterosalpingography and two-dimensional sonography. Ultrasound Obstet Gynecol. 1995;5:233-7.
14. Raine-Fenning N, Campbell B, Collier J, Brincat M, Johnson I. The reproducibility of endometrial volume acquisition and measurement with the VOCAL-imaging program. Ultrasound Obstet Gynecol. 2002;19:69-75.
15. Alcazar JL. New rendering techniques in 3D USG. Ultrasound Obstet Gynecol. 2019;54(5):689-96.
16. Timor-Tritsch LE, Lerner JP, Monteagudo A, Santos R. Transvaginal ultrasonographic characterization of ovarian masses by means of color flow-directed Doppler measurements and a morphologic scoring system. Am J Obstet Gynecol. 1993;168(3 Pt 1):909-13..
17. Tekay A, Martikainen H, Jouppila P. Blood flow changes in uterine and ovarian vasculature, and predictive value of transvaginal pulsed colour Doppler ultrasonography in an in-vitro fertilization programme. Hum Reprod. 1995;10:688-93.
18. Turkgeldi E, Urman B, Ata B. Role of three-dimensional ultrasound in gynecology. J Obstet Gynaecol India. 2014;65(3):146-54.
19. Soares SR, dos Reis MM, Camargos AF. Diagnostic accuracy of sonohysterography, transvaginal sonography, and hysterosalpingography in patients with uterine cavity diseases. Fertil Steril. 2000;73: 406–11.
20. Serrano González L, Pérez-Medina T, Bueno Olalla B, Royuela A, De La Cuesta MLR, Saéz de la Mata D, et al. Is hysterosalpingo-foam sonography (HyFoSy) more tolerable in terms of pain and anxiety than hysterosalpingography (HSG)? A prospective real-world setting multicentre study. BMC Womens Health. 2022;22(1):41.
21. Mishra VV, Agarwal R, Sharma U, Aggarwal R, Choudhary S, Bandwal P. Endometrial

and subendometrial vascularity by three-dimensional (3D) power Doppler and its correlation with pregnancy outcome in frozen embryo transfer (FET) cycles. J Obstet Gynaecol India. 2016;66:521-7.

22. Emanuel MH. HyCoSy and HyFoSy: innovations in tubal patency testing. Reprod Biomed Online. 2019;39(3):345-52.
23. Strobel D, Bernatik T, Blank W, Schuler A, Greis C, Dietrich CF, et al. Diagnostic accuracy of CEUS in the differential diagnosis of small (≤ 20 mm) and subcentimetric (≤ 10 mm) focal liver lesions in comparison with histology: results of the DEGUM multicenter trial. Ultraschall Med. 2011;32:593-7.

SECTION 3

Emerging Biological Insights

8. **Unexplained Infertility: Folate Pathway Variants, Epigenetic Mechanisms, Immune Dysregulation**
Himanshu Roy, Indira Prasad

CHAPTER 8

Unexplained Infertility: Folate Pathway Variants, Epigenetic Mechanisms, Immune Dysregulation

Himanshu Roy, Indira Prasad

INTRODUCTION

Unexplained infertility (UI) accounts for a substantial proportion of infertility diagnoses after routine evaluations (ovulatory function, tubal patency, semen analysis, uterine anatomy) are normal. Understanding molecular contributors beyond standard testing is essential for developing targeted diagnostics and therapies. One-carbon (folate) metabolism supplies methyl groups and nucleotides critical for DNA synthesis and methylation; epigenetic processes govern gene expression during gametogenesis and early development; and immune tolerance at the maternal–fetal interface is required for implantation and early placentation. These systems interact: Methyl donor availability influences epigenetic programming, which in turn modulates immune cell differentiation and function. This interdependence provides biologic plausibility for a role in UI, while clinical evidence remains incomplete and, in some areas, conflicting.

FOLATE AND ONE-CARBON METABOLISM: BIOCHEMISTRY AND REPRODUCTIVE ROLES

Overview of Pathway Function

One-carbon metabolism (OCM) integrates folate, methionine and homocysteine cycles and requires dietary folate (or folic acid), vitamins B12 and B6, and multiple enzymes to generate S-adenosylmethionine (SAM), the universal methyl donor for DNA, RNA, and protein methylation, and to supply nucleotides for DNA replication and repair. OCM therefore underpins both macromolecular synthesis and epigenetic methylation during periods of high cellular proliferation and epigenetic reprogramming (e.g., gametogenesis, preimplantation development). Refer to **Figure 1** for pathway flowchart.

Key Enzymes and Genetic Variation

Methylenetetrahydrofolate reductase (MTHFR) catalyzes the conversion of 5,10-methylene-THF to 5-methyl-THF (5-MTHF), the predominant circulating folate form used for remethylation of homocysteine to methionine. Common polymorphisms (C677T, A1298C) reduce enzyme activity to varying degrees and can be associated with higher homocysteine concentrations in the absence of adequate folate/B12 status. However, carriage of these variants alone is not a definitive cause of infertility; clinical interpretation should incorporate biochemical measures (folate, RBC folate, homocysteine, B12) rather than genotype alone.

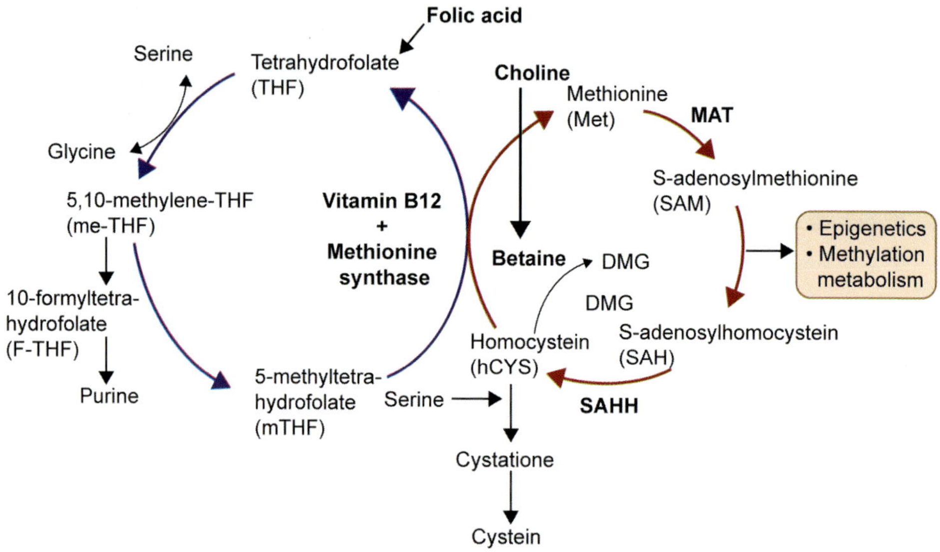

Fig. 1: Folate and one-carbon metabolism.
Source: Paro R, Grossniklaus U, Santoro R, Wutz A. Introduction to Epigenetics. Cham (CH): Springer; 2021. Fig. 9.6 [One-carbon metabolism. SAM is produced.]

Roles in Reproduction

Gametogenesis: Folate is necessary for nucleotide synthesis during germ-cell proliferation and for establishment of methylation marks during germ-line epigenetic programming. Animal studies and human observational data support a requirement for adequate methyl donor availability for gamete quality and imprint establishment.[1,2]

Early embryo: Preimplantation embryos rely on OCM for nucleotide supply and de novo methylation patterns; disturbances in methyl donor supply can alter methylation and embryo development in model systems.

Implantation/placentation: Adequate methylation and redox balance are implicated in appropriate decidualization and trophoblast invasion.

Box 1 summarizes relevance of folate and one-carbon metabolism in fertility.

BOX 1: Folate and one-carbon metabolism in fertility.

- *Folate deficiency* → impaired DNA synthesis, poor oocyte quality
- *High homocysteine levels* → oxidative stress, poor embryo viability
- *MTHFR gene polymorphisms* → reduced folate conversion, lower fertility outcomes
- *Impaired methylation* → disrupted gene expression in gametes and embryos
- *Poor endometrial receptivity* → compromised implantation

EPIGENETICS IN REPRODUCTION

Mechanisms and Dynamics

Epigenetic regulation—DNA methylation, histone post-translational modifications, chromatin remodeling, and noncoding RNAs—controls gene expression without changing DNA sequence. Germ cells and early embryos undergo waves of genome-wide demethylation followed by sex-specific remethylation to establish imprinting marks

TABLE 1: Role of epigenetics in human reproduction.

Aspect	*Epigenetic mechanism*	*Impact on reproduction*
Gamete development	DNA methylation, histone modification	Regulates gene expression during spermatogenesis and oogenesis; affects gamete quality
Fertilization	Genomic imprinting	Ensures correct parent-of-origin gene expression; errors can lead to developmental failure
Embryo development	Epigenetic reprogramming	Resets epigenetic marks post fertilization; crucial for normal embryogenesis
Implantation	Endometrial methylation patterns	Influences endometrial receptivity and successful implantation
Placental function	Chromatin remodeling, methylation	Controls nutrient transport and fetal growth; abnormalities linked to preeclampsia
Pregnancy outcomes	Noncoding RNAs, histone acetylation	Affects fetal development and maternal adaptation; linked to miscarriage and complications
Infertility disorders	Aberrant methylation in reproductive tissues	Associated with PCOS, endometriosis, and unexplained infertility
Environmental influence	Epigenetic changes via toxins, diet	Lifestyle and exposures can alter reproductive epigenome; transgenerational effects noted
ART	Epigenetic sensitivity during IVF	ART procedures may disrupt imprinting and methylation; linked to altered birth outcomes

(ART: assisted reproductive technology; IVF: in vitro fertilization; PCOS: polycystic ovary syndrome)

and lineage-specific gene expression patterns; selective protection of imprinted loci is critical for normal development.[2] **Table 1** describes the role of epigenetics in human reproduction.

Dysregulation and Reproductive Outcomes

Aberrant methylation or epigenetic programming may impair gamete competence, embryonic viability, implantation, and placentation. Some imprinting disorders (e.g., Beckwith–Wiedemann syndrome) have been observed more frequently, though still rarely, in assisted reproductive technology (ART)-conceived children, raising concern about sensitive windows for epigenetic perturbation.[2] Nutritional status (folate and other methyl donors), environmental exposures, and maternal metabolic health can influence epigenetic marks during critical windows.

IMMUNE REGULATION IN EARLY REPRODUCTION

Maternal–Fetal Immune Balance

Pregnancy requires maternal immune adaptations to tolerate the semiallogeneic conceptus while preserving host defense. Uterine natural killer (uNK) cells, regulatory T cells (Tregs), antigen-presenting cells, and macrophages orchestrate a tolerant, proangiogenic uterine environment necessary for implantation and spiral artery remodeling.[3,4]

Key Immune Cell Roles and Dysfunction

uNK cells: They predominate in the decidua during early pregnancy and regulate

TABLE 2: Immune dysregulation in human reproduction.

Reproductive stage	*Normal immune role*	*Dysregulation effects*
Gamete formation	Immune privilege in gonads prevents attack on sperm/egg antigens	Antisperm antibodies, autoimmune oophoritis, impaired gametogenesis
Fertilization	Tolerance to paternal antigens	Fertilization failure due to immune rejection or inflammation
Implantation	Controlled inflammation and immune cell recruitment	Poor endometrial receptivity, implantation failure, recurrent pregnancy loss
Pregnancy maintenance	Maternal–fetal tolerance via Tregs, cytokine balance	Preeclampsia, miscarriage, IUGR
Male reproductive tract	Blood–testis barrier maintains immune privilege	Orchitis, epididymitis, viral persistence (e.g., Zika, HIV), infertility
Female reproductive tract	Mucosal immunity and cytokine signaling	Chronic endometritis, altered cytokine profiles, infertility
Environmental influence	Immune system adapts to stressors	Toxins, infections, and aging disrupt immune balance, affecting fertility
ART	Immune modulation during IVF and embryo transfer	Increased risk of immune rejection, altered cytokine milieu, lower success rates

(ART: assisted reproductive technology; IUGR: intrauterine growth restriction)

trophoblast invasion and vascular remodeling; functional imbalance [e.g., proinflammatory cytokine secretion or abnormal interactions with trophoblast human leukocyte antigen (HLA) molecules] may impede implantation.[3]

Tregs: They are central to maternal tolerance; reductions in Treg number or function are associated with implantation failure and pregnancy loss in preclinical and human observational studies.[4]

Autoimmune and prothrombotic states: Well-defined conditions such as antiphospholipid syndrome (APS) cause recurrent pregnancy loss via thrombosis and impaired placental function and have evidence-based management strategies.

Clinical Testing and Controversies

Many immune assays are available—peripheral NK cell counts/functional tests, endometrial NK-cell immunophenotyping, cytokine panels, and autoantibody testing. Professional bodies caution against routine use of many of these tests for UI because thresholds are not standardized and predictive utility is unproven.

Table 2 portrays how dysruption of immune regulation makes fertility challenging.

INTERSECTIONS: HOW FOLATE/OCM, EPIGENETICS, AND IMMUNE REGULATION INTERACT

SAM and methylation: OCM-derived SAM is consumed during DNA and histone methylation; thus, folate/methyl donor availability can directly influence the epigenetic landscape in gametes, embryos, and endometrial/immune cells.

Immune epigenetics: Differentiation and stability of immune cell subsets—particularly Tregs—are regulated by DNA methylation and histone modifications (e.g., FOXP3 locus methylation). Nutritional modulation of methyl donor availability can therefore influence immune tolerance mechanisms.[4,5]

Homocysteine and inflammation: Elevated homocysteine levels may promote endothelial dysfunction and a proinflammatory state, potentially impairing implantation and placentation; homocysteine metabolism also impacts redox balance and nitric oxide signaling.

Microbiome: Gut microbial folate production and interactions with host immunity are emerging as factors that may modify systemic folate availability and immune development; this is an active area of investigation.

CLINICAL EVIDENCE LINKING THESE MECHANISMS TO UNEXPLAINED INFERTILITY

Folate and Fertility Outcomes

Periconceptional folic acid reduces neural tube defect incidence and is standard practice.[1] Observational studies associate higher folate intake or RBC folate with improved ovulatory function and, in some cohorts, better ART outcomes, though randomized trials specifically targeting UI outcomes are lacking.

MTHFR Variants and Reproductive Outcomes

Studies assessing MTHFR C677T and A1298C polymorphisms yield inconsistent associations with infertility and recurrent pregnancy loss; many carriers have normal biochemical profiles when adequately supplemented, underscoring the need to interpret genotype in the biochemical context rather than as an isolated causal factor.

Epigenetic Findings

Human data showing altered methylation patterns in gametes, embryos, or placental tissues from some infertile couples are largely associative; causality in UI remains unproven. ART-related epigenetic perturbations have been reported, but absolute risks of imprinting disorders are small.

Immune Factors and Therapies

Certain immune causes of infertility/recurrent loss (e.g., APS) have clear diagnostic and therapeutic pathways supported by trials and guidelines (antiplatelet + heparin therapy improves live birth rates in obstetric APS). For many other immune markers and therapies [e.g., peripheral NK-cell testing, empiric immunotherapy with intravenous immunoglobulin (IVIG), glucocorticoids, intralipid], evidence of efficacy in UI is weak or conflicting and their routine use is not recommended by major professional societies.

DIAGNOSTIC AND THERAPEUTIC CONSIDERATIONS

Diagnostic Approach (Practical Recommendations)

Ensure completion of standard infertility evaluation (ovulation, tubal patency, semen analysis, uterine cavity assessment).

Measure serum or RBC folate and vitamin B12; consider plasma homocysteine if history suggests metabolic risk (recurrent loss, thrombosis, family history) or if folate/B12 levels are suboptimal.

Reserve MTHFR genotyping for selected clinical scenarios (e.g., persistent hyperhomocysteinemia or recurrent pregnancy loss) and interpret alongside biochemical measures.

Screen for antiphospholipid antibodies when the history suggests recurrent pregnancy loss or thrombosis.

Avoid routine, nonvalidated immune testing (peripheral NK cell counts, unstandardized cytokine panels) for UI outside research settings.

Therapeutic Strategies

Folate supplementation: Universal periconceptional folic acid (0.4–0.8 mg/day) is recommended to reduce neural tube defects; higher doses (4 mg/day) are indicated for women at high risk for neural tube defects. Some clinicians use 5-MTHF formulations, particularly when MTHFR variants are present or when individuals report intolerance to folic acid; high-quality evidence that 5-MTHF improves fertility outcomes over standard folic acid is limited.

B12 and B6: Correct Deficiencies to Optimize OCM.

- *Homocysteine lowering:* In cases of hyperhomocysteinemia, treatment with folate, B12 and B6, and lifestyle interventions may normalize levels; whether this improves fertility outcomes is not definitively established but is biologically plausible.
- *Immune therapies:* For obstetric APS, low-dose aspirin plus low-molecular-weight heparin improves live birth rates and is guideline-recommended. Empiric use of corticosteroids, IVIG, intralipid, or lymphocyte immunotherapy for isolated UI is not supported by consistent evidence and should be limited to clinical trials or selected cases after informed discussion of risks and uncertain benefit.
- *Vitamin D:* Correct deficiency given its immunomodulatory roles; evidence for improving UI outcomes is inconclusive.

Counseling and Safety

Avoid overtesting and unproven, potentially risky therapies. Counsel patients clearly about the strength of evidence for any recommended test or treatment and prioritize evidence-based interventions (nutritional optimization, targeted therapy for clearly defined disorders such as APS).

GUIDELINES AND PROFESSIONAL STATEMENTS

Professional societies recommend individualized, evidence-based approaches: Routine periconceptional folic acid supplementation is universally endorsed; targeted testing and treatment are recommended for well-defined conditions (e.g., APS); and routine use of many immunologic assays and empiric immunotherapies for UI is not recommended in the absence of validated predictive value and randomized trial evidence.

RESEARCH PRIORITIES AND KNOWLEDGE GAPS

- Randomized trials of targeted methyl donor therapy (including 5-MTHF) and of interventions to normalize homocysteine in populations with biochemical abnormalities, with fertility outcomes as primary endpoints
- Longitudinal human mechanistic studies linking folate metabolites, gamete/embryo and endometrial methylation profiles, and immune cell epigenomes to clinical reproductive outcomes
- Standardization and validation of immune assays predictive of implantation or therapeutic response
- Integration of microbiome, metabolome, and epigenome data to define novel mechanistic pathways and targets for intervention

- Development of personalized strategies combining genomic, epigenetic, and immunologic phenotyping for patient stratification in clinical trials

CONCLUSION

One-carbon metabolism, epigenetic regulation, and immune tolerance are interdependent systems essential to reproductive success. While perturbations in these pathways may contribute to UI for some couples, definitive causal links and evidence-based targeted treatments remain limited. Routine optimization of nutritional status (including folate and B12), avoidance of environmental insults, and evidence-based management of defined immune disorders represent sound clinical practice. Translational and clinical trial research is needed to convert mechanistic insights into validated diagnostics and therapies that improve outcomes for couples with UI.

REFERENCES

1. Medical Research Council Vitamin Study Research Group. Prevention of neural tube defects: results of the Medical Research Council Vitamin Study. Lancet. 1991;338(8760):131-7.
2. Reik W, Dean W, Walter J. Epigenetic reprogramming in mammalian development. Science. 2001;293(5532):1089-93.
3. Moffett A, Colucci F. Uterine natural killer cells: active regulators at the maternal–fetal interface. Nat Rev Immunol. 2014;14(10):1-12.
4. Aluvihare VR, Kallikourdis M, Betz AG. Regulatory T cells mediate maternal tolerance to the fetus. Nat Immunol. 2004;5(3):266-71.
5. Soubry A. Epigenetic inheritance and the intergenerational transfer of information in humans. Nat Rev Endocrinol. 2015;11(5):213-27.

SECTION 4

Artificial Reproductive

9. **Fertility Preservation Technologies**
Amreen Singh, Akansha Mishra

10. **Embryo Selection: Artificial Intelligence-driven Multimodal Grading and Explainability**
Snigdha Soni, Gunupuru Gayatri Swetha

11. **Noninvasive and Minimally Invasive Preimplantation Genetic Testing and Advances in Next-generation Sequencing**
Priyanka Rai, Shruti P Shirodkar, Divya MB

12. **Ethical and Clinical Debates: Preimplantation Genetic Screening, Blastocyst Transfer, and BMI Limits**
Rohit Gutgutia, Gayatri Satpathy

CHAPTER 9

Fertility Preservation Technologies

Amreen Singh, Akansha Mishra

INTRODUCTION

The field of fertility preservation encompasses diverse interventions—including medical treatments, surgeries, and psychological support—aimed at safeguarding the reproductive potential of individuals facing threats to future fertility. Despite being created initially for cancer patients receiving gonadotoxic treatments, fertility preservation is today used in a broader variety of situations, such as nononcologic illnesses, genetic predispositions, care that is gender affirming, and deliberate fertility delay.[1,2]

This chapter reviews the biological principles, clinical indications, available techniques, outcomes, counseling strategies, ethical and legal considerations, and future directions relevant to clinicians, trainees, and policymakers.

BIOLOGICAL AND CLINICAL RATIONALE

Reproductive potential depends on age, baseline gonadal reserve, genetic factors, and exposures such as chemotherapy, radiation, gonadotoxic surgery, or environmental toxins. As women age, the number and quality of eggs naturally decrease, which significantly affects fertility compared to men. In contrast, male fertility is typically more resilient but remains vulnerable to cytotoxic therapy, gonadectomy, or endocrine disruption.[3]

Preservation strategies focus on banking gametes or tissues prior to anticipated damage or on minimizing harm during the treatment process.

FERTILITY PRESERVATION INDICATOR

Recent research has shown that fertility preservation now is not limited to only cancer treatments but is also expanding in fields of nonmalignant conditions, genetic factors, and also social considerations.[4]

These developments reflect a shift in how reproductive health is approached, encouraging earlier discussions about fertility options, especially for younger individuals who may be confronted with therapies or conditions that could lead to sterilization.

Malignant and Gonadotoxic Conditions

The potential for loss of fertility to cancer treatments has been a reason for considering fertility preservation; however, recent studies highlight the diverse effects depending on the particular therapies employed and the patient's age.

- *Chemotherapy:* Certain chemotherapy drugs, particularly alkylating agents used before stem cell transplants, can severely affect fertility. For prepubertal patients and those requiring immediate treatment, ovarian tissue cryopreservation (OTC) remains the sole option.[5]

- *Radiotherapy:* Exposure to radiation in the abdominal areas or pelvic can harm the ovaries or testes (gonads). Moreover, radiation directed toward the brain may hinder with hormonal signals crucial for reproduction. In female patients, technique such as ovarian transposition (relocation of the ovaries) can shade them from pelvic radiation, although the uterus may still sustain damage.
- *Surgery:* Surgical treatment such as hysterectomy (removal of the uterus), bilateral oophorectomy (both ovaries removed), or orchiectomy (removal of a testicle) can lead to infertility. Fertility-cautious surgical techniques are being employed for early-stage gynecological cancers, including ovarian, cervical, and endometrial cancers.[6]
- *Specific cancers:* Breast cancer serves as a major indication for fertility preservation since a large number of younger women are affected by it, along with the gonadotoxic nature of chemotherapy and prolonged endocrine therapy.
- Considerable risk also includes hematological malignancies, such as leukemia and lymphoma.

Benign Gynecological Conditions

Increasing evidence indicates the importance of fertility preservation in cases of benign gynecological disorders that may compromise ovarian function or necessitate multiple surgical interventions.

- *Endometriosis and endometriomas:* The presence of these conditions, along with their surgical management, has the potential to harm the ovarian reserve. Cryopreservation is especially recommended for individuals with bilateral ovarian endometriomas or those who are likely to undergo repeated ovarian surgeries.
- *Benign ovarian tumors or cysts:* The occurrence of multiple or recurrent benign cysts may require surgical procedures that can adversely affect healthy ovarian tissue, thereby warranting preemptive fertility preservation measures.
- *Recurrent adnexal torsion:* This medical condition, characterized by the twisting of the ovary which restricts its blood supply, can result in the deterioration of ovarian function. Fertility preservation options may be considered, particularly in cases where only one ovary remains.

Autoimmune Diseases

Autoimmune diseases can adversely affect fertility, either directly or indirectly through treatment effects. Research highlights the importance of discussing preservation options with patients of reproductive age.

- *Systemic lupus erythematosus (SLE):* Patients suffering from severe SLE, especially those with nephritis, may receive treatment involving gonadotoxic agents such as cyclophosphamide. The disease itself, along with the administration of high-dose steroids for treatment, elevates the risk of primary ovarian insufficiency (POI).
- *Rheumatoid arthritis (RA) and other diseases:* Conditions such as RA and various systemic autoimmune diseases are linked to a heightened risk of POI and can impact fertility in both males and females. The use of gonadotoxic chemotherapy for severe cases, in addition to certain immunosuppressants, serves as a significant indication for fertility preservation.

Genetic Conditions

Specific genetic syndromes and mutations that elevate the likelihood of primary ovarian insufficiency (POI) are increasingly acknowledged as valid reasons for fertility preservation.

- *Turner syndrome:* This disorder is marked by gonadal dysgenesis and POI. Traditionally, treatment involved the use of donor eggs; however, recent advancements in preservation methods provide an opportunity for younger patients with mosaicism and some ovarian functionality to cryopreserve their own ovarian tissue or oocytes.
- *Fragile X (FMR1) premutation:* Women who possess this premutation are at a 20% risk of experiencing POI and early ovarian failure. They may opt for fertility preservation through oocyte cryopreservation, frequently accompanied by preimplantation genetic testing (PGT) to prevent the transmission of the mutation.
- *BRCA1/2 mutations:* Individuals with these mutations are at a significantly increased risk for breast and ovarian cancer and often undergo preventive oophorectomy, which reduces their reproductive timeframe. For younger carriers who have not yet completed their families, options such as egg or embryo cryopreservation become crucial.

Additionally, genetic testing is available to screen embryos for the presence of the mutation.

Elective or Social Reasons

Elective fertility preservation has become increasingly important for those who intend to delay parenthood due to personal, professional, or various social factors.

- *Advanced maternal age:* Women experience a notable decrease in both the quantity and quality of eggs after the age of 35 years, making it advantageous to freeze eggs at a younger age to maximize the likelihood of a successful pregnancy in the future.
- *Transgender individuals:* The pretransition cryopreservation of gametes (sperm and eggs) or gonadal tissue is an essential component of healthcare for transgender individuals who are undergoing gender-affirming hormone therapy or surgical procedures that could jeopardize their fertility.

FERTILITY PRESERVATION TECHNIQUE

Vitrification, a technique that rapidly cools cells to ultra-low temperatures, has revolutionized fertility preservation. Fertility preservation can be achieved through several procedures, which include cryopreservation of oocytes, embryos, and ovarian tissue.

- Oocyte cryopreservation is a choice for women undergoing treatment for age-related loss in fertility, and in the majority of cases in women for fertility preservation for medical indications.
- Embryo cryopreservation is a long-established and widely used technique where an embryo or blastocyst is cryopreserved for future use.
- Ovarian tissue cryopreservation is considered when there is less time for ovarian stimulation (OS) and also for the cases of prepubertal girls.

In vitro maturation (IVM) can be a choice where a small number of immature oocytes are achieved and then are matured in vitro by a number of methods and media.

Ovarian transposition in women scheduled for pelvic radiotherapy is also discussed.

OVARIAN STIMULATION FOR FERTILITY PRESERVATION

Before any oocyte or embryo cryopreservation, the initial steps for any patient are OS. It is a pharmaceutical treatment for developing multiple follicles, with the goal to achieve multiple oocytes (eggs) for assisted reproductive technique (ART) procedure or fertility preservation **(Flowchart 1)**.

Ovarian stimulation in cases of fertility preservation becomes a case of urgency, efficacy, and safety, and the collection of an adequate number of oocytes in the restricted time, with the safety issue of complication of ovarian hyperstimulation syndrome (OHSS), persisting risk of malign or benign disease. Approaches such as random start stimulation and stimulation related to estrogen sensitive cancer are taken.

Specialized Stimulation Approaches for Fertility Preservation[7-9]

Fertility preservation requires adaptations of conventional OS to meet urgent timelines, minimize hormonal risks, and optimize outcomes in often complex clinical settings such as oncology.

Random-start Stimulation Protocols

Traditionally, OS begins in the early follicular phase, which may delay cancer therapy initiation. In random-start protocols, stimulation can begin at any stage of the menstrual cycle, helping to avoid treatment delays.

Flowchart 1: Schematic overview of the options for female fertility preservation.

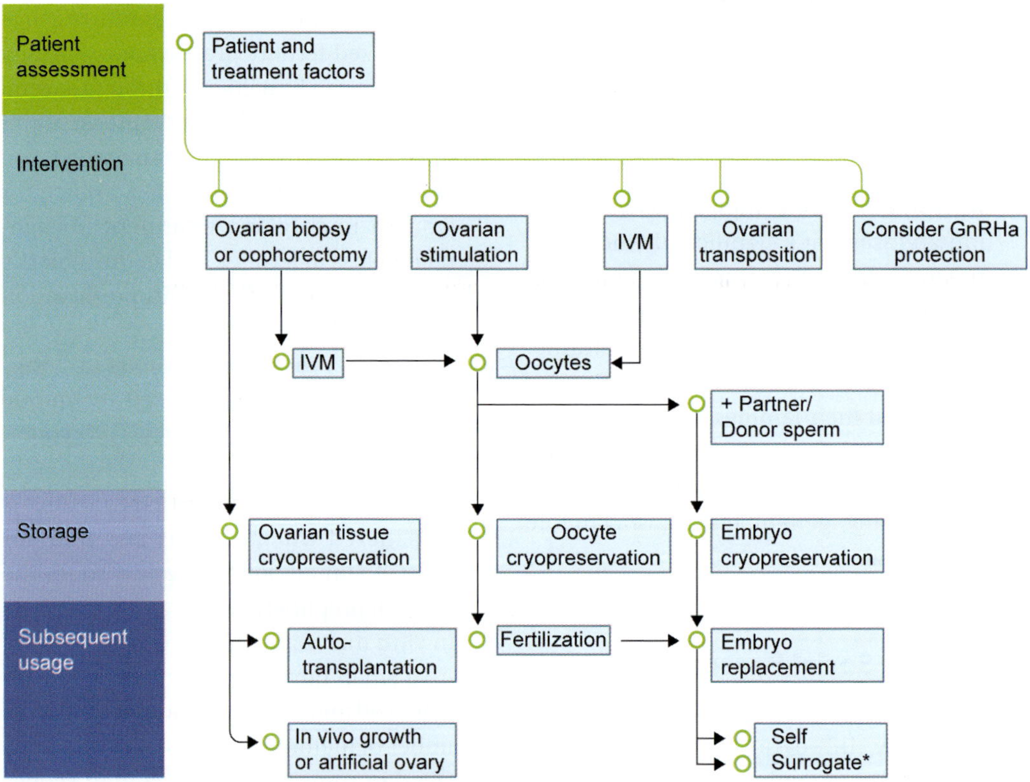

(GnRHa: gonadotropin-releasing hormone agonist; IVM: in vitro maturation)[7]

Source: Anderson DM, Rees DI, Sabia JJ. Anderson et al. respond. Am J Public Health. 2015;105(4):e8-9.

Clinical evidence confirms comparable oocyte yield, maturity, and developmental potential to conventional start protocols, making this a pivotal advancement for oncofertility patients.

Progestin-primed Ovarian Stimulation

Progestin-primed ovarian stimulation (PPOS) employs oral progestins in lieu of gonadotropin-releasing hormone (GnRH) antagonists to suppress premature luteinizing hormone (LH) surge. This approach simplifies treatment, reduces cost, and enhances patient convenience while maintaining similar oocyte retrieval rates and maturity outcomes to traditional antagonist protocols. It is particularly useful where antagonist availability or affordability poses challenges.

Aromatase Inhibitor-based Protocols

In women with hormone-sensitive malignancies—most notably estrogen receptor-positive breast cancer—traditional stimulation can transiently elevate systemic estradiol levels, theoretically risking tumor stimulation. Incorporating aromatase inhibitors (AIs) such as letrozole into the stimulation regimen effectively suppresses estrogen biosynthesis, maintaining estradiol levels near physiologic or minimally elevated ranges. This allows safe stimulation with preserved oocyte yield and favorable maturity profiles. Long-term follow-up data demonstrate no increase in cancer recurrence rates, underscoring the safety and efficacy of AI-based stimulation in this population.

Dual Stimulation

Dual stimulation (DuoStim) entails two consecutive stimulation cycles within the same menstrual cycle—one in the follicular phase and a second in the luteal phase. This intensive approach is particularly valuable for poor responders or patients with limited time before cancer therapy, as it maximizes oocyte yield over a condensed timeframe.

Cryopreservation is a process that makes cells stabilize at cryogenic temperature, which allows study of life at low level. Many advances in cryopreservation technology have led to the development of methods that allow for low-temperature maintenance of a variety of cell types including male and female gametes, small multicellular organisms, and even more complex organisms such as embryos.

Vitrification is a technique of cryopreservation for oocytes or embryos that is able to generate an extremely fast cooling rate, preventing formation of ice crystals during the process.

Oocyte Cryopreservation

When keeping in mind age-related fertility loss, cryopreservation of mature oocytes through vitrification has been showing its efficacy in banking the oocytes. This technique has been increasing day by day compared to embryo preservation, as it gives women without a male partner an option to bank oocytes.

Method

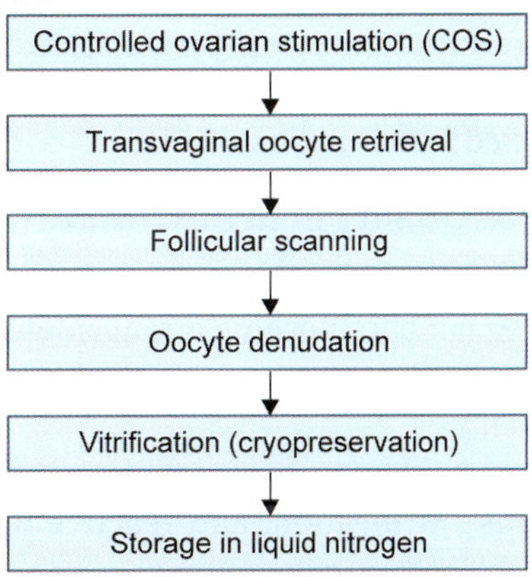

Embryo Cryopreservation

Embryos are formed from the contribution of male sperm and female oocytes and from the earlier time, embryo cryopreservation has been a technique for adult women for fertility preservation, and it is available....

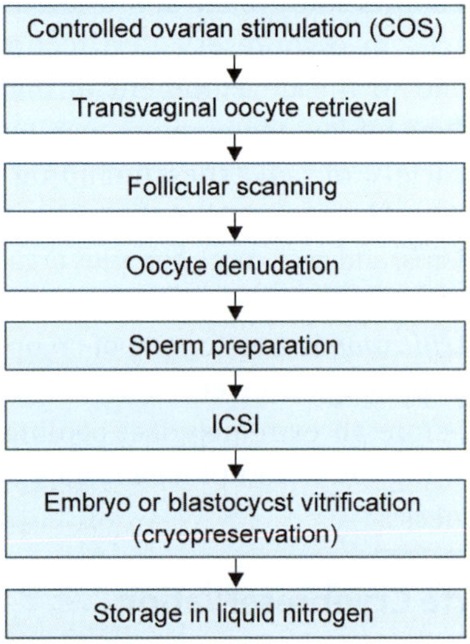

In Vitro Maturation

Mostly considered for women with polycystic ovary syndrome (PCOS) to decrease risk of OHSS. In IVM, cumulus-oocyte complexes (COCs) are retrieved at germinal vesicle (GV) stage with or without previous exogenous gonadotropin administration followed by maturation to metaphase II (MII) oocytes and vitrification or fertilization for embryo cryopreservation. GV oocyte is arrested at the diplotene stage of prophase I, which is later subjected to maturation till MII.

Oocyte Quality in In Vitro Maturation

- Oocytes matured in vitro often show irregular chromosome arrangements and spindle abnormalities, which may reduce quality.
- Zona hardening due to in vitro manipulations, vitrification, and reactive oxygen species (ROS) generation
- Poor cytoplasmic maturation
- Abnormal organelle distribution
- Inadequate cortical granules
- Risk of aneuploidy

Possible Causes

- Lack of in vivo environment
- Oxidative stress
- Improper culture conditions
- Poor understanding of oocyte maturation processes

Pros

- Low-cost treatment
- Avoids frequent injections
- Avoids repeated sonography
- Avoids health risk
- Preserves future fertility of cancer affected girls/women

Cons

- Lower fertilization rate
- Less number of oocytes
- Nonphysiological conditions
- Imprinting errors in IVM born babies
- Nonsynchronization of oocyte maturity and endometrial receptivity.

Ovarian Tissue Cryopreservation

Ovarian tissue cryopreservation is a technique, which is still in experimental stage to preserve reproductive potential in young patient who are at risk of POI. Despite being the experimental technique in some countries the American Society for Reproductive Medicine (ASRM) suggested to consider OTC as an established option for selected patient who are at risk of infertility like cancer therapy. Other indications include benign conditions that potentially affect the ovarian reserve either due to the disease itself, such as genetic disorders (Turner syndrome and galactosemia), or due to gonadotoxic treatments, such as alkylating agents for autoimmune disorders [systemic lupus erythematous (SLE)] or as a conditioning regimen before hematopoietic stem cell transplantation (HSCT) (in sickle cell anemia and thalassemia).[5]

Ovarian tissue cryopreservation has a bigger advantage than other of being feasible within short or less time frame for both post- and prepubertal patient's and no preceding drug is required for the same and for the same reason is becoming a good alternative for oocyte/embryo cryopreservation. OTC requires high-quality control assurance including laboratory training distinct from the standard medically assisted reproduction (MAR).

Technique: There can be two ways for storing tissue by storing an ovarian cortex biopsy (the location of the primordial follicle pool) or one whole ovary can be retrieved at any time during the menstrual cycle and the cortex cryopreserved for future restoration of ovarian function.

1. *Cortical ovarian biopsy:* A cortical ovarian biopsy is a surgical procedure that involves the removal of a small sample from the outer layer (cortex) of the ovary, typically performed using laparoscopy, in order to safeguard fertility or for research purposes.
2. *Whole ovary:* A whole ovary biopsy is generally not a typical or recommended procedure. But any of these can be freezed.
    - Ovarian cortex strips
    - Whole ovary
    - Single follicle

- *Method:*

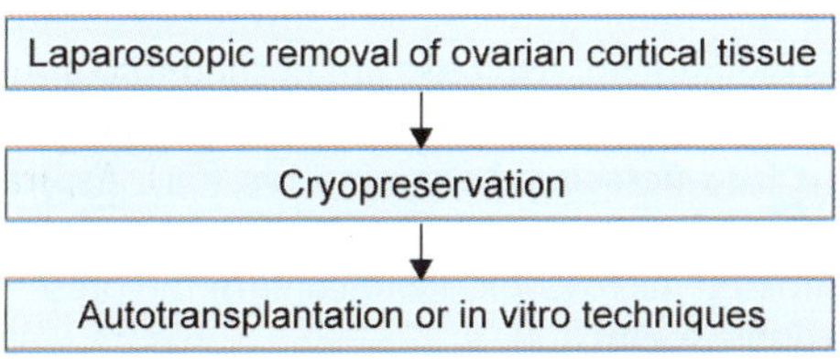

- *Strengths:* Increasingly successful, some study reported similar success rates in terms of fertility restoration for OTC and oocyte vitrification in younger patients.[10]
- *Limitations:* Risk of reintroducing malignant cells in certain cancers; still developing infrastructure.

Ovarian Suppression with GnRH Analogs

- *Method:* Use of GnRH agonists/antagonists during chemotherapy.
- *Indications:* As adjunctive protection during specific chemotherapy regimens (e.g., breast cancer).
- *Strengths/limitations:* It is not a proven standalone preservation method, but may reduce POI in some settings.

Testicular Sperm Cryopreservation

Sperm cryopreservation has been a technique used widely for men to preserve fertility undergoing treatments and allow making it possible for conception in infertile couple. The method of collection for sperm for banking remains masturbation, but for some cases, other methods can also be used one such as disposal penile vibratory stimulation device which is simple and noninvasive. Cases where there is disruption of the ejaculatory reflex arc such as in spinal cord injury, electro-ejaculation can be used under general anesthesia. And in an anticipated low-sperm yield, surgical sperm retrieval technique such as epidermal sperm aspiration and testicular sperm extraction (TESE) can be done.

Indications for Sperm Freezing

- Men risk of infertility due to older ages
- Men planning to have a vasectomy

- Men consider specific medical interventions such as chemotherapy which can impair fertility potential
- Men undergoing surgeries, such as prostrate cancer surgery
- Men in life-endangering occupations, such as military personnel
- Men who are considering IVF.

Sperm Cryopreservation

Method:

Sample is collected in a container and after liquefaction the sample is then washed using density gradient centrifugation (DGC) method to remove debris, dead sperm, or any unwanted material from sperm

↓

Once washed sample and overlayed with 0.5 media, the sample is then introduced to cryoprotectant by drop-by-drop method maintaining 1:1 ratio for both sample and media

↓

Transfer the above mixture into a labeled sterile cryovial

↓

Keep the cryovial in the LN2 vapor phase for 20 minutes and then plunge in LN2

Testicular Sperm Extraction and Cryopreservation

Several sperm retrieval methods have been developed to collect sperm from the epididymis or the testis of azoospermic men. Surgically-retrieved spermatozoa can be used to induce pregnancy through ARTs, i.e., in vitro fertilization associated with intracytoplasmic sperm injection (ICSI).

Percutaneous sperm retrieval methods: Percutaneous retrievals are usually undertaken under local anesthesia only or in association with intravenous sedation. Percutaneous sperm retrieval can be either diagnostic or therapeutic. In the former, it is used to confirm the presence of viable spermatozoa prior to ICSI. In the latter, it is carried out on the same day of oocyte retrieval or the day before.

- *Percutaneous epididymal sperm aspiration (PESA)*
- *Testicular sperm aspiration (TESA)*

Microsurgical sperm retrieval techniques: Microsurgical sperm retrieval can be performed under either local anesthesia in association with intravenous sedation or epidural anesthesia. Operating microscope and microsurgery techniques are used throughout the procedures **(Figs. 2 and 2)**.

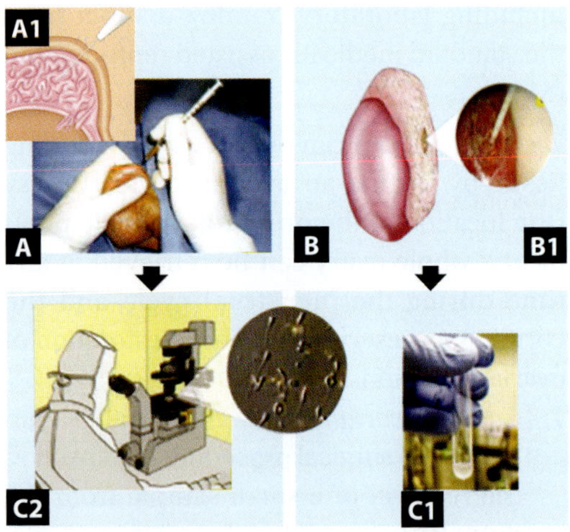

Figs. 1A to C: Epididymal sperm retrieval techniques. (A) Percutaneous epididymal sperm aspiration (PESA). Epididymis is stabilized between the index finger, thumb, and forefinger. A needle attached to a tuberculin syringe is inserted into the epididymis through the scrotal skin (A1), and fluid is aspirated; (B) Microsurgical epididymal sperm aspiration (MESA). After epididymis exposure, a dilated epididymal tubule is microdissected and opened. Fluid emanating from the epididymal tubule is aspirated using an angiocatheter attached to a tuberculin syringe (B1); and (C) Laboratory sperm handling. Aspirates are flushed into a tube containing HEPES-buffered sperm medium and sent for microscope examination (C1). Aspirate aliquots are spread onto a Petri dish and are examined microscopically to confirm the presence of motile sperm (C2).

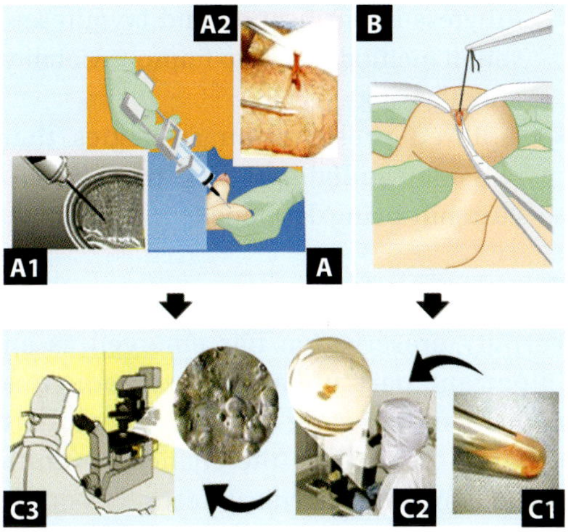

Figs. 2A to C: Testicular sperm retrieval techniques. (A) Percutaneous testicular sperm aspiration (TESA). A needle attached to a syringe is percutaneously inserted into the testis. Negative pressure is created and the tip of the needle is moved within the testis to disrupt the seminiferous tubules and sample different areas (A1). A piece of testicular tissue is aspirated, and a forceps is used to remove the seminiferous tubules that exteriorize from the scrotal skin; (B) Conventional testicular sperm extraction (TESE). A 1–2 cm skin incision is made to allow opening of scrotal layers down to the albuginea. Testicle is not exteriorized from scrotum. A small incision is made in an avascular area of the albuginea to expose testicular parenchyma. A fragment of approximately 5 × 5 mm is excised. Additional fragments may be taken from the same incision or from different testicular poles using multiple incisions; and (C) Laboratory sperm handling. Testicular specimens are flushed into a tube containing sperm medium (C1), and the tube is transferred to the laboratory for tissue processing. Testicular fragments are washed-free from blood clots, and seminiferous tubules are mechanically dispersed using needled-tuberculin syringes until no intact tubules are seen (C2). Testicular homogenates are microscopically examined to confirm the presence of spermatozoa (C3).

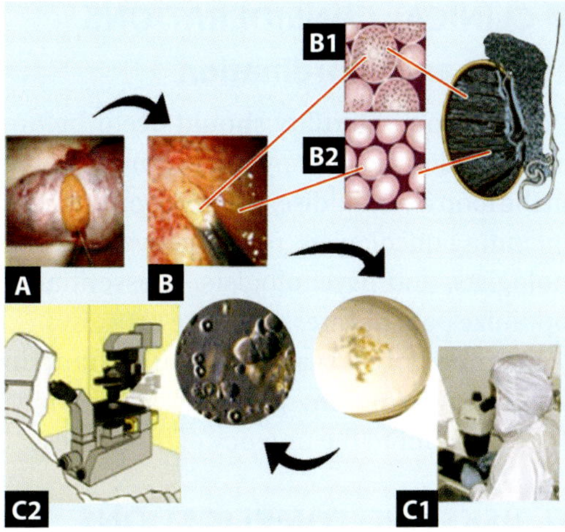

Figs. 3A to C: Microsurgical testicular sperm extraction (micro-TESE). Operating microscope and microsurgical technique are used throughout the procedures. After testis exteriorization, a single and large incision is made in an avascular area of the albuginea to expose testicular parenchyma (A). Microdissection of seminiferous tubules is carried out to identify and remove large tubules that are most likely to contain germ cells and active spermatogenesis. A photograph taken at x40-magnification indicates enlarged and nonenlarged seminiferous tubules (B). Enlarged tubules may contain active spermatogenesis, as illustrated in the transversal section of a histopathology specimen (B1). Nonenlarged tubules are more likely to contain no active spermatogenesis (B2). Excised testicular specimens are sent to the laboratory for processing and examination. Seminiferous tubules are mechanically dispersed using needled-tuberculin syringes (C1). Testicular homogenates are microscopically examined to confirm the presence of spermatozoa (C2).

- *Microsurgical Epididymal Sperm Aspiration (MESA)*
- *Conventional Testicular Sperm Extraction (TESE)*
- *Microsurgical Testicular Sperm Extraction (micro-TESE)* **(Figs. 3A to C)**
  - *Method:* Surgical retrieval of sperm for azoospermic men or inability to produce ejaculate.
  - *Indications:* Severe male factor infertility or pretreatment where ejaculation is not possible.

CLINICAL CONSIDERATIONS

Timing and Coordination

Preservation of fertility should occur before any gonadotoxic therapy has begun. Keeping in the loop for multidisciplinary coordination, including oncologists, reproductive endocrinologists, and psychologists, is essential to optimize patient care.

Hence, preservation should happen before initiating any gonadotoxic therapy, keeping in mind the urgency of the process.[1]

RISKS AND COMPLICATIONS

- Delaying cancer treatment for OS for retrieval.
- Risks like bleeding, anesthesia effect, and mild pain are related to the surgical procedure.
- Psychological stress and burden due to the uncertainty of fertility outcomes in the future.

ETHICAL AND LEGAL ASPECTS

- Obtaining informed consent is essential, particularly when dealing with minors or vulnerable groups (Ethics Committee of the ASRM, 2013).
- Local laws dictate the duration of storage, ownership rights, and the disposal of gametes or tissue.
- Providing realistic counseling regarding success rates, associated risks, and available alternatives is required (Practice Committee of ASRM, 2013).

FUTURE DIRECTIONS

- The in vitro maturation of gametes, along with the development of artificial ovarian and testicular constructs, presents significant potential for enhancing outcomes
- Progress in vitrification and cryopreservation methods seeks to improve viability after thawing
- Tailored preservation strategies that consider individual risk profiles are currently being developed.

CONCLUSION

Fertility preservation has emerged as an important part of modern reproductive and oncologic care, offering individuals a way to hold on to the chance of future parenthood when medical treatments or life situations threaten fertility. What began as a supportive option for patients undergoing cancer treatment has now expanded to include benign medical conditions, genetic and autoimmune disorders, gender-affirming care, and personal choices such as delayed childbearing. New techniques in cryopreservation, ovarian stimulation, and surgical procedures have significantly improved outcomes and accessibility. Yet fertility preservation is not only about technology. Early conversations, timely referrals, and sensitive counseling play a crucial role in helping patients feel informed and supported during difficult decisions. Ethical awareness and clear communication are especially important when caring for adolescents and vulnerable individuals. As research continues to progress, integrating fertility preservation into routine care reflects a commitment to treating patients as whole individuals—preserving not just reproductive potential, but also hope, autonomy, and quality of life for the future.

REFERENCES

1. Practice Committee of the American Society for Reproductive Medicine. Electronic address: asrm@asrm.org. Fertility preservation in patients undergoing gonadotoxic

therapy or gonadectomy: a committee opinion. Fertil Steril. 2019;112(6):1022-33.

2. Henry L, Berek JS, Diaz I, Feldberg D, Mocanu E, Niederberger CC, et al. FIGO statement: Fertility preservation. Int J Gynaecol Obstet. 2023;163(3):790-4.
3. Huleihel M, Lunenfeld E. Approaches and Technologies in Male Fertility Preservation. Int J Mol Sci. 2020;21(15):5471.
4. Lambertini M, Del Mastro L, Pescio MC, Andersen CY, Azim HA Jr, Peccatori FA, et al. Cancer and fertility preservation: international recommendations from an expert meeting. BMC Med. 2016;14:1.
5. Donnez J, Martinez-Madrid B, Jadoul P, Van Langendonckt A, Demylle D, Dolmans MM. Ovarian tissue cryopreservation and transplantation: a review. Hum Reprod Update. 2006;12(5):519-35.
6. Vinolas C, Raad J, Sonigo C, Sifer C, Sermondade N, Grynberg M. Medical techniques of fertility preservation in the male and female. J Visc Surg. 2018;155 Suppl 1:S3-S9.
7. ESHRE. ESHRE guideline female fertility preservation. [online] Available from https://www.eshre.eu/Guidelines-and-Legal/Guidelines/Female-fertility-preservation [Last accessed December, 2025].
8. Eftekhar M, Miraj S, Mortazavifar Z. The effect of luteal phase gonadotropin-releasing hormone antagonist administration on IVF outcomes in women at risk of OHSS. Int J Reprod Biomed. 2016;14(8):507-10.
9. Su HI, Lacchetti C, Letourneau J, Partridge AH, Qamar R, Quinn GP, et al. Fertility preservation in people with cancer: ASCO guideline update. J Clin Oncol. 2025;43(12):1488-515. doi:10.1200/JCO-24-02782.
10. Doungkamchan C, Orwig KE. Recent advances: fertility preservation and fertility restoration options for males and females. Fac Rev. 2021;10:55.

CHAPTER 10

Embryo Selection: Artificial Intelligence-driven Multimodal Grading and Explainability

Snigdha Soni, Gunupuru Gayatri Swetha

INTRODUCTION

Selecting the embryo with the highest implantation potential remains one of the most critical and challenging aspects of in vitro fertilization (IVF). Traditionally, embryologists have relied on visual morphological grading, which involves assessing the appearance of the embryo under a microscope, to guide embryo selection.[1] This approach, however, is subjective and prone to interobserver variability, often leading to inconsistent outcomes.[1] Despite over four decades since the first IVF success, live birth rates per transfer have plateaued around 30%.[2] With single embryo transfer now the standard to minimize multiple pregnancies, there is an urgent need for objective and precise methods to assess embryo viability.[3] This chapter explores how multimodal embryo grading, which integrates diverse data sources such as imaging, time-lapse development videos, and genetic testing, can improve embryo selection. It also examines the development of explainable artificial intelligence (AI) tools to assist clinicians, outlining their clinical applications, technical foundations, and the regulatory frameworks that ensure transparency in the era of AI-assisted reproductive medicine.

EMBRYO ASSESSMENT MODALITIES IN CLINICAL PRACTICE

Conventional Morphological Grading

Embryo evaluation in IVF has traditionally relied on morphological grading at defined developmental stages and is typically done on day 3 (cleavage stage) and day 5 (blastocyst stage). Key parameters include cell number, symmetry, fragmentation, and, for blastocysts, the quality of the inner cell mass (ICM) and trophectoderm (TE).[4] Good-quality embryos exhibit a regular cell arrangement and minimal fragmentation, correlating with a better developmental potential. This method is noninvasive and quick, but it is inherently subjective and heavily dependent on the embryologist's expertise and vulnerable to interobserver variability. Moreover, static morphological assessment provides only a single snapshot in time, overlooking dynamic developmental processes that may be equally critical for predicting implantation success.

Time-lapse Imaging and Morphokinetic Analysis

Time-lapse imaging (TLI) involves culturing embryos in incubators equipped with built-in cameras that capture images at frequent intervals, enabling continuous observation of embryo development without removing the embryos from controlled culture conditions. This approach provides detailed morphokinetic data on key developmental milestones including timing of cell divisions (e.g., time to 2-cell, 4-cell stage, and blastulation) that are often missed during routine once-daily evaluations. Continuous monitoring also means that embryos remain undisturbed in optimal culture conditions, thereby avoiding the stress of being removed for observation.[5] Clinically, certain morphokinetic parameters such as early cleavage timing or synchrony of cell division have been linked to higher implantation rates,[6] improved blastocyst formation[7] and even differences in aneuploidy risk. TLI systems allow ranking embryos based on algorithms that combine these time-based markers with morphology. However, despite these theoretical advantages, studies to date have not definitively shown that time-lapse selection yields higher live birth rates than conventional methods. A 2017 meta-analysis of RCTs concluded there was insufficient evidence that TLI improves clinical outcomes over standard morphology-based selection.[5] Nonetheless, time-lapse technology offers practical benefits, including the ability to combine evaluation of morphology and morphokinetic characteristics to identify the most viable embryos for transfer and improving the workflow in the laboratory by reducing the need to handle embryos.

Preimplantation Genetic Testing

Preimplantation genetic testing (PGT) incorporates a genetic component in the process of embryo selection. By biopsying a few cells from the developing day-5 blastocyst and analyzing them, clinicians can identify euploid embryos and screen out those with aneuploidies or specific genetic disorders.[8] Since chromosomal abnormalities are a major cause of implantation failure and miscarriage, PGT-A (for aneuploidy) can improve implantation and live birth rates, particularly in older women or those with recurrent implantation failure, by ensuring that only euploid embryos are transferred.[9] In clinical practice, PGT is often used in conjunction with morphological assessment, as in among embryos with good morphology, the euploid embryo is prioritized for transfer. This integration of genetic and visual data represents one of the earliest forms of multimodal selection. However, PGT is invasive and adds cost and time to the IVF cycle and carries a small risk of embryo damage due to biopsy. A promising alternative is offered by the emergence of noninvasive preimplantation genetic testing (niPGT), which analyzes cell-free DNA in spent culture media to infer chromosomal status,[10] potentially combining the genetic insight of PGT with the safety of noninvasive monitoring.

Artificial Intelligence

Advances in AI, particularly deep learning have transformed embryo assessment by enabling automated, high-accuracy analysis of images and time-lapse videos.

Convolutional Neural Networks (CNNs) are designed to process images by detecting visual patterns such as texture, boundaries, and cellular features that correlate with embryo quality.

Recurrent Neural Networks (RNNs) process sequential or time-series data, making them ideal for analyzing developmental sequences captured through TLI, allowing the model to interpret the dynamic timing and synchrony of cell divisions.

Transformer-based architectures, originally developed for language processing, have been adapted to handle both spatial and temporal information in embryo videos by focusing attention on the most informative visual or kinetic features.

Using these architectures, AI-systems can identify subtle morphological and dynamic cues often imperceptible to the human eye. CNN models trained on thousands of labeled embryo images have achieved classification accuracies exceeding 80–85%, comparable to experienced embryologists. Similarly, transformer models can extract morphokinetic trajectories automatically, identifying patterns such as asynchronous cleavage or suboptimal timing that predict implantation failure. One such system, IVFormer developed by Wang et al.,[1] demonstrated reliable performance in predicting euploidy and live birth across diverse clinical settings. AI-assisted embryo selection significantly increased live birth rates compared with conventional grading and matched the accuracy of invasive PGT-A, while providing a noninvasive, flexible scoring system adaptable to different clinical goals. Building on this foundation, Deep Neural Networks (DNNs) have been developed for morphological grading and implantation prediction using static images.[11,12] More recent systems have also been trained to predict embryo ploidy,[13,14] blastulation and implantation outcomes[11] from time-lapse frames. A major strength of AI-based evaluation lies in its consistency, eliminating observer variation by applying uniform criteria to every embryo. However, training such models requires large well-annotated datasets, which can prove to be a challenge in domains such as prediction of ploidy and determination of live birth rates.

Integrating Multiple Modalities for Embryo Selection

Multimodal embryo grading combines information from multiple sources, including, morphological scores, time-lapse metrics, genetic results, and even patient-specific factors, to make a more informed selection. In routine IVF practice, embryologists already apply this concept intuitively, weighing an embryo's appearance, PGT result, and morphokinetic behavior to decide which to transfer. The goal is to leverage the complementary strengths of each modality. For example, an embryo might have average morphology but being the only euploid embryo; another might look excellent morphologically but show abnormal cleavage pattern on time-lapse.

Integrating multiple data types (images, time-series data, genetic results, patient demographics, etc.) is an area of ongoing research with multimodal AI-driven scoring systems being developed to assist in this by quantifying and standardizing this data. Multimodal AI models often consist of separate feature extractors for each data source, which are then combined. For instance, one component of the model might be a CNN analyzing the *static* morphology of the blastocyst, while another component like a temporal convolution or transformer network processes the *time-lapse sequence*. Yet another could incorporate *clinical data* including patient age, hormone levels, etc. via techniques like fully connected networks or embedding layers.[2] Extracted features are then merged either through simple concatenation or through attention mechanisms to produce a unified prediction, such as implantation probability or embryo ranking **(Fig. 1)**. Two complementary strategies are typically employed:

1. *Data fusion*, which merges raw or embedded data before prediction; and
2. *Model fusion*, which combines the outputs of separate models trained on individual modalities.

The key challenge lies in ensuring how much each modality should contribute to outcome prediction.

Evidence and Performance

Early research demonstrates that multimodal approaches outperform single-modality models in terms of predictive accuracy. In a study by Salih et al.,[2] a deep learning model integrating embryo images with clinical data achieved an accuracy of 82.4% for pregnancy prediction, compared with 66.9% for images alone and 81.8% for clinical data alone. The authors suggested that integrating clinical information enables AI to contextualize and interpret visual embryo features such as morphology, developmental patterns, and cellular dynamics. Similarly, AI models that incorporate both static images and time-lapse sequences of embryos demonstrate more consistent grading and better outcome prediction than traditional methods. By fusing modalities, we can potentially identify embryos that have both the required genetic normalcy and developmental competence

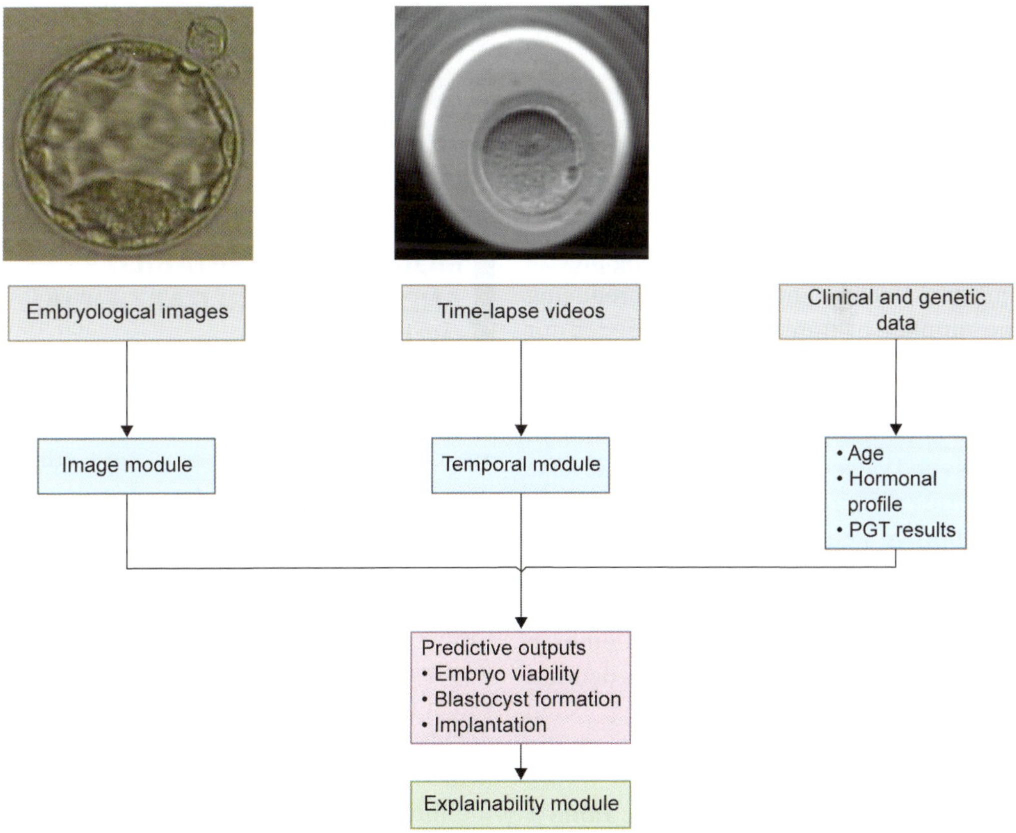

Fig. 1: AI-driven multimodal embryo assessment pipeline.
(AI: artificial intelligence; PGT: preimplantation genetic testing)

TABLE 1: Comparison of different embryo selection techniques.

Method	*Data*	*Invasiveness*	*Assessment*	*Advantages*	*Limitations*
Morphological grading	Embryo appearance (cell number, symmetry, and fragmentation)	Noninvasive	Structural	Simple, widely used, and inexpensive	Subjective, limited predictive accuracy, and interobserver variability
Morphokinetic grading	Time-lapse imaging and cell-division parameters	Noninvasive	Functional and developmental dynamics	Objective, provides continuous development data	Requires specialized equipment, variable interpretability, and increased cost
PGT	Genetic analysis (PGT-A, PGT-M, PGT-SR)	Invasive (biopsy)	Genetic/aneuploidy status	Direct assessment of genetic health	Invasive, costly, potential for mosaicism, and diagnostic error
Multimodal grading	Integrated morphology, morphokinetics, genetic, and clinical data	Mixed (mostly noninvasive, biopsy if PGT used)	structural, functional, and genetic	Leverages complementary data; higher predictive accuracy; supports single embryo transfer	Complex implementation, requires advanced AI systems; interpretability and regulatory challenges; regulatory higher cost

(PGT: preimplantation genetic testing)

for successful implantation, enabling precise embryo selection and potentially reducing the number of transfer cycles needed for pregnancy.

However, a continuing challenge lies in the heterogeneity of the data as embryo images and videos are obtained using diverse platforms and protocols across IVF centers. To improve generalizability, researchers are exploring self-supervised learning and visual-temporal contrastive frameworks that can learn robust multimodal embryo representations from heterogeneous datasets without extensive manual labeling.[1] Such approaches promise to enhance both the scalability and interpretability of future AI systems for embryo selection. **Table 1** summarizes the different embryo selection methods that are currently in use.

MODEL INTERPRETABILITY AND EXPLAINABLE ARTIFICIAL INTELLIGENCE

As AI models become integral to embryo selection, explainability and transparency are essential to ensure trust and ethical use. Two key aspects of transparency are: (1) understanding *why* a particular decision was made and (2) being aware *when and how* AI is used in the decision process. Clinicians and patients must understand *why* an algorithm makes a recommendation, which is challenging when systems function as "black boxes". This essentially means that while their input and output is observed, the internal reasoning behind decisions is opaque.[15,16] Explainable AI (XAI) techniques aim to bridge this gap by highlighting key visual or morphological features influencing predictions. For example, heatmaps can highlight image regions that most affected an embryo's score, such as fragmented areas or the ICM region, and providing clear and interpretable justifications like optimal cleavage timing or absence of fragmentation. Some AI tools provide explanations in text-based outputs with interpretable summaries like, "embryo #3 was ranked highest because it had optimal cell division timing and absence of fragmentation, and it is predicted to be euploid". Transparency can be achieved either through the development of inherently simpler and interpretable models or feature post hoc explanations integrated into the user interface, allowing embryologists to compare AI outputs with raw embryo data. Ensuring transparency is not only an ethical imperative but also a practical necessity as it enhances clinician confidence, supports patient autonomy, and fosters clinical adoption.

CLINICAL IMPLEMENTATION AND APPLICATIONS

Emerging Tools and Systems for Multimodal Embryo Selection

Several AI-driven embryo assessment platforms have recently entered clinical use, reflecting rapid progress in the field. Life Whisperer,[17] a cloud-based AI system, analyzes uploaded embryo images to predict viability and likelihood of euploidy. In a multicenter study by Diakiw et al.[17] involving over 15,000 embryos across 10 IVF centers, the model trained on 5,050 labeled images with corresponding PGT-A results, achieved an accuracy of 65.3 % and sensitivity of 74.6 % on a blind test dataset. This improved to 77.4% after excluding poor quality or mislabeled images. The AI score correlated strongly with the euploidy rate; with top-scoring embryos twice as likely to be euploid than those with the lowest scores. Therefore, this tool can assist in selecting high quality embryos for fresh transfer, cryopreservation, or PGT-A, and can help prioritize among multiple euploid embryos. Fairtility's "Chloe EQ",[18] integrates time-lapse morphokinetics and AI-based scoring to rank embryos by implantation potential and euploidy probability, combining quantitative prediction with a transparent, explainable interface. Similarly, Vitrolife's *iDAScore*, automatically analyzes time-lapse videos captured in EmbryoScope incubators, and offers automated scoring of embryos that matches or exceeds embryologist accuracy in multicenter studies. Several research-grade systems have also been developed in this field. ERICA (Embryo Ranking Intelligent Classification Algorithm)[19] and STORK-A[20] apply deep learning to microscopy images and morphokinetic data, achieving 70–75% accuracy for ploidy prediction and strong generalizability across centers. Other newer systems such as Embryo Predict (Alife Health),[21] Ubar (Embryonics),[22] and FiTTE (Japan)[23] extend these principles by incorporating clinical parameters and time-lapse data into predictive frameworks for implantation and fetal heartbeat outcomes. **Table 2** summarizes some of the major AI-based embryo assessment systems. Collectively, these systems exemplify how embryo selection is evolving into a truly multimodal data-driven process, where visual, developmental, genetic information, and clinical insights converge through AI to provide consistent, transparent, and evidence-based guidance for clinicians and embryologists.

TABLE 2: Summary of major artificial intelligence-based embryo assessment systems.

AI system	*Primary inputs*	*Predicted outputs*	*Reported performance*
Life whisperer	Static embryo images (days 5–6)	Viability and ploidy	Accuracy up to 77% for euploidy prediction; top-rank embryo euploid in 82% of cohorts
Chloe EQ	Time-lapse videos (EmbryoScope)	Gestational sac	AUC: 0.68–0.70; ~9% higher accuracy than embryologists
iDAScore	Time-lapse videos (EmbryoScope)	Fetal heartbeat	AUC: 0.67–0.70
ERICA	Static images	Euploidy prediction and ranking	Accuracy 70%; AUC: 0.74
STORK-A	Static images + morphokinetic data + maternal age	Blastocyst grade and ploidy prediction	ROC-AUC: 0.72–0.74; accuracy 63–68%
Embryo Predict	Static images + patient age	Fetal heartbeat	ROC-AUC: 0.62–0.64; 3–17% gain over embryologists
Ubar	Time-lapse videos (EmbryoScope)	Gestational sac	AUC: 0.70; 20% accuracy gain
FiTTE	Static images	hCG + fetal heartbeat	ROC-AUC: 0.68; accuracy 62.7%

(AUC: area under the curve; hCG: human chorionic gonadotropin; ROC: receiver operating characteristic)

Impact on Clinical Outcomes and Efficiency

Early clinical experience with these AI systems suggests measurable benefits in both treatment outcomes and laboratory efficiency. Studies show that AI-assisted grading can improve the likelihood of identifying a viable embryo in the first transfer, potentially reducing the number of IVF cycles.[24] ERICA (IVF 2.0, UK), which is an AI system trained on static day-5 images, predicts ploidy and pregnancy probability and has demonstrated accuracy comparable to or exceeding that of experienced embryologists[19] Similarly, Life Whisperer's viability model demonstrated higher predictive accuracy for pregnancy than manual grading in a multicenter trial, while a fully automated deep-learning tool outperformed semiautomated systems and provided reliable predictions within 30 hours post-fertilization.[25] Bernstein et al.[26] evaluated iDAScore v1.0 model, trained on over 115,000 embryos from 18 clinics. This model achieved an area under the curve (AUC) of 0.67 for transferred embryos with known outcomes, maintaining consistent performance across patient ages, insemination methods, and clinic settings (AUC: 0.60–0.75). It also correlated strongly with key morphological features such as ICM, TE grade, and blastulation timing, demonstrating that deep learning can reproduce and even enhance traditional morphokinetic scoring, without manual annotation. These improvements have meaningful clinical and practical implications. Higher implantation rates per transfer shorten the time to pregnancy and reduce the emotional and financial burden for patients. Automated analysis streamlines workflows and minimizes observer variability and supports continuous quality monitoring. However, long-term prospective validation remains essential before such tools can function as standalone decision systems.

Clinical Implementation and Regulatory Considerations

Integrating AI-based grading into the IVF workflow requires practical adjustments and regulatory oversight. In most laboratories, embryo images and videos from time-lapse incubators are automatically captured and analyzed by AI software, either locally or via secure cloud platforms. Embryologists review AI-generated embryo scores through integrated dashboards linked to electronic laboratory records, using them to complement rather than replace manual grading. Successful adoption depends on seamless data integration, staff training, and contingency planning for system downtime.

As these tools influence clinical decisions, they are classified as software as a medical device (SaMD) and are regulated for safety and effectiveness. Frameworks differ by region: in the United States, the Food and Drug Administration (FDA) reviews AI-based systems for risk and clinical performance, while in Europe, CE marking is required under EU medical device regulations. The Eeva system was among the first FDA-approved embryo assessment tool, approved as a Class II device for adjunctive use alongside morphology grading.[27] More recently, platforms such as Fairtility's Chloe EQ (CE-marked in 2022) and systems from AiVF/Embryonics[28] have gained approval for clinical use. Regulatory evaluation requires evidence from clinical studies demonstrating that the tool's use improves or at least does not compromise outcomes. Post-market surveillance and algorithm monitoring are essential to detect performance drift, bias, or safety concerns as adoption expands.

Validation, Performance, and Data Security

Even with regulatory clearance, each clinic must independently validate AI-based embryo assessment tool to ensure reliable performance in its specific setting. Accuracy may vary across centers due to differences in patient demographics, laboratory protocols, and imaging systems. Initial implementation should involve parallel testing, which includes using AI alongside standard grading, to confirm that its recommendations align with clinical judgment and outcomes. Key performance metrics for validation include sensitivity, specificity, and calibration with periodic re-evaluation recommended after software updates to prevent algorithmic drift.

Because multimodal grading systems process sensitive reproductive and genetic data, robust privacy and security safeguards are essential. Clinics must comply with applicable data protection regulations and ensure that cloud-based platforms use strong encryption and secure data transfer protocols to maintain confidentiality and prevent unauthorized access.

ETHICAL AND SOCIETAL CONSIDERATIONS

Transparency and Explainability in Decision-making

A frequently cited ethical concern in AI-assisted embryo selection is transparency. Deep learning models, often function as "black boxes". This lack of interpretability can erode clinician and patient trust, hinder shared decision-making, and create accountability gaps when outcomes are suboptimal. It is ethically imperative to provide a clear rationale, why a particular embryo was chosen by the AI model. The lack of interpretability also makes it difficult to detect confounders or erroneous reasoning in the algorithm.

Transparent or "glass-box" models are therefore preferred, as they enhance confidence, enable the detection of confounders, and support patient autonomy.[16]

If an AI model leads to a poor outcome, its opaque nature creates a "responsibility gap", making it challenging to determine whether the fault lies with the clinician, the developer, or the AI system itself. Clinics should document AI-assisted decisions in the medical record and disclose to patients when AI tools are used, ideally through interfaces that show both raw embryo data and AI-derived reasoning.

Algorithmic Bias and Fairness

Artificial intelligence systems learn from historical data, and therefore, can learn and perpetuate hidden biases. Biases can arise from various sources, including demographic variation in datasets and clinical practices. Such bias risks propagating systemic inequities or inadvertently prioritizing certain embryo characteristics correlated with sex or ethnicity. To promote fairness, models must be trained and validated on diverse, representative datasets across clinics and populations. Algorithms should be routinely audited for performance discrepancies among different subgroups.

Preserving Human Oversight and Responsibility

Artificial intelligence should augment, not replace, clinician judgment. Concerns about the "dehumanization" of reproduction arise when decision-making is ceded entirely to machine. While AI tools can standardize grading and reduce variability, the ultimate responsibility for embryo selection rests with the treating physician and embryologist. Overreliance on AI risks "machine paternalism",[29] where clinicians defer to automated outputs without critical review, and "deskilling",[16] where manual expertise erodes over time. To prevent this, AI must be used prudently, with clinicians critically reviewing its recommendations. Training programs should continue to emphasize traditional embryology skills while integrating AI as a teaching aid, can reinforce learning as well.

FUTURE DIRECTIONS

- *Continuous improvement of AI models:* With access to increasingly large and global datasets, next-generation AI systems are expected to achieve higher predictive accuracy and incorporate newer such as metabolomic and transcriptomic profiling. Importantly, next-generation models will emphasize *explainability by design*, integrating data-driven learning with embryology expertise for transparent and interpretable decision rules.
- *Prospective clinical trials:* Well-designed trials comparing AI-assisted versus conventional embryo selection are essential to establish clinical benefit and cost-effectiveness. Outcomes such as cumulative live birth rate, time to pregnancy, and patient burden should guide evidence-based adoption.
- *Regulation and standards:* As AI becomes integral to IVF laboratories, regulatory and professional frameworks must evolve in parallel.

CONCLUSION

The integration of imaging, time-lapse, genetic, and clinical data marks a pivotal shift in embryo selection in modern IVF. By uniting these complementary modalities, multimodal AI systems have the potential to enhance objectivity, consistency, and predictive accuracy, addressing the limitations of traditional assessment methods. Early clinical evidence is encouraging, but, there is a need for rigorous validation, transparency, and ethical oversight before the successful adoption of these technologies. Ensuring that AI systems remain explainable, equitable, and patient-focused which will allow their integration to enhance, rather than compromise, the quality of reproductive care.

REFERENCES

1. Wang G, Wang K, Gao Y, Chen L, Gao T, Ma Y, et al. A generalized AI system for human embryo selection covering the entire IVF cycle via multi-modal contrastive learning. Patterns (N Y). 2024;5(7):100985.
2. Salih M, Austin C, Mantravadi K, Seow E, Jitanantawittaya S, Reddy S, et al. Deep learning classification integrating embryo images with associated clinical information from ART cycles. Sci Rep. 2025;15(1):17585.
3. Gleicher N, Kushnir VA, Barad DH. Is it time for a paradigm shift in understanding embryo selection? Reprod Biol Endocrinol. 2015;13:3.
4. Nasiri N, Eftekhari-Yazdi P. An overview of the available methods for morphological scoring of pre-implantation embryos in in vitro fertilization. Cell J. 2015;16(4):392-405.
5. Chen M, Wei S, Hu J, Yuan J, Liu F. Does time-lapse imaging have favorable results for embryo incubation and selection compared with conventional methods in clinical in vitro fertilization? A meta-analysis and systematic review of randomized controlled trials. PloS One. 2017;12(6):e0178720.
6. Basile N, Vime P, Florensa M, Aparicio Ruiz B, García Velasco JA, Remohí J, et al. The use of morphokinetics as a predictor of implantation: a multicentric study to define and validate an algorithm for embryo selection. Hum Reprod. 2015;30(2):276-83.
7. Kirkegaard K, Kesmodel US, Hindkjær JJ, Ingerslev HJ. Time-lapse parameters as predictors of blastocyst development and pregnancy outcome in embryos from good prognosis patients: a prospective cohort study. Hum Reprod. 2013;28(10):2643-51.
8. Simopoulou M, Sfakianoudis K, Maziotis E, Tsioulou P, Grigoriadis S, Rapani A, et al. PGT-A: who and when? A systematic review and network meta-analysis of RCTs. J Assist Reprod Genet. 2021;38(8):1939-57.
9. Practice Committees of the American Society for Reproductive Medicine and the Society for Assisted Reproductive Technology. Electronic address: asrm@asrm.org. The use of preimplantation genetic testing for aneuploidy: a committee opinion. Fertil Steril. 2024;122(3):421-34.
10. Layek SS, Kanani S, Doultani S, Gohil T, Patil S, Sudhakar A, et al. Analyzing Cell-free Genomic DNA in Spent Culture Media: Noninvasive Insight into the Blastocysts. Glob Med Genet. 2024;11(3):227-32.
11. Leahy BD, Jang WD, Yang HY, Struyven R, Wei D, Sun Z, et al. Automated Measurements of Key Morphological Features of Human Embryos for IVF. Med Image Comput Comput Assist Interv. 2020;12265:25-35.
12. Silver DH, Feder M, Gold-Zamir Y, Polsky AL, Rosentraub S, Shachor E, et al. Data-driven prediction of embryo implantation probability using IVF time-lapse imaging. arXiv preprint arXiv:2006.01035. 2020.
13. Huang B, Tan W, Li Z, Jin L. An artificial intelligence model (euploid prediction algorithm) can predict embryo ploidy status based on time-lapse data. Reprod Biol Endocrinol. 2021;19(1):185.
14. Jiang VS, Kandula H, Thirumalaraju P, Kanakasabapathy MK, Cherouveim P, Souter I, et al. The use of voting ensembles to improve the accuracy of deep neural networks as a non-invasive method to predict embryo ploidy status. J Assist Reprod Genet. 2023;40(2):301-8.
15. Luong TMT, Le NQK. Artificial intelligence in time-lapse system: advances, applications,

and future perspectives in reproductive medicine. J Assist Reprod Genet. 2024; 41(2):239-52.

16. Koplin JJ, Johnston M, Webb ANS, Whittaker A, Mills C. Ethics of artificial intelligence in embryo assessment: mapping the terrain. Hum Reprod. 2025;40(2):179-85.
17. Diakiw SM, Hall JMM, VerMilyea MD, Amin J, Aizpurua J, Giardini L, et al. Development of an artificial intelligence model for predicting the likelihood of human embryo euploidy based on blastocyst images from multiple imaging systems during IVF. Hum Reprod. 2022;37(8):1746-59.
18. Erlich I, Hariharan R, Har-Vardi I, Tran M, Karavani G, Levitas E, et al. Chloe EQ™ Effectively and Automatically Predicts Embryo Implantation Across all Patient age groups by Combining Morphokinetic and Morphology Algorithms Over Culture Time. Fertil Steril. 2022;118(4):e114.
19. Chavez-Badiola A, Flores-Saiffe-Farías A, Mendizabal-Ruiz G, Drakeley AJ, Cohen J. Embryo Ranking Intelligent Classification Algorithm (ERICA): artificial intelligence clinical assistant predicting embryo ploidy and implantation. Reprod Biomed Online. 2020;41(4):585-93.
20. Barnes J, Brendel M, Gao VR, Rajendran S, Kim J, Li Q, et al. A non-invasive artificial intelligence approach for the prediction of human blastocyst ploidy: a retrospective model development and validation study. Lancet Digit Health. 2023;5(1):e28-40.
21. Loewke K, Cho JH, Brumar CD, Maeder-York P, Barash O, Malmsten JE, et al. Characterization of an artificial intelligence model for ranking static images of blastocyst stage embryos. Fertil Steril. 2022;117(3):528-35.
22. Fordham DE, Rosentraub D, Polsky AL, Aviram T, Wolf Y, Perl O, et al. Embryologist agreement when assessing blastocyst implantation probability: is data-driven prediction the solution to embryo assessment subjectivity? Hum Reprod. 2022;37(10): 2275-90.
23. Enatsu N, Miyatsuka I, An LM, Inubushi M, Enatsu K, Otsuki J, et al. A novel system based on artificial intelligence for predicting blastocyst viability and visualizing the explanation. Reprod Med Biol. 2022;21(1): e12443.
24. Cohen J, Silvestri G, Paredes O, Martin-Alcala HE, Chavez-Badiola A, Alikani M, et al. Artificial intelligence in assisted reproductive technology: separating the dream from reality. Reprod Biomed Online. 2025;50(4):104855.
25. Erlich I, Ben-Meir A, Har-Vardi I, Grifo J, Wang F, Mccaffrey C, et al. Pseudo contrastive labeling for predicting IVF embryo developmental potential. Sci Rep. 2022;12(1):2488.
26. Berntsen J, Rimestad J, Lassen JT, Tran D, Kragh MF. Robust and generalizable embryo selection based on artificial intelligence and time-lapse image sequences. PloS One. 2022;17(2):e0262661.
27. De Novo classification request for Eeva™ System. [online] Available from https://www.accessdata.fda.gov/cdrh_docs/reviews/den120015.pdf [Last accessed December, 2025].
28. Gilboa D, Garg A, Shapiro M, Meseguer M, Amar Y, Lustgarten N, et al. Application of a methodological framework for the development and multicenter validation of reliable artificial intelligence in embryo evaluation. Reprod Biol Endocrinol. 2025;23(1):16.
29. Aufieri R, Mastrocola F. Balancing Technology, Ethics, and Society: A Review of Artificial Intelligence in Embryo Selection. Information. 2025;16(1):18.

CHAPTER 11

Noninvasive and Minimally Invasive Preimplantation Genetic Testing and Advances in Next-generation Sequencing

Priyanka Rai, Shruti P Shirodkar, Divya MB

INTRODUCTION

Preimplantation genetic testing (PGT) has become a key component in contemporary in vitro fertilization (IVF), which enables healthy embryo transfer. The terms preimplantation genetic diagnosis (PGD) and preimplantation genetic screening (PGS) have been replaced with preimplantation genetic testing (PGT).[1] PGT is a procedure used for studying deoxyribonucleic Acid (DNA) from oocytes (polar bodies) or embryos (blastocyst, cleavage stage, and trophectoderm) in order to perform human leukocyte antigen (HLA) typing or identify genetic defects. Results of the test are further classified into PGT for aneuploidy (PGT-A), PGT for monogenic/single gene defects (PGT-M), and PGT for chromosomal structural rearrangements (PGT-SR). Traditionally, PGT was performed by extracting a few embryonic cells and subjecting them to whole-genome amplification (WGA) followed by molecular analysis. Concerns remain about biopsy-related risks, such as reduced post-biopsy embryo survival, the need for prolonged culture, expense, and interpretive constraints such as mosaicism. These concerns have driven interest in non-invasive PGT (niPGT) using cell-free DNA (cfDNA) in spent culture medium (SCM), and minimally invasive sampling such as blastocoel fluid (BF) aspiration. In parallel, next-generation sequencing (NGS) methods and single-cell/WGA innovations have transformed data quality, enabling higher resolution copy-number calls, combined haplotyping, and better handling. This chapter reviews the clinical workflow from basics to cutting-edge advances, critically appraises non-/minimally invasive approaches, and highlights where NGS is taking the field next.[2-4]

TRADITIONAL PREIMPLANTATION GENETIC TESTING

Embryonic biopsy: Prior to transfer, one or more embryonic cells are carefully removed for genetic analysis. The main goal is to preserve embryo viability while acquiring enough genetic material. Polar body (PB) biopsy, the least invasive option, can be performed sequentially—first PB before insemination (about 4 hours post-retrieval) and second PB after fertilization (16–18 hours post-insemination)—or simultaneously, with both PBs collected at 16 hours; this approach provides information only about maternal pathogenic variants, meiotic aneuploidies, or genetic makeup.[5]

Blastomere biopsy is performed at the 6–8 cell stage (around 72 hours post-insemination); although two-cell biopsy improves diagnostic accuracy, it removes nearly 30% of the embryo, potentially reducing viability, whereas single-cell biopsy carries a risk of misdiagnosis.[6] Trophectoderm biopsy, performed at the blastocyst stage (day 5–6), allows more cells to be sampled thus improving mosaicism detection but requires significant expertise and may slightly compromise implantation potential. TE biopsy can be done by early zona drilling before expansion, laser hatching at full expansion to protect the inner cell mass, or post-expansion zona opening with TE herniation, which combines the advantages of both approaches but adds cost and technical complexity.[6] A significant disadvantage of this approach is that the cells only come from the trophectoderm, which means that the mosaic inner cell mass is not identified.

The traditional workflow of PGT is mentioned in **Figure 1**.

Analytical platforms: Earlier platforms used array CGH (comparative genomic hybridization) or SNP (single nucleotide polymorphism) arrays for copy-number and linkage analysis. NGS (next-generation sequencing) now predominates, typically via low-pass genome sequencing (low coverage with binning for copy-number) for PGT-A and targeted/amplicon-based or haplotype-based approaches for PGT-M/PGT-SR. Low-pass WGS on WGA (whole genome amplification) products has been clinically validated and allows detection of whole-chromosome and many segmental events.[7] Various analytical methods used in PGT are mentioned in **Table 1**.

Interpretive challenges: Mosaicism (the presence of two or more karyotypically distinct lineages) complicates interpretation and clinical decision-making, prompting guidance from ESHRE, ASRM, and PGDIS on thresholds, reporting, and transfer policies **(Table 2)**.[9]

WHY PURSUE NON-/MINIMALLY INVASIVE STRATEGIES?

- *Avoiding biopsy:* Even if biopsy-related harm is rare in experienced hands, it requires skill, infrastructure, and cost.
- *Improving representativeness:* Sampling cfDNA released into medium or BF could integrate signals from across the embryo.
- *Scalability and access:* A cheaper, simpler test could broaden PGT availability.

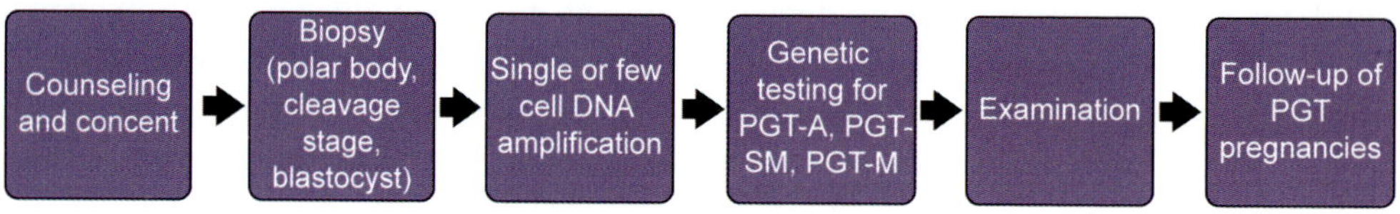

Fig. 1: Traditional workflow in preimplantation genetic testing (PGT).

TABLE 1: Comparison of various analytical methods used in preimplantation genetic testing (PGT).[8]

Method	*Principle*	*Applications*	*Limitations/notes*
FISH (fluorescence in situ hybridization)	Determines the copy number at certain chromosomal loci using target-specific DNA probes that have been labelled with haptens or fluorochromes	Detects chromosome imbalances due to meiotic segregation errors in structural rearrangements; screens for sporadic aneuploidies to improve ART outcomes	Limited predictive value, because of a restricted number of chromosomes evaluated, it is not advised for routine clinical use

Contd...

Contd...

Method	*Principle*	*Applications*	*Limitations/notes*
aCGH (array comparative genomic hybridization)	A DNA microarray chip that represents the entire genome is co-hybridized with patient and control DNA that has been tagged with distinct fluorescent dyes (green for sample, red for control). Relative fluorescence intensities are measured by a scanner	Detects minor chromosomal duplications or deletions and provides genome-wide detection of DNA copy number gains and losses	Provides comprehensive coverage but cannot detect balanced rearrangements; relatively costly
NGS (next-generation sequencing)	Precise quantification of chromosomal copy number using parallel sequencing of the genome	Improves embryo selection, implantation, and IVF pregnancy rates, particularly in cases of recurrent implantation failure (RIF); detects mosaicism, euploidy, and aneuploidy	Requires advanced infrastructure and expertise, more time- and data-intensive than FISH/aCGH but provides higher resolution

TABLE 2: Comparing mosaic embryo guidelines of ESHRE, ARM, and PGDIS.

Aspect	*ASRM (2024)*	*ESHRE (2023)*	*PGDIS (2021)*
Definition	Mosaicism diagnosed via intermediate copy number signals in trophectoderm biopsy	Same definition, emphasizes platform validation and biological interpretation	Same, highlights segmental vs. whole chromosome mosaicism
Reporting standards	Labs should disclose classification schemes and thresholds; standardization is needed	Reports must include type, level (% abnormal cells), and diagnostic confidence	Recommends reporting mosaic level (low <30%, moderate 30–50%, high >50%) and affected chromosomes
Transfer considera-tion	Transfer may be considered when no euploid embryos are available, individualized decision-making advised	Transfer allowed with prior-itization based on risk (e.g., low-level, single chromo-some mosaic preferred)	Supports transfer of low/moderate mosaic embryos if no euploid options; discourages high-level mosaic transfer
Counseling	Genetic counseling strongly recommended before transfer	Mandatory counseling with informed consent; risks and uncertainties must be clearly explained	Strongly recommends counselling; patients must understand risks, limitations, and follow-up needs
Follow-up	Prenatal testing (e.g., amniocentesis) recommended after mosaic embryo transfer	Same recommendation; emphasizes post-transfer monitoring	Same; recommends invasive prenatal diagnosis after mosaic embryo transfer
Policy requirement	Clinics should maintain written policies on mosaic embryo disposition	Not explicitly stated, but transparency in reporting and decision-making is emphasized	Encourages clear lab policies and documentation of mosaic classification and transfer criteria

These potential benefits must be weighed against analytical obstacles—especially low DNA quantity, maternal/culture contaminants, variable embryonic fraction, and stochastic WGA/NGS noise.[3]

MINIMALLY INVASIVE AND NON-INVASIVE PREIMPLANTATION GENETIC TESTING

Blastocoel Fluid Deoxyribonucleic Acid (Minimally Invasive Preimplantation Genetic Testing)

In certain procedures, blastocoel fluid (BF) aspiration during aided hatching or before vitrification can aid in the extraction of DNA with possibly greater embryonic specificity than SCM. BF is a less intrusive source of PGT-A and can be employed for exploratory biomarkers of embryo competence, even though its DNA quantity is still low and fluctuates. The technique does not remove any cells, although it does require micromanipulation. BF aspiration during aided hatching or before vitrification can aid in the extraction of DNA with possibly greater embryonic specificity than SCM. BF is a less intrusive source of PGT-A and can be employed for exploratory biomarkers of embryo competence, even though its DNA quantity is still low and fluctuates. The technique does not remove any cells, although it does require micromanipulation.[10] BF is sampled on the other side of the inner cell mass, causing the embryo to collapse completely. The BF's aspiration has no effect on the architecture of the embryo; both embryos with good and poor morphology have high survival rates.[10] Lower mosaic rates, more precision, and greater implantation rates are among the benefits; nevertheless, DNA originating from necrotic or apoptotic cells, higher false positive and false negative results, variances in technical expertise, and the possibility of embryo harm are the drawbacks. The advantages and disadvantages of blastocoel fluid aspiration are mentioned in **Table 3**.

TABLE 3: Advantages and disadvantages of blastocel fluid aspiration.

Advantages	*Disadvantages*
• Simple method • Less invasive • Low rates of mosaicism • Improved accuracy	• Costly • Risk of damage to embryo • DNA may originate from necrotic or apoptotic cells • High false positive and negative results

Spent Culture Medium (SCM) cfDNA (Noninvasive Preimplantation Genetic Testing)

Embryos release cfDNA into culture media via apoptosis, necrosis, exosomes, or active secretion. There are studies that show that SCM cfDNA can be sequenced and compared to TE biopsy results.[11] Reported similarity with TE/whole embryo varies widely across laboratories due to differences in culture systems, media changes, timing of collection, and DNA extraction. **Table 4** explains in detail the stepwise process involved in preimplantation genetic testing using spent culture medium. At present, a cautious consensus is that niPGT-A may serve as a "backup" or adjunct, not a replacement for TE biopsy in most clinical settings due to the following drawbacks:[12]

- *Contamination and embryonic fraction:* A central limitation is maternal DNA contamination, like residual cumulus/corona cells, follicular fluid DNA, which can dominate low-quantity samples and give false positive results. Methylation and Machine-learning-based deconvolution methods and improved laboratory

TABLE 4: Steps of preimplantation genetic testing (PGT) using spent culture medium (SCM).

Step	*Process*	*Details and requirements*	*Documentation*
1	*SCM collection timing*	• Collect SCM at 90–120 hours postfertilization (Day 5) • Use ≤5 µL media per embryo drop • Avoid oil overlay carryover • Store at –20°C (≤7 days) or –80°C (long-term)	Record embryo ID, collection time, operator initials in LIMS
2	*Negative control setup*	• Include one blank media drop per batch (processed same as SCM) • Include reagent-only control during extraction/WGA • Include no-template control during qPCR/NGS prep	Log control IDs and results in QC section of LIMS
3	*WGA method and validation*	• Use validated WGA kit (MDA/PTA recommended) • *Annual validation:* >95% amplification efficiency, >80% genome coverage, <10% allelic dropout • Record lot-to-lot QC	Upload validation data and QC reports to central lab records
4	*DNA quantification and QC*	• Quantify DNA yield post-WGA • Compare yield to negative controls • Check for abnormal allele fractions or poor amplification	Document results and flag abnormal samples in LIMS
5	*Contamination thresholds*	• >3× DNA yield vs. negative control = potential contamination • *Low-level (<5%):* Report with caution + recommend prenatal confirmatory testing • *Moderate/High (>5–10%):* Mark inconclusive, request recollection if possible	Record contamination status, escalate to laboratory director if recurrent

practices such as thorough denudation, media change schedules, and separate drops are emerging to mitigate this.[13] Based on the observation that a mammalian preimplantation embryo's DNA methylation level reaches its lowest point during the blastocyst stage, the reasoning is supported. Thus, it is possible to select blastocyst DNA over nonembryonic DNA by choosing hypomethylated readings.

- *Standardization:* The following techniques should be standardized for better generalization of outcomes:
  - Timing of SCM collection—collection should be done often, just before vitrification at D5-D7.[14]
  - Media volume and drop isolation to prevent crosstalk.
  - Reporting channels that monitor embryonic fraction and contamination.[15]

Another noninvasive method for assessing embryos is metabolomic profiling. This method specifically looks at the metabolic waste products produced by growing embryos.[16] The chemical makeup of the culture material used to nurture an embryo can provide researchers with further information on its metabolic processes. Similar to this method, morphokinetic analysis evaluates the morphological characteristics and the kinetics of embryonic development. SCM's benefits include greater selection, less fetal harm, and less mosaicism's influence; its drawbacks include higher levels of noise and pollutants, reduced susceptibility, problems with standardization, failure

TABLE 5: Advantages and disadvantages of spend culture medium.

Advantages	*Disadvantages*
• Non-inasive • Less danger to fetus • Broader selection • Enhanced efficiency	• High contaminants and noise • Unable to identify cell ploidy • Limitations due to technology • High false positive and negative results

to identify ploidy, and limitations on embryo representation. Advantages and disadvantages of spent culture medium are mentioned in **Figure 5**.

NEXT GENERATION SEQUENCING IN PREIMPLANTATION GENETIC TESTING

- *Low-pass genome sequencing for PGT-A:* The mainstay for PGT-A is low-pass WGS (e.g., ~0.05–0.5×) with genomic binning and GC correction. Genomic binning is a computational method used to group DNA fragments, called contigs, into clusters (or "bins"). This process helps to reconstruct individual genomes from complex and deficient samples. GC correction refers to adjusting for biases caused by uneven guanine-cytosine (GC) content across the genome during sequencing. It can detect numerous segmental copy-number changes as well as whole-chromosome changes. With niPGT, these factors are more significant because of the reduced input and contamination.[7]
- *Higher-resolution copy number variations (CNV) and combined assays:* Higher resolution and high throughput PGT-A can identify incidental patient-level variations and minor CNVs, which need further reporting and counseling. In an effort to decrease batching and turnaround, combined platforms (a single workflow for PGT-A/PGT-M/PGT-SR) are becoming more common (e.g., "KaryoSeq").[17]
- *Haplotype-based PGT-M and structural rearrangements:* PGT-M can be detected even for difficult variants and in certain proband-independent situations because of genome-wide haplotyping, also known as karyomapping, which connects disease alleles to parental haplotypes. PGT-SR's phasing and breakpoint mapping are enhanced by long-read or virtual long-read techniques that assemble short reads into longer fragments.[5,18]
- *Single-cell WGA innovations:* The conventional WGA techniques (DOP-PCR, MDA, and MALBAC) vary in terms of their compatibility with downstream tests, consistency, and allelic dropout (ADO). Primary template-directed amplification (PTA) provides better uniformity and coverage for small cell inputs. This makes it useful for limited TE biopsies and may also be useful for low-input niPGT libraries.[19]
- *Mosaicism:* NGS has revealed that embryo mosaicism is common; however, its prevalence and clinical significance vary across laboratories, thresholds, and analytical pipelines. Updated ASRM and PGDIS guidance outline embryo transfer priority schemes and counseling around false positives/negatives and pregnancy outcomes following mosaic embryo transfer.[20] Recent data interrogate whether fine-grained mosaic calls improve outcomes or risk discarding viable embryos.[2,9,21]

PRACTICAL WORKFLOW FOR niPGT AND BF-PGT

Laboratory Preanalytics

- *Denudation and washing:* Carefully remove cumulus and corona cells before ICSI to ensure clean and uncontaminated samples.
- *Culture strategy:* Use single-embryo microdrops under barrier oil, with scheduled media refreshes to minimize carry-over. Collect SCM just before cryostorage to maintain sample integrity.
- *Quality controls:* Include blank media controls and adjacent-well controls to catch any potential aerosol contamination or crosstalk between samples.
- *DNA extraction and whole genome amplification (WGA):* Use of kits validated for very small (picogram-level) inputs. Choose WGA methods such as MDA or PTA that recognize bias and always run negative controls to rule out contamination.
- *Bioinformatics:* Apply pipelines that estimate the fraction of embryonic DNA and use contamination deconvolution techniques such as methylation-guided or machine learning-based approaches to improve the accuracy and specificity of results[22] **(Flowchart 1)**.

Flowchart 1: Sampling strategies for embryonic DNA—classical TE biopsy, noninvasive spent culture medium cfDNA, and minimally invasive blastocoel fluid aspiration are among the sampling methods used for PGT. Each route feeds into WGA and NGS, after which it undergoes route-specific bioinformatics.

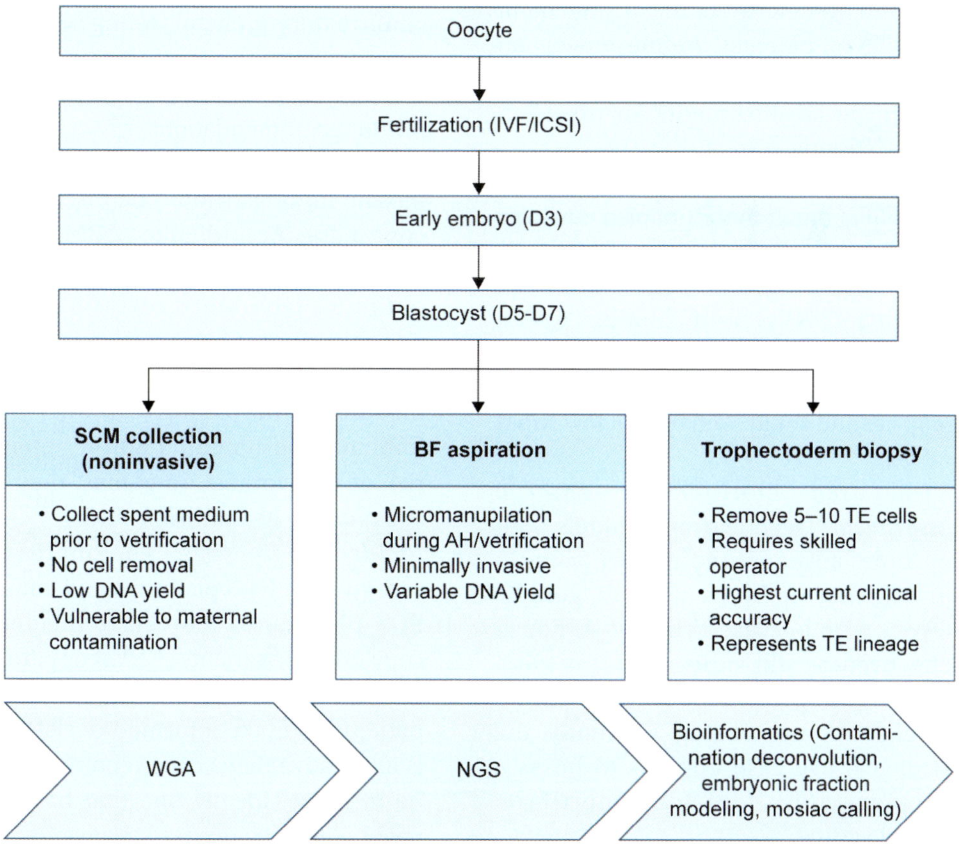

ADVANCES IN NEXT GENERATION SEQUENCING

- *Integrated assays:* Modern workflows can now combine PGT-A, PGT-M, and PGT-SR in a single test. This lowers the possibility of accumulating errors and speeds up turnaround times. Platforms such as KaryoSeq, which combine low-pass genome sequencing with targeted or haplotype-based analysis, are examples.[17]
- *Long-read and virtual long-read sequencing:* These methods enhance our capacity to identify repeat-rich regions or complex chromosomal rearrangements, as well as phase variations. They could make it possible for proband-independent haplotyping (which uses DNA from a known affected family member, known as the proband, to determine the arrangement of alleles on parental chromosomes) and even direct mapping of breakpoints, two significant advancements for precision embryo testing.[23]
- *Improved whole genome amplification:* PTA offers much more uniform coverage and reduces allelic dropout. This leads to better detection of single-nucleotide variants (SNVs) and smaller CNVs, which is crucial when working with very small samples such as trophectoderm biopsies and could even benefit low-input niPGT.[24,25]
- *AI-assisted noninvasive embryo assessment:* Deep learning models built on time-lapse embryo photos assist in prioritizing embryos without genetic testing or to forecasting ploidy. Although effectiveness still varies, and it is not a complete replacement for PGT-A, the results are encouraging. Currently, the strongest use case appears to be as a supplementary tool for cohort-level embryo rating.[26,27]
- *Contamination deconvolution using methylation or single-cell signals:* The accuracy of niPGT may be raised by novel methods that use single-cell methylation data or embryo-specific methylation patterns to help distinguish actual embryonic DNA from maternal contamination and enable methylation-informed CNV inference from SCM.[9,21]

COUNSELING POINTS AND ETHICAL CONSIDERATIONS

- *Screening versus diagnosis:* Patients should be reminded that PGT-A is a screening test, not a definitive diagnostic tool. A normal (euploid) result does not completely eliminate the risk of chromosomal abnormalities.[28] Therefore, confirmatory prenatal testing (e.g., CVS, amniocentesis) remains appropriate when clinically indicated, consistent with ASRM recommendations.[20,29]
- *Mosaic results:* The uncertainty of mosaic findings should be discussed in counseling. According to ASRM, PGDIS, and ESHRE recommendations, this entails outlining laboratory reporting limits, possible clinical outcomes, and center-specific embryo transfer rules. Although mosaic embryos have a decreased implantation potential and a potential risk of unfavorable outcomes, they can still produce healthy live babies.[2,9]
- *Incidental findings:* The increasing sensitivity of NGS platforms and coupled PGT procedures may make incidental copy number variants (CNVs) or parental genetic results visible. In order for patients to make informed decisions, it is imperative that a clear reporting policy be in place, ideally one that has been negotiated and approved in advance.[30]

- *Equity and access:* If proven and standardized, emerging non-invasive PGT (niPGT) methods might significantly reduce costs and increase access.[31] This brings up significant issues about equitable access, especially in resource-constrained environments, and emphasizes the necessity of strong quality control to guarantee dependable outcomes prior to broad adoption.[22,32]

CONCLUSION

Preimplantation genetic testing techniques that are non-invasive or minimally invasive offer a compelling vision for precise embryo genetics without the need for cell removal. Early long-read applications, robust haplotyping, enhanced WGA (PTA), low-pass WGS, and ML-based decontamination have all helped to close some of the gaps in the past 10 years. However, TE biopsy with NGS is still the clinical gold standard for accuracy today, and niPGT/BF-PGT are best suited as triage tools or adjuncts until protocols and analytics are developed. AI-guided imaging to rank embryos, niPGT to filter, TE-PGT for confirmation in specific scenarios, and unified NGS that combines PGT-A/M/SR are expected to be hybrid techniques in the near future. Non-/minimally invasive methods may advance from promise to reality in a way that genuinely expands safe access to embryo genetic screening with strict standardization, external quality evaluation, and prospective outcome trials.

REFERENCES

1. Zegers-Hochschild F, Adamson GD, Dyer S, Racowsky C, de Mouzon J, Sokol R, et al. The International Glossary on Infertility and Fertility Care, 2017. Hum Reprod Oxf Engl. 2017;32(9):1786-801.
2. Carvalho F, Coonen E, Goossens V, Kokkali G, Rubio C, Meijer-Hoogeveen M, et al. ESHRE PGT Consortium good practice recommendations for the organisation of PGT. Hum Reprod Open. 2020 May 29;2020(3):hoaa021.
3. Sousa LN, Monteiro PB. Non-invasive preimplantation genetic testing: a literature review. JBRA Assist Reprod. 2022;26(3): 554-8.
4. Cimadomo D, de los Santos MJ, Griesinger G, Lainas G, Le Clef N, McLernon DJ, et al. ESHRE good practice recommendations on recurrent implantation failure. Hum Reprod Open. 2023;2023(3):hoad023.
5. Giuliano R, Maione A, Vallefuoco A, Sorrentino U, Zuccarello D. Preimplantation Genetic Testing for Genetic Diseases: Limits and Review of Current Literature. Genes. 2023;14(11):2095.
6. Greco E, Litwicka K, Minasi MG, Cursio E, Greco PF, Barillari P. Preimplantation Genetic Testing: Where We Are Today. Int J Mol Sci. 2020;21(12):4381.
7. Xia Y, Katz M, Chandramohan D, Bechor E, Podgursky B, Hoxie M, et al. The first clinical validation of whole-genome screening on standard trophectoderm biopsies of preimplantation embryos. FS Rep. 2024;5(1):63-71.
8. Moustakli E, Zikopoulos A, Skentou C, Bouba I, Dafopoulos K, Georgiou I. Evolution of Minimally Invasive and Non-Invasive Preimplantation Genetic Testing: An Overview. J Clin Med. 2024;13(8):2160.
9. Leigh D, Cram DS, Rechitsky S, Handyside A, Wells D, Munne S, et al. PGDIS position statement on the transfer of mosaic embryos 2021. Reprod Biomed Online. 2022;45(1):19-25.
10. Chen S, Wang L, Hu Y, Yao Y, Gao F, Chang C, et al. Noninvasive preimplantation genetic testing for aneuploidy using blastocyst spent culture medium may serve as a backup of trophectoderm biopsy in conventional preimplantation genetic testing. BMC Med Genomics. 2025;18(1):34.

11. Chen Y, Huang J, Tang F, Wen L, Qiao J. A computational DNA methylation method to remove contaminated DNA from spent embryo culture medium for noninvasive preimplantation genetic testing. eBioMedicine. 2025;114:105669.
12. Li J, Liu Y, Qian Y, Zhang D. Noninvasive preimplantation genetic testing in assisted reproductive technology: current state and future perspectives. J Genet Genomics Yi Chuan Xue Bao. 2020;47(12):723-6.
13. Awaga H. Cell-free DNA Analysis of Spent Embryo Culture Media as a Non-invasive Approach for Preimplantation Genetic Diagnosis. Report No.: NCT07076719. [online] Available from https://clinicaltrials.gov/study/NCT07076719 [Last accessed December 2025].
14. Zheng W, Zhang S, Gu Y, Gong F, Kong L, Lu G, et al. Non-invasive Metabolomic Profiling of Embryo Culture Medium Using Raman Spectroscopy with Deep Learning Model Predicts the Blastocyst Development Potential of Embryos. Front Physiol. 2021;12:777259.
15. Campos G, Nel-Themaat L. Blastocoel fluid as an alternative source of DNA for minimally invasive PGT and biomarker of embryo competence. Reprod Biomed Online. [online] Available from: https://www.rbmojournal.com/article/S1472-6483%2824%2900511-X/fulltext?utm_source=chatgpt.com [Last accessed December 2025].
16. Chen SU, Lee TH, Lien YR, Tsai YY, Chang LJ, Yang YS. Microsuction of blastocoelic fluid before vitrification increased survival and pregnancy of mouse expanded blastocysts, but pretreatment with the cytoskeletal stabilizer did not increase blastocyst survival. Fertil Steril. 2005;84 Suppl 2:1156-62.
17. Li S, Chang C, Bai H, Qian W, Zou Y, Wu D, et al. A Novel and Comprehensive Whole-Genome Sequencing-Based Preimplantation Genetic Testing Approach for Different Genetic Conditions. J Mol Diagn. 2025;27(5):395-404.
18. Kim MJ, Park SO, Hong YS, Han G, Park EA, Lee KA, et al. PGT-M Strategy Using Genome-Wide Haplotype Karyomapping Analysis for Patients With De Novo Mutations. Fertil Steril. 2022;118(4):e253-4.
19. Volozonoka L, Miskova A, Gailite L. Whole Genome Amplification in Preimplantation Genetic Testing in the Era of Massively Parallel Sequencing. Int J Mol Sci. 2022;23(9):4819.
20. Asrm.org. (2024). The use of preimplantation genetic testing for aneuploidy: a committee opinion. [online] Available from https://www.asrm.org/practice-guidance/practice-committee-documents/the-use-of-preimplantation-genetic-testing-for-aneuploidy-a-committee-opinion-2024/ [Last accessed December 2025].
21. Springer.com. (2025). Changes in sequencing technology used for preimplantation genetic testing for aneuploidy. [online] Available from: https://link.springer.com/article/10.1007/s10815-025-03576-5?utm_source=chatgpt.com [Last accessed December 2025].
22. Layek SS, Kanani S, Doultani S, Gohil T, Patil S, Sudhakar A, et al. Analyzing Cell-free Genomic DNA in Spent Culture Media: Noninvasive Insight into the Blastocysts. Glob Med Genet. 2024;11(3):227-32.
23. Zhao Y, Tsuiko O, Jatsenko T, Peeters G, Souche E, Geysens M, et al. Long-read whole-genome sequencing-based concurrent haplotyping and aneuploidy profiling of single cells. Nucleic Acids Res. 2025;53(6):gkaf247.
24. Gonzalez-Pena V, Natarajan S, Xia Y, Klein D, Carter R, Pang Y, et al. Accurate genomic variant detection in single cells with primary template-directed amplification. Proc Natl Acad Sci U S A. 2021;118(24):e2024176118.
25. Xia Y, Gonzales-Pena V, Klein DJ, Luquette JJ, Puzon L, Siddiqui N, et al. Genome-Wide Disease Screening in Early Human Embryos with Primary Template-Directed Amplification. bioRxiv. 2021;2021.07.06.451077.
26. Zou Y, Pan Y, Ge N, Xu Y, Gu R, Li Z, et al. Can the combination of time-lapse parameters and clinical features predict embryonic ploidy status or implantation? Reprod Biomed Online. 2022;45(4):643-51.

27. Munné S, Horcajadas JA, Seth-Smith ML, Perugini M, Griffin DK. Non-invasive selection for euploid embryos: prospects and pitfalls of the three most promising approaches. Reprod Biomed Online. 2025;51(5):105077.
28. Volovsky M, Scott RT Jr, Seli E. Non-invasive preimplantation genetic testing for aneuploidy: is the promise real? Hum Reprod. 2024;39(9):1899-908.
29. Roman IC, Coull G, Knowlton N, Doherty-Eagles T, Ozturk O, Michielsen A, et al. Limitations of ploidy prediction by time-lapse morphokinetics and artificial-intelligence-based embryo selection algorithms: trisomies fly under the radar. Reprod Biomed Online. 2025;51(1):104828.
30. Leahy D, Marin D, Xu J, Eccles J, Treff NR. High-resolution PGT-A results in incidental identification of patients with small pathogenic copy number variants. J Assist Reprod Genet. 2024;41(1):121-6.
31. Bakalova DN, Navarro-Sánchez L, Rubio C. Non-Invasive Preimplantation Genetic Testing. Genes (Basel). 2025;16(5):552.
32. Chen K, Hu Z, Lian Y, Han Y, Zhou X, Li Y, et al. The diagnostic accuracy of preimplantation genetic testing (PGT) in assessing the genetic status of embryos: a systematic review and meta-analysis. Reprod Biol Endocrinol RBE. 2025;23:39.

CHAPTER 12

Ethical and Clinical Debates: Preimplantation Genetic Screening, Blastocyst Transfer, and BMI Limits

Rohit Gutgutia, Gayatri Satpathy

INTRODUCTION

Preimplantation genetic testing (PGT) is an early form of prenatal genetic diagnosis where abnormal embryos are identified, and only genetically normal embryos are transferred into a woman's uterus. The purpose of PGT is to improve embryo implantation thereby improving pregnancy and live birth rates and also reduces the time to pregnancy. PGT is few steps ahead of the routine morphological grading of the embryos as it gives information on the embryo's genetic health and has garnered a lot of attention becoming an integral part of assisted reproductive technology (ART) procedures.

There are three different types of PGT: (1) for aneuploidy (PGT-A), such as Down Syndrome and Turner Syndrome; (2) for monogenic/single gene defects (PGT-M), such as myotonic dystrophy and thalassemia; (3) and for chromosomal structural rearrangements (PGT-SR). PGT-SR includes reciprocal and Robertsonian translocations, insertional translocations, deletions, duplications, and inversions.[1]

The technique of PGT has evolved over the years starting with a polar body biopsy to biopsy of two or three cells from a cleavage stage embryo to biopsy of 6–10 trophoectoderm cells from a blastocyst or a day 5 embryo. The technique has also utilized several cytogenetics molecular techniques beginning with fluorescence in situ hybridization technique (FISH) to comparative genomic hybridization (CGH), array-comparative genomic hybridization (aCGH), single-nucleotide polymorphism (SNP) array, quantitative-polymerase chain reaction (q-PCR), and next-generation sequencing (NGS).[2]

Through PGT not only the DNA is analyzed but also the human leukocyte antigen (HLA)-typing is possible of the biopsied cells with PGT-M. For couples with a previous child affected with disease that can benefit with hematopoietic stem cell transplantation, PGT-M can be employed. Such diseases include genetic diseases affecting the hematopoietic system (e.g., β-thalassemia, sickle cell anemia), acquired diseases impacting the immune system (e.g., leukemia) as well as some rare metabolic diseases (e.g., adrenoleukodystrophy.[3,4] PGT-M selects a suitable embryo with HLA type matched to the sick child, who can be subsequently treated by harvesting and transplanting hematopoietic stem cells (HSCs) from the umbilical cord blood of the newborn. In case the cord blood is insufficient, bone marrow transplantation may also be offered.

Preimplantation genetic testing is indicated in various scenarios like in cases of male infertility, advanced maternal age, recurrent miscarriage, and recurrent implantation failure.

Preimplantation genetic testing test helps in better embryo selection, thereby allowing for single embryo transfer (which has a better pregnancy outcome for both the mother and her newborn), reducing miscarriage rates and improving take home baby rates; especially in women of advanced age.[5]

Preimplantation genetic testing empowers couples to avoid the challenging decision of pregnancy termination in cases of embryos affected by serious genetic conditions. Thus, with PGT the risk of conceiving a child with genetic disorders is reduced thereby reducing the rates of elective pregnancy termination for fetal/embryo abnormalities as the indication.

Preimplantation genetic testing offers a benefit to the society at large by reducing the burden of genetic and hereditary disorders.

Lastly there are certain countries (UAE, Mexico, United States of America) that allow for non-medical sex selection using PGT allowing it for "family balancing".

CLINICAL DEBATES WITH PREIMPLANTATION GENETIC TESTING

Preimplantation genetic testing is slowly starting to become a routine add-on for IVF to improve clinical outcomes worldwide.[6] While the benefits of PGT-M and PGT-SR are well accepted, the same does not apply to PGT-A. There needs to be clear cut guidelines in place for whom to offer PGT-A.

A multicenter, randomized, blinded clinical trial (STAR study) suggested that using morphological criteria alone to select single embryos for transfer in good-prognosis patients can be as effective as PGT-A highlighting that for good-prognosis women (especially younger women with more embryos), PGT-A did not provide a substantial benefit in improving pregnancy outcomes.[7] Another multicenter randomized controlled trial randomly assigned subfertile women between 20 and 37 years with three or more good-quality blastocysts to undergo either PGT-A or conventional IVF. At the end of 1-year conventional IVF treatment was non-inferior to PGT-A and resulted in a higher cumulative live-birth rate in women with a good prognosis for a live birth.[8]

The current PGT procedures that are extensively studied and routinely practiced rely on "invasive" embryo biopsy that may pose a theoretical risk to the growing embryo. It has always been emphasized that embryologists should exercise care and caution while using LASER and perform embryo biopsy with adequate skill and expertise.[9]

Another point of concern is the lack of clinical validation and high false-positive rate with PGT.[10] A single trophoectoderm biopsy may not be representative of the actual genetic composition of the inner cell mass which will actually form the fetus during pregnancy.

Reproductive medicine (ASRM) defines a mosaic embryo in PGT as "presence of more than one chromosomally distinct cell line in a single sample originating from one individual".[11] The prevalence of mosaic embryo after PGT testing varies from 2 to 40%.[12-14] After exhausting and expensive IVF and PGT procedures, clinical decisions around transferring a mosaic embryo can be challenging, particularly when no chromosomally normal embryo is available.

In circumstances where a PGT gives inconclusive results and embryo is transferred despite a result of "not a euploid" embryo, prenatal diagnosis is advised.[15] In such cases there is an extra charge that the couple need to bear for "invasive pre-natal genetic tests" such as Chorionic villus sampling or amniocentesis in case they conceive with these embryos. Not only this creates concern and anxiety in the couple who are awaiting the procedure or the final confirmatory results but also they need to spend an extra cost for these procedures along with a potential risk for miscarriage and maternal complications.

Particularly in women with very low ovarian reserve, culturing the embryos till day 5, relying on PGT-A and then discarding the embryos based on an aneuploidy/mosaic report (which may be false-positive) may further deprive them of their minimal chance to a healthy pregnancy (which they might have achieved with their discarded or unused embryos).[16] Failure to reach embryo transfer because of poor or arrested embryo development is more likely in extended culture (till the blastocyst stage) compared with cleavage-stage embryo transfer, especially in women with few day 3 cleavage-stage embryos.[17] A retrospective cohort study in women with only one viable embryo on day 3 suggested that transferring that embryo on that day doubled the pregnancy rate over exposing the day 3 embryo to culture till blastocyst stage and transfer at that stage.[18] PGT-A procedure is costly, time-consuming and loss of embryos either due to the extended culture, biopsy, freezing or false positive report can potentially downsize the presumed benefits of PGT-A of selecting euploid embryos.

Trophectoderm biopsy in PGT exhibits variability in detecting abnormal fragments, with 40% of these fragments being euploid upon re-biopsy.[19]

Preimplantation genetic testing also comes with technical limitations, such as contamination and preferential amplification (because the copy number of short DNA fragments is always more than that of long fragments) which will unavoidably cause false positive or negative results. This risks either the wastage or discarding of an euploid embryo (with a false positive result) or transfer of an aneuploid embryo (with a false negative result).[8]

Non-invasive PGT (niPGT) and minimally invasive PGT (miPGT) are the new kids on the block that examine the cfDNA (cell-free DNA). NiPGT focusses on the use of spent blastocyst medium whereas miPGT uses blastocoel fluid. The advantage with these techniques is that they demand lesser skill and there is a lower risk to embryos when compared to PGT.[20]

Although it seems promising, niPGT comes with its own unique challenges before it can fully replace the existing PGT. These include differences in results obtained from niPGT compared to results obtained from biopsy samples, maternal DNA contamination, fetal mosaicism, the relatively low abundance of DNA present in spent culture medium and significant variability in results.[21-23]

ETHICAL DEBATES WITH PREIMPLANTATION GENETIC TESTING

This debate exists as PGT-A is built on misconceptions. A single trophoectoderm biopsy is presumed to represent the whole embryo. Moreover, human embryos have the ability to self-correct downstream from blastocyst stage further questioning the utility of PGT-A. Thus, if we get a PGT-A report suggesting mosaicism or aneuploidy, the likelihood of the report being false-positive is high. In 2015, a study reported that embryos diagnosed as mosaic by TE-biopsy were successfully implanted, resulting in healthy live births.[24]

The likelihood of a false positive or a false negative report with PGT-A is the reason why PGT-A is not found to be beneficial in an unselected IVF population with no clear increase in the pregnancy or live birth rates in comparison to conventional IVF without PGT. Moreover, the value of PGT-A to lower the risk of clinical miscarriage is also unclear.[5] Ethical concerns arise about disposal of large numbers of human embryos (with probably normal pregnancy potential) based on the results of PGT-A testing, which may not be perfectly accurate.

While PGT-A is designed to select for healthy embryos, concerns exist that it could evolve into selecting for non-medical traits, leading to "designer babies" and creating social inequalities.

When PGT is used to select embryos for HLA matching so that a "savior sibling" is born (example in conditions such as Fanconi's anemia or thalassemia), there are ethical dilemmas that can arise. On one hand there is a concern that these children are born primarily to provide therapy for their elder siblings and are not valued in their own right. On the other hand, the opponents may argue that these children may be more valued as they have contributed to the health of a sibling.

Couples who would benefit from PGT but have health risks to the female partner from ovarian stimulation, oocyte retrieval or pregnancy should re-consider not to opt for PGT preferring the health of the female partner over reproducing at any cost.

While PGT is ethically justified for preventing severe sex-linked genetic diseases, its use for elective sex selection (e.g., "family balancing") is ethically controversial, with concerns that it could lead to population-level sex ratio imbalances, reinforce harmful gender stereotypes, expose women to invasive treatments that are not deemed medically necessary, potential risks to offspring associated with ART and divert expensive technology from genuine medical needs. This raises complex questions about social equity, individual rights and the appropriate use of advanced reproductive technologies.[2] PGT-A is a costly procedure, raising ethical concerns about access and equity, as it may only be available to those who can afford it, creating a divide in reproductive healthcare.

Lastly with PGT obtaining truly informed consent is complex, as the process and its implications are intricate. Patients may not fully understand the potential risks and benefits or the broader ethical issues involved.

GENETIC COUNSELING AND INFORMED CONSENT

Before PGT, comprehensive genetic and psychological counseling should be provided to prospective parents to clarify the scope, limitations, and implications of the test. Patients need to have appropriate expectations for PGT, especially in cases where infertility is not the underlying reason for afforded care. Prenatal testing is imperative during follow-up care, considering the test limitations for PGT. Patients with well-documented counseling records and consent should voluntarily select the test.

Because of patient demand and financial incentives for IVF centers (and testing industry, i.e., genetic laboratories), widespread utilization of PGT-A will likely continue, unless a regulatory body/professional organization is in place demanding transparency and clear information to the patients opting for PGT including situations where inconsistent results arise.

Because the practice of PGT for sex selection remains ethically controversial, IVF centers are encouraged to draft written policies setting forth whether and under what circumstances non-medical sex selection will be available.

CONCLUSION

Thus, there exist both ethical and clinical dilemmas with advanced reproductive technologies such as PGT. Although proposed for embryo selection based on the genetic makeup, PGT comes with its technical challenges such as embryo damage during biopsy and possibility of mosaicism and misdiagnosis. Much thought to be given to the ethical concerns such as "designer babies" and "non-medical sex selection" which could be viewed as potential misuses of PGT. Other issues that need consideration before routinely going ahead with these advanced technologies are the emotional strain that the couples have to endure, the lack of long-term outcome data for some PGT types and the unclear benefit of PGT-A for certain patient groups. This emphasizes the need for more data on cost-effectiveness, need for informed consent, comprehensive genetic counseling, and ethical dialogue before offering these technologies to our patients.

REFERENCES

1. ESHRE PGT Consortium Steering Committee, Carvalho F, Coonen E, Goossens V, Kokkali G, Rubio C, et al. ESHRE PGT Consortium good practice recommendations for the organisation of PGT. Hum Reprod Open. 2020;2020(3):hoaa021.
2. Burks C, Van Heertum K, Weinerman R. The technological advances in embryo selection and genetic testing: a look back at the evolution of aneuploidy screening and the prospects of non-invasive PGT. Reprod Med. 2021;2(1):26-34.
3. Shenfield F, Pennings G, Cohen J, Devroey P, Tarlatzis B. Taskforce 9: the application of preimplantation genetic diagnosis for human leukocyte antigen typing of embryos. Human Reproduction. 2005;20(4):845-7.
4. Tur-Kaspa I, Jeelani R. Clinical guidelines for IVF with PGD for HLA matching. Reprod BioMed Online. 2015;30(2):115-9.
5. Orvieto R. The use of preimplantation genetic testing for aneuploidy: a committee opinion. Fertility and Sterility. 2024;122(3):555.
6. Theobald R, SenGupta S, Harper J. The status of preimplantation genetic testing in the UK and USA. Human Reproduction. 2020;35(4):986-98.
7. Munné S, Kaplan B, Frattarelli JL, Child T, Nakhuda G, Shamma FN, et al. Preimplantation genetic testing for aneuploidy versus morphology as selection criteria for single frozen-thawed embryo transfer in good-prognosis patients: a multicenter randomized clinical trial. Fertility and sterility. 2019;112(6):1071-9.
8. Yan J, Qin Y, Zhao H, Sun Y, Gong F, Li R, et al. Live birth with or without preimplantation genetic testing for aneuploidy. N Engl J Med. 2021;385(22):2047-58.
9. Soni N, Mantravadi KC, Gedala DR, Bandari H. P-102 Can embryo biopsy technique in a PGT-A cycle affect foetal well-being in-utero and neo-natal health?. Hum Reprod. 2025;40(Supplement_1):deaf097-411.
10. Yang H, DeWan AT, Desai MM, Vermund SH. Preimplantation genetic testing for aneuploidy: challenges in clinical practice. Human Genomics. 2022;16(1):69.
11. Gleicher N, Barad DH, Ben-Rafael Z, Glujovsky D, Mochizuki L, Modi D, et al. Commentary on two recently published formal guidelines on management of "mosaic" embryos after preimplantation genetic testing for aneuploidy (PGT-A). Reprod Biol Endocrinol. 2021;19(1):23.

12. Munné S, Grifo J, Wells D. Mosaicism: "survival of the fittest" versus "no embryo left behind". Fertil Steril. 2016;105(5):1146-9.
13. Fragouli E, Munne S, Wells D. The cytogenetic constitution of human blastocysts: insights from comprehensive chromosome screening strategies. Hum Reprod Update. 2019;25(1):15-33.
14. Rodrigo L, Clemente-Císcar M, Campos-Galindo I, Peinado V, Simón C, Rubio C. Characteristics of the IVF cycle that contribute to the incidence of mosaicism. Genes. 2020;11(10):1151.
15. Muñoz E, Bronet F, Lledo B, Palacios-Verdú G, Martinez-Rocca L, Altmäe S, et al. To transfer or not to transfer: the dilemma of mosaic embryos–a narrative review. Reproductive BioMedicine Online. 2024;48(3):103664.
16. Deng J, Hong HY, Zhao Q, Nadgauda A, Ashrafian S, Behr B, et al. Preimplantation genetic testing for aneuploidy in poor ovarian responders with four or fewer oocytes retrieved. J Assist Reprod Genet. 2020;37(5):1147-54.
17. Glujovsky D, Retamar AM, Sedo CR, Ciapponi A, Cornelisse S, Blake D. Cleavage-stage versus blastocyst-stage embryo transfer in assisted reproductive technology. Cochrane database of systematic reviews. 2022;5(5):CD002118.
18. Xiao JS, Healey M, Talmor A, Vollenhoven B. When only one embryo is available, is it better to transfer on Day 3 or to grow on?. Reprod Biomed Online. 2019;39(6):916-23.
19. Navratil R, Horak J, Hornak M, Kubicek D, Balcova M, Tauwinklova G, et al. Concordance of various chromosomal errors among different parts of the embryo and the value of re-biopsy in embryos with segmental aneuploidies. Molecul Human Reprod. 2020;26(4):269-76.
20. Cinnioglu C, Glessner H, Jordan A, Bunshaft S. A systematic review of non-invasive preimplantation genetic testing for aneuploidy. Fertil Steril. 2023;120(2):235-9.
21. Kang X, Wen M, Zheng J, Peng F, Zeng N, Chen Z, et al. Influence of the number of washings for embryos on non-invasive preimplantation chromosome screening results. Frontiers in Endocrinology. 2024;15:1363851.
22. Hu Z, Li Y, Chen K, Li M, Tian M, Xiang L, et al. The comparison of two whole-genome amplification approaches for noninvasive preimplantation genetic testing (ni-PGT) and the application scenario of ni-PGT during the fresh cycle. The Journal of Molecular Diagnostics. 2023;25(12):945-56.
23. Rubio C, Navarro-Sánchez L, García-Pascual CM, Ocali O, Cimadomo D, Venier W, et al. Multicenter prospective study of concordance between embryonic cell-free DNA and trophectoderm biopsies from 1301 human blastocysts. American journal of obstetrics and gynecology. 2020;223(5):751-e1.
24. Greco E, Minasi MG, Fiorentino F. Healthy babies after intrauterine transfer of mosaic aneuploid blastocysts. N Engl J Med. 2015;373(21):2089-90.

SECTION 5

Special Causes and Populations

13. **Endometriosis-associated Infertility: Mechanisms and Clinical Pathways**
Apurba Kumar Dutta

14. **Polycystic Ovary Syndrome and Anovulation**
Rajeev Agarwal, Ankita Kaushal

15. **Age-related Ovarian Decline and Poor Ovarian Response**
Neha Priyadarshini, Shivani Jha

16. **Male Infertility: Emerging Diagnostics and Microsurgical Approaches**
Gunupuru Gayatri Swetha, Snigdha Soni, Rekha Ramappa

17. **Impact of Cancer Treatment on Fertility and Preservation Strategies**
Prachi Singh, Varsha Agrawal

CHAPTER 13

Endometriosis-associated Infertility: Mechanisms and Clinical Pathways

Apurba Kumar Dutta

INTRODUCTION

Endometriosis is an estrogen-dependent benign inflammatory disease characterized by the presence of ectopic endometrial implants.[1] Implants typically occur in the pelvis but have also been seen in the upper abdomen, peripheral and axial skeleton, lungs, diaphragm, and central nervous system. The most common sites of endometriosis, in decreasing order, are the ovaries, anterior/posterior cul-de-sac, broad ligaments and uterosacral ligaments, uterus, fallopian tubes, sigmoid colon, and appendix.

Because the growth of the implants is dependent on ovarian-produced steroids, it is a disease that most severely affects women aged 25–35 years.[2] Patients can present with a wide range of symptoms, ranging from being asymptomatic to being infertile. In addition to infertility, it is commonly associated with symptoms such as dyspareunia, dysmenorrhea, bladder/bowel symptoms, and chronic pelvic pain.

PATHOGENESIS OF ENDOMETRIOSIS

Retrograde Menstruation

In this theory, endometrial tissue is transported in a retrograde fashion through patent fallopian tubes into the peritoneal cavity. The endometrial cells then attach to the peritoneal mesothelial cells, establish a blood supply, proliferate, and produce endometrial implants.

Coelomic Metaplasia and Metastatic Spread

In this theory, the peritoneum contains undifferentiated cells that can differentiate into endometrial cells. Another theory argues that menstrual tissue travels from the endometrial cavity through lymphatic channels and veins to distant sites, which could attribute for implants found outside the pelvic cavity.

Altered Immunity

Women with endometriosis have altered immunity, preventing them from clearing the refluxed endometrial cells/fragments that appear in retrograde menstruation.[3] This would help explain why some women with retrograde menstruation develop endometriosis while others do not. Cell-mediated immunity is thought to be deficient in patients with the disease; leukocytes are unable to recognize that the endometrial tissue is not in its normal location.

Stem Cells

It is presumed that de novo development of endometrial tissue occurs from endogenous stem cells in the endometrium.[4,5] Over the last decade, we have studied the possibility that bone marrow-derived cells may also differentiate into endometrial cells, and pertinently, may be implicated in the development of ectopic endometrial implants.

Genetics

For over 20 years, it has been known that endometriosis has a familial tendency. Women who have a first-degree relative affected by the disease have a seven times higher risk of developing endometriosis than women who do not have a family history of the disease.[6] Familial aggregation has also been shown in studies of monozygotic twins and studies involving nonhuman primates.[7,8] Genetic polymorphisms may lead to aberrantly expressed genes identified in the endometrium of both human and nonhuman primates, but their contribution to the etiology of endometriosis is not yet well defined. Alternatively, these alterations in gene expression are more likely acquired and indeed are seen in animal models of the disease, where normal endometrium (without genetic predisposition to the disease) is transplanted to the peritoneal cavity.

ENDOMETRIOSIS ASSOCIATED INFERTILITY

The current evidence and proposed mechanisms of how endometriosis adversely impacts fertility. It is clear how severe disease can cause infertility. Pelvic anatomy becomes distorted, and fecundity is reduced via mechanical disruptions such as pelvic adhesions. These disruptions impair oocyte release or pick-up, alter sperm motility, cause disordered myometrial contractions, as well as impair fertilization and embryo transport. Infertile women are more likely to have advanced stages of the disease. However, there is still much speculation about the proposed mechanisms by which mild disease impacts fertility. Inflammatory cytokines, growth and angiogenic factors, and aberrantly expressed genes are all being explored as potential etiologic factors of endometriosis-associated infertility.

Effect on Gametes and Embryo

Altered ovulation and oocyte production are seen in endometriosis and are associated with the increased inflammatory cells in the peritoneal fluid and endometriomas. Inflammatory effects resulting from the presence of endometriomas have been shown to affect both oocyte production and ovulation in the affected ovary.[9] There is also a luteal phase disruption in endometriosis that may result from progesterone receptor dysregulation as well as an effect on progesterone target genes, which in turn leads to decreased endometrial receptivity.[1,9] Sperm quality or function is also decreased and has been proposed to be from the inflammatory/toxic effects of the peritoneal fluid and increased activated macrophages.[10] The increased number of inflammatory cells in the peritoneal fluid not only damages the oocytes and sperm but also has been shown to have toxic effects on the embryo.[11] In addition, studies have shown aberrant expression of glutathione peroxidase and catalase in the endometrium of patients with endometriosis, and it can be suspected that there is also an increase in endometrial free radicals and subsequently a negative effect on embryo viability.

Effect on Fallopian Tube and Embryo Transport

Gamete transport is also affected by the inflammatory environment and increased cytokines found in endometriosis;

inflammation impairs tubal function and decreases tubal motility. Disordered myometrial contractions associated with endometriosis can also impair gamete transport and embryo implantation.

Effect on the Endometrium

In addition to the above-mentioned inflammatory effects of endometriosis, there is increasing evidence supporting that endometriosis affects the eutopic endometrium and causes implantation failure; however, the mechanism of cellular or molecular signaling from the lesion to the uterus is unknown. As described above, numerous genes are aberrantly expressed in the endometrium of women with endometriosis, many known to be necessary for endometrial receptivity. The mechanism and specific signal that leads to alterations in the endometrium of women with endometriosis is not well characterized. We recently published data demonstrating that cells migrate from ectopic endometrial implants to the eutopic endometrium. Experimental endometriosis was established by implanting endometrial tissue from green fluorescent protein (GFP) mice into the peritoneal cavity of DS-Red mice. The study showed that GFP+ cells were found in the eutopic endometrium, preferentially the basalis layer, of mice with experimental endometriosis. In addition, gene expression profiling of the GFP+ cells showed increased expression of pan-epithelial markers and, more interestingly, upregulation of Wnt7A expression along with 17 other genes in the *wingless pathway*. Wnt7a is essential to estrogen-mediated uterine growth and implantation in mice, likely by signaling between the epithelium and stroma. It has been theorized by Liu et al. that aberrant activation of the Wnt pathway disturbs endometrial development during the implantation window. We theorize that the increased expression of ectopic Wnt7a outside of the gland likely disrupts the normal epithelial-stromal polarity required for normal fertility. There is likely bidirectional movement of cells between the eutopic and ectopic endometrial tissue. The reprogrammed and abnormally located cells likely that have "returned" to the endometrium, generate the signal that leads to aberrant gene expression and implantation failure.

There are several other studies proposing that aberrant gene expression in eutopic and ectopic endometrium may be related to infertility or the establishment of the disease.

An example of aberrant gene expression is the *Hoxa10/HOXA10* gene. This gene is directly involved in the embryogenesis of the uterus and subsequently in endometrial regeneration in each menstrual cycle. Expression of this gene is necessary for endometrial receptivity. Mice with a targeted disruption of the *Hoxa10* gene show complete loss of endometrial receptivity. Similarly, women with lower levels of expression of HOXA10 have lower implantation rates. In women, cyclical endometrial expression of this gene peaks during the window of implantation in response to estrogen and progesterone. Women with endometriosis, however, do not exhibit the midluteal rise as would be expected, which may partially explain their infertility.

Aromatase, the enzyme that converts androstenedione and testosterone to estrone and estradiol, has also been extensively studied in endometriosis. It has been shown that abnormal levels of aromatase are present in both endometriotic implants as well as eutopic endometrium, where it is normally absent, resulting in increased estradiol production. The role of aromatase in the pathophysiology of endometriosis is clear, given that it is an estrogen-dependent disease; increased estrogen production in the endometrium may also affect endometrial development and receptivity.

Progesterone resistance and dysregulation of progesterone receptors also appear to play a role in implantation failure. Because progesterone induces endometrial decidualization during the luteal phase, its presence is crucial for a normal pregnancy. Progesterone receptors have been shown to be dysregulated in both eutopic and ectopic endometrium. Downregulation of receptors is seen before implantation in normal endometrium, but is delayed in the endometrium of endometriosis. In addition, both eutopic and ectopic endometrium have been shown to be resistant to progesterone, causing an unopposed estrogen state, which is likely not suitable for implantation.

There is a well-established association between endometriosis and infertility; however, as evidenced above, it appears to be multifactorial, involving mechanical, molecular, genetic, and environmental causes. As newer research identifies alterations in gene expression and genetic defects, it is appropriate to consider testing of endometrial adequacy to diagnose and treat endometriosis-associated infertility.

CONCLUSION

- Endometriosis is an estrogen-dependent disease that affects between 10 and 15% of reproductive-aged women.
- There is a well-established association between endometriosis and infertility; however, as evidenced above, it appears to be multifactorial, involving mechanical, molecular, genetic, and environmental causes.

REFERENCE

1. Kennedy S, Bergqvist A, Chapron C, D'Hooghe T, Dunselman G, Saridogan E, et al. ESHRE guideline on the diagnosis and management of endometriosis. Hum Reprod. 2005;20(10):2698-2704.
2. Rock JA, Markham SM. Pathogenesis of endometriosis. Lancet. 1992;340:1264-67.
3. Giudice LC, Kao LC. Endometriosis. Lancet. 2004;364(9447):789-799.
4. Counsellor VS. Endometriosis. A clinical and surgical review. Am J Obstet Gynecol. 1938;36:877.
5. Hummelshoj L, Prentice A, Groothuis P. Update on endometriosis. Womens Health (Lond Engl) 2006;2(1):53-6.
6. Simoens S, Hummelshoj L, D'Hooghe T. Endometriosis: cost estimates and methodological perspective. Hum Reprod Update. 2007;13:394-404.
7. Vercellini P, Trespidi L, Giorgi O, Cortesi I, Parazzini F, Crosignani PG. Endometriosis and pelvic pain: relation to disease stage and localization. Fertil Steril. 1996;65:299-304.
8. Gruppo italiano per lo studio dell' endometriosi Prevalence and anatomical distribution of endometriosis in women with selected gynaecological conditions: results from a multicentric Italian study. Hum Reprod. 1994;9(6):1158-62.
9. Berube S, Marcoux S, Maheux R. Characteristics related to the prevalence of minimal or mild endometriosis in infertile women. Canadian Collaborative Group on Endometriosis. Epidemiology. 1998;9:504-10.
10. Vessey MP, Villard-Mackintosh L, Painter R. Epidemiology of endometriosis in women attending family planning clinics. BMJ. 1993;306:182–184.
11. ACOG Practice Bullettin No 51 Chronic pelvic pain. Obstet Gynecol. 2004;103(3):589–605.

CHAPTER 14

Polycystic Ovary Syndrome and Anovulation

Rajeev Agarwal, Ankita Kaushal

INTRODUCTION

Anovulation is defined when an egg does not release, absence of ovulation in a menstrual cycle. Polycystic ovarian syndrome (PCOS) is a common endocrine disorder[1] affecting 10–13% of women of reproductive age. One of the most common causes (~75%) of anovulatory infertility. It impacts women of all age groups, from adolescents to postmenopausal women.

Polycystic ovarian syndrome is defined as a complex endocrine and metabolic disorder, typically characterized by anovulation, infertility, obesity, insulin resistance (IR), and polycystic ovaries. Other risk factors predisposing women with PCOS at risk of anovulation are lifestyle management, obesity, diet, gut dysbiosis, neuroendocrine alterations, and environmental pollutants.

The etiology for PCOS is not clear and is recognized as a heterogeneous disorder that results in high levels of androgens due to overproduction. Primary sites are from the ovary and are associated with IR.[1] The Rotterdam 2003 criteria define PCOS as the incidence of any two of the three key criteria.

- Oligo ovulation and/or anovulation
- Excess androgen activity
- Polycystic ovarian morphology (PCOM) on ultrasound.[1,2]

Resulting in:

- Hyperinsulinemia
- Hyperandrogenism
- Oxidative stress
- Impaired folliculogenesis
- Irregular menstrual cycle
- Upstaging PCOS-associated metabolic syndrome.

What is clear is that anovulation in women with PCOS is characterized by arrest of antral follicle development before the mature to preovulatory stage.

If anovulation is the only underlying problem, the diagnosis of PCOS becomes important.

Polycystic ovarian syndrome should be diagnosed using the 2018 International Evidence-based Guideline criteria, which were built on the consensus-based 2003 Rotterdam criteria.

Presence of any two:

- Clinical/biochemical hyperandrogenism
- Ovulatory dysfunction
- Polycystic ovaries on ultrasound (≥12 follicles measuring 2–9 mm in diameter and/or an ovarian volume >10 mL in at least one ovary).[3]
- In 2023, alternatively, anti-Mullerian hormone (AMH) can now be used instead of ultrasound, with the exclusion of other etiologies.

Persistent hyperandrogenism, associated pathology, is due to:

- Luteinizing hormone (LH) hypersecretion.
- Aberrant oocyte maturation.
- Impaired hypothalamic-pituitary feedback.
- Premature granulosa cell luteinization and premature arrest of activated primary follicles.

The basic etiology of PCOS is still unclear, and the molecular basis of its progression is still a puzzle.

If we look at pathways involved in PCOS pathophysiology, these are multifactorial.[4]

- *Androgen excess:* Ovary and adrenal (hyperandrogenism)
- IR, hyperinsulinemia, and the β-cell
- Metabolic syndrome
- Developmental hypothesis/fetal origins
- Microbiome
- Genetics
  - *Androgen excess:* The Hallmark feature of PCOS is hyperandrogenism. It impacts ovulation, leads to anovulation. Genetic and clinical heterogeneity associated with hyperandrogenic conditions indicate the possible involvement of abnormalities in the steroid synthesis pathway.[5] Ovaries and adrenals, both lead to excess androgen production. Recent studies indicate that the hyperandrogenic phenotype is familial.[6] Maternal inheritance is postulated, affecting genes particularly governing steroid hormone biosynthesis. Altered expression of genes involved, governing synthesis of androgen in PCOS, leads to excess androgen exposure in utero. This leads to hypersecretion of LH, alteration in differentiation of thecal cells, and male-type fat distribution in female offspring.[7,8]

Clinical features include:

- *Hirsutism:* Diagnosed on the basis of the modified Ferriman–Gallway (mFG) score. The score defines hirsutism as the overgrowth of male-type hair in the nine androgen-sensitive areas of a woman's body: the upper lip, chin, chest, upper and lower back, upper and lower abdomen, upper arm, and thighs.[9] The score starts from 0 (no terminal hair growth) to 4 (male pattern hair growth) in each of the nine areas and requires a minimum score of 8 to diagnose hirsutism. A diagnostic dilemma regarding using the mFG score for clinical hyperandrogenism diagnosis has arisen, because the score is examiner-dependent and has been shown to have decent intraobserver reliability, but inadequate interobserver reliability.[10] Clinical signs are not always present in hyperandrogenism PCOS; here, biochemical assessment of androgens becomes important. Testosterone of ovarian origin, high levels of androstenedione, or increased levels of adrenal androgens dehydroepiandrosterone and dehydroepiandrosterone-sulfate.[11] Biochemical assessment is not useful in women on oral contraceptive pills for two main reasons. Oral contraceptive pills (OCPs) have an impact on sex hormone-binding globulin (SHBG), and they distort gonadotropin-dependent androgen production.[12]
  - Androgenic acne.
  - Alopecia (male pattern baldness)
- *IR, hyperinsulinemia, and the β-cell:* IR is a pathological condition, defined by decreased responsiveness or decreased sensitivity to the metabolic actions of insulin.[13] Women with PCOS have intrinsic IR, 12–60%, regardless of degree of obesity or androgen levels.[14]

This is mainly due to a defect in insulin receptors resulting from excessive serine phosphorylation and decreased tyrosine phosphorylation, which leads to a decrease in insulin activation of the phosphatidylinositol-3-kinase signaling pathway that activates glucose transport and consequently increases glucose levels.[15] Increased insulin secretion directly triggers the pituitary gland to release luteinizing hormone, which triggers androgen secretion and affects the development and growth of ovarian follicles.[16,17] Both elevated insulin and androgen levels inhibit SHBG secretion, which leads to an increase in free and bioactive androgens.[18] BMI impact on IR is greater in PCOS than in controls, irrespective of visceral fat, prioritizing lifestyle intervention and the need for effective therapeutic interventions to address intrinsic IR and prevent diabetes in this high-risk population.[18]

With respect to anovulation, IR can lead to anovulation by causing the body to produce more insulin (hyperinsulinemia), which in turn increases androgen production in the ovaries. This excess of androgens interferes with the normal development and maturation of follicles, preventing ovulation and leading to an irregular or absent menstrual cycle.

Another mechanism by which hyperinsulinemia causes anovulation is due to hyperinsulinemia, luteinizing hormone induces an early response on granulosa cells of small follicles and causes premature differentiation of theca cells. As a result, hyperinsulinemia causes anovulation. Insulin-sensitizing agents are useful for the improvement of anovulation due to hyperinsulinemia.[19,20]

- *AMH:* Women with a diagnosis of PCOS have higher AMH levels. This elevation is due to an increase in preantral follicles and small antral follicles, leading to increased secretion within each of these follicles. There has been no clear explanation found about the overproduction of AMH in PCOS cases; a correlation has been found between androgens and AMH expression.[21] AMH has been postulated as an ovarian reserve marker; it has not yet been postulated as a diagnostic marker for polycystic ovarian morphology, and hence anovulation. Whether the AMH value has any clinical role in the diagnosis of anovulation requires more clinical studies.
- *Metabolic syndrome:* The modified American Heart Association/National Heart Lung and Blood Institute AHA/NHLBI (ATP III 2005) defined metabolic syndrome as having three or more of the following metabolic symptoms: (1) Obesity (waist circumference of ≥88 cm), (2) hypertension (blood pressure ≥130/85 mm Hg), (3) dyslipidemia (high-density lipoprotein (HDL) of ≤50 mg/dL), and (4) hyperglycemia (fasting blood sugar of ≥100 mg/dL). The prevalence of metabolic syndrome among women with PCOS was 45.8%, as found by Madhusudaran et al.;[22] 46%, as reported by Glueck et al.;[23] and 43.4%, as reported by Ishak A, et al.[24]

It was more prevalent in hyperandrogenic PCOS phenotypes in comparison to normal androgenic phenotypes.

The metabolic symptoms of PCOS seem to be connected; androgen excess is the beginning of a vicious cycle of metabolic disorders in PCOS patients.

A positive correlation was observed between PCOS diagnosis in women and overweight and abdominal fat deposition.[25] A study in 2017 by Melal et al. included 1,387 women previously diagnosed with PCOS and reported that at least 52% of them were struggling with obesity,[26] Hyperglycemia is yet another metabolic disorder associated with PCOS. Findings from longitudinal cohort studies have reported that developing hyperglycemia is significantly more common in PCOS-diagnosed women within the age group of 15–49 years old compared to non-PCOS control women.[27,28] Dyslipidemia, reflected by high triglycerides and low HDL cholesterol, is one of the most common metabolic disorders identified in females with PCOS.[29,30] In multiple cross-sectional studies, PCOS has been linked to significantly higher blood pressure compared to normal controls, independently of weight/obesity.[31,32]

- *Reproductive problems:* women with PCOS are prone to hormonal imbalances leading to anovulation, poor quality of oocytes, elevated serum LH, and hyperinsulinemia associated with miscarriages.[33] Multiple studies conducted show that PCOS is the most common trigger for female infertility.[34] In a cross-sectional study conducted by Joham et al., infertility was recorded in 72% of women with PCOS compared to 16% in women without PCOS. In addition, the study discovered significantly higher use of hormonal fertility treatments among women with PCOS.[16]
- Further postulated pathologies for polycystic ovarian disease (PCOD) and anovulation:
  - *Leptin:* It originates in fat cells, regulates glucose homeostasis. Obese patients have elevated leptin levels, reduced sensitivity to leptin, and developed leptin resistance. Follicular functions are impacted due to elevated leptin levels, leading to anovulation and fertility issues that are linked to PCOS.[17,35,36] Leptin also has a role in the impairment of inulin sensitivity. It leads to the accumulation of triglycerides in adipose tissue, liver, and pancreas, leading to IR.[37] Peng et al demonstrated that women with PCOS have higher leptin levels, which results in hyperandrogenism and I. This association needs more concrete studies to consider it a satisfactory marker for PCOS and anovulation.[34,35]
  - *Adiponectin:* Adiponectin is an adipocytokine, present in adipose tissue, which affects IR, type 2 diabetes mellitus, obesity, and metabolic disorders.[38] It has an inhibitory effect on both LH secretion and gonadotropin-releasing hormone secretion. Bokshy et al.[39] demonstrated low levels of adiponectin in PCOS women as compared to controls. Another study by Onyegbule et al. demonstrated low levels of adiponectin in obese women and women with higher body mass index (BMI) with PCOS than in women with normal weight and PCOS.[40] More insights are needed to consider this as a biomarker for PCOS.
  - *Genetic:* One gene, the location of DENN domain-containing protein 1A (*DENND1A*) gene, has a role in ovarian steroid origin. All aspects of genetic factors for diagnosing PCOS in the future are under extensive research.[41]
  - *Neuroendocrine:* Alteration in the hypothalamic–ovarian–pituitary axis is one of the known causes of anovulation and other hormonal problems in PCOS. Elevated LH

levels, follicle-stimulating hormone (FSH) cells are hypofunctional. There are steady low levels of FSH, which keep on recruiting more follicles, but not growing up to maturation. The presence of atretic follicles creates dense ovarian stroma, which, under LH stimulation, produces more androgens.

- *Luteinizing hormone/FSH ratio* >2.5 is the result of either increased sensitivity pituitary gland or hypothalamic secretion of GnRH, nor an alteration in the secretion pattern of GnRH by the pituitary.[42,43]

Higher circulating levels of estrone (E1) and estradiol (E2) cause anovulation. Elevated E1 levels are associated with two biochemical mechanisms:

- Peripheral conversion of androgens (aromatization of androgens in adipose tissue and skin).
- Increased androgen-dependent aromatase activity of granulosa ovarian cells.
- Inversion of the E1:E2 ratio due to peripheral aromatization of androstenedione to estrone, especially in adipose tissue. This increases the risk of endometrial cancer due to endometrial proliferation.
- Anovulation is one of the ovulatory disturbances associated with PCOS. But it is the most common one associated with PCOS and infertility.
- Ovulation induction with oral ovulogens and/or gonadotropins is the way forward. Establishing ovulatory cycles is of utmost importance, where lifestyle modifications also play a big role.
- Chronic anovulation also leads to a decrease in progesterone levels. This leads to unopposed estradiol action, causing hyperplastic changes in the endometrium.
- One of the main challenges in the diagnostic–therapeutic course of PCOS is the identification of the phenotype and the main cause of the anovulatory disorder.
- Establishing ovulatory cycles is the mainstay of treatment for anovulation caused by PCOS in women trying for conception.
- Ovulation induction with oral ovulogens and gonadotropins stimulates follicles by crossing the FSH threshold of the ovary.
- Simultaneously, IR and hyperandrogen also need to be treated along with ovulation.
- Lifestyle changes, 5% of weight loss is recommended for better outcomes of treatment strategies in PCOS with anovulation.

REFERENCES

1. Azziz R, Woods KS, Reyna R, Key TJ, Knochenhauer ES, Yildiz BO. The prevalence and features of the polycystic ovary syndrome in an unselected population. J Clin Endocrinol. Metab. 2004;89(6): 2745-49.
2. Rotterdam ESHRE/ASRM-Sponsored PCOS Consensus Workshop Group. Revised 2003 consensus on diagnostic criteria and long-term health risks related to polycystic ovary syndrome. Fertil. Steril. 2004;81(1): 19-25.
3. Jonard S, Robert Y, Cortet-Rudelli C, Pigny P, Decanter C, Dewailly D. Ultrasound examination of polycystic ovaries: is it worth counting the follicles? Hum Reprod. 2003;18(3):598-603.
4. Witchel SF, Oberfield SE, Peña AS. Polycystic Ovary Syndrome: Pathophysiology, Presentation, and Treatment with Emphasis on Adolescent Girls. 2019;3(8): 1545-73.
5. Reddy KR, Deepika MLN, Supriy K, Latha KP, Rao SSL, Rani VU, et al. CYP11A1

microsatellite (tttta)n polymorphism in PCOS women from South India. J Assist Reprod Genet. 2014;31(7):857-63.
6. Prapas N, Karkanaki A, Prapas I, Kalogiannidis I, Katsikis I, Panidis D (2009) Genetics of polycystic ovary syndrome. Hippokratia. 2009;13(4):216-23.
7. Xita N, Tsatsoulis A. Review: fetal programming of polycystic ovary syndrome by androgen excess: evidence from experimental, clinical, and genetic association studies. J Clin Endocrinol Metabol. 2006;91(5):1660-6.
8. Xita N, Lazaros L, Georgiou I, Tsatsoulis A. CYP19 gene: a genetic modifier of polycystic ovary syndrome phenotype. Fertil Steril. 2010;94(1):250-4.
9. Kahraman FC, Erdoğan SS. Grading of hirsutism: A practical approach to the modified Ferriman-Gallwey scoring system. Adv. Postepy Dermatol Alergol. 2022;39(4):744-48.
10. Wild RA, Vesely S, Beebe L, Whitsett T, Owen W. Ferriman Gallwey self-scoring I: performance assessment in women with polycystic ovary syndrome. J Clin Endocrinol Metab. 2005;90(7):4112-4.
11. Abruzzese GA, Silva AF, Velazquez ME, Ferrer MJ, Motta AB. Hyperandrogenism and Polycystic ovary syndrome: Effects in pregnancy and offspring development. WIREs Mech. Dis. 2022;14(5):e1558.
12. Teede HJ, Misso ML, Costello MF, Dokras A, Laven J, Moran L, et al. Recommendations from the international evidence-based guideline for the assessment and management of polycystic ovary syndrome. Hum. Reprod. 2018;33(9):1602-18.
13. Zeng X, Xie YJ, Liu YT, Long SL, Mo ZC. Polycystic ovarian syndrome: Correlation between hyperandrogenism, insulin resistance and obesity. Clin Chim Acta. 2020;502:214-21.
14. Kim JJ, Hwang KR, Oh SH, Chae SJ, Yoon SH, Choi YM. Prevalence of insulin resistance in Korean women with polycystic ovary syndrome according to various homeostasis model assessment for insulin resistance cutoff values. Fertil Steril. 2019;112(5):959-66.e1.
15. Dunaif A, Finegood DT. Beta-cell dysfunction independent of obesity and glucose intolerance in the polycystic ovary syndrome. J Clin Endocrinol Metab. 1996;81(3):942-47.
16. Stepto NK, Cassar S, Joham AE, Hutchison SK, Harrison CL, Goldstein RF, et al. Women with polycystic ovary syndrome have intrinsic insulin resistance on euglycaemic-hyperinsulaemic clamp. Hum Reprod. 2013;28(3):777-84.
17. Karnatak R, Agarwal A, Asnani M, Singh R. The Effect of Insulin Resistance on Ovulation Induction With Clomiphene Citrate in Non-polycystic Ovary Syndrome (PCOS) Women. Cureus. 2022;14(7):e27433.
18. Assens M, Dyre L, Henriksen LS, Brocks V, Sundberg K, Jensen LN, et al. Menstrual pattern, reproductive hormones, and transabdominal 3D ultrasound in 317 adolescent girls. J Clin Endocrinol Metab. 2020;105(9):e3257-66.
19. Jonard S, Dewailly D. The follicular excess in polycystic ovaries, due to intra-ovarian hyperandrogenism, may be the main culprit for the follicular arrest. Hum Reprod Update. 2004;10(2):107-17.
20. Madusudhanan RR, Nambisan B, Brahmanandan M, Radha S. Study on the prevalence and characteristics of metabolic syndrome in women of reproductive age group with polycystic ovarian syndrome. J South Asian Fed Obstet Gynaecol. 2016;9(4):341-7.
21. Glueck CJ, Papanna R, Wang P, Goldenberg N, Sieve-Smith L. Incidence and treatment of metabolic syndrome in newly referred women with confirmed polycystic ovarian syndrome. Metabolism. 2003;52(7):908-15.
22. Ishak A, Kadir AA, Hussain NHN, Ismail SB. Prevalence and Characteristics of Metabolic Syndrome among Polycystic Ovarian Syndrome Patients in Malaysia. Int J Collab Res Intern Med. Public Health. 2012;4(8):1577-91.

23. Rantakallio JSS, Nevalainen JE, West SI, Ollila MM, Puukka K, Bloigu AH, et al. Association of self-reported polycystic ovary syndrome, obesity, and weight gain from adolescence to adulthood with hypertensive disorders of pregnancy: a community-based approach. Hypertension. 2021;77(3):1010-19.
24. Gibson-Helm M, Teede H, Dunaif A, Dokras A. Delayed diagnosis and a lack of information associated with dissatisfaction in women with polycystic ovary syndrome. J Clin Endocrinol Metab. 2017;102(2):604-12.
25. Ng NYH, Jiang G, Cheung LP, Zhang Y, Tam CHT, Luk AOY, et al. Progression of glucose intolerance and cardiometabolic risk factors over a decade in Chinese women with polycystic ovary syndrome: A case-control study. PLoS Med. 2019; 16(10):e1002953.
26. Tehrani RF, Montazeri SA, Hosseinpanah F, Cheraghi L, Erfani H, Tohidi M, et al. Trend of cardio-metabolic risk factors in polycystic ovary syndrome: A population-based prospective cohort study. PLoS ONE. 2015;10(9):e0137609.
27. Guo F, Gong Z, Fernando T, Zhang L, Zhu X, Shi Y. The lipid profiles in different characteristics of women with PCOS and the interaction between dyslipidemia and metabolic disorder states: A retrospective study in Chinese population. Front Endocrinol (Lausanne). 2022;13, 892125.
28. Cander S, Gül OO, Şişman P. Evaluation of Insulin Resistance and Vitamin D Levels in Patients with Polycystic Ovary Syndrome. Turk J Intern Med. 2022;4(2):66-72.
29. Joham AE, Boyle JA, Zoungas S, Teede HJ. Hypertension in reproductive-aged women with polycystic ovary syndrome and association with obesity. Am J Hypertens. 2015;28(7):847-51.
30. Zachurzok-Buczynska A, Szydlowski L, Gawlik A, Wilk K, Malecka-Tendera E. Blood pressure regulation and resting heart rate abnormalities in adolescent girls with polycystic ovary syndrome. Fertil. Steril. 2011;96(6):1519-25.
31. Louwers YV, Laven JS. Characteristics of polycystic ovary syndrome throughout life. Ther Adv Reprod Health. 2020;14: 2633494120911038.
32. Deshpande PS, Gupta AS. Causes and prevalence of factors causing infertility in a public health facility. J Hum Reprod Sci. 2019;12(4):287-93.
33. Joham AE, Teede H, Ranasinha S, Zoungas S, Boyle J. Prevalence of infertility and use of fertility treatment in women with polycystic ovary syndrome: Data from a large community-based cohort study. J Womens Health (Larchmt). 2015;24(4): 299-307.
34. Khomami MB, Joham AE, Boyle JA, Piltonen T, Silagy M, Arora C, et al. Increased maternal pregnancy complications in polycystic ovary syndrome appear to be independent of obesity-A systematic review, meta-analysis, and meta-regression. Obes Rev. 2019;20(5):659-74.
35. Peng Y, Yang H, Song, J, Feng, D, Na, Z, Jiang, H, Meng, Y, Shi, B, Li, D. Elevated Serum Leptin Levels as a Predictive Marker for Polycystic Ovary Syndrome. Front Endocrinol. 2022;13:845165.
36. Nikolettos K, Nikolettos N, Vlahos N, Pagonopoulou O, Asimakopoulos B. Role of leptin, adiponectin, and kisspeptin in polycystic ovarian syndrome pathogenesis. Minerva Obstet. Gynecol. 2023;75(5): 460-7.
37. Yadav A, Kataria MA, Saini V, Yadav A. Yadav, A. Role of leptin and adiponectin in insulin resistance. Clin Chim Acta. 2013;417:80-4.
38. Beyazit F, Hiz MM, Turkon H, Unsal MA. Serum spexin, adiponectin and leptin levels in polycystic ovarian syndrome in association with FTO gene polymorphism. Ginekol Polska. 2021;92(10):682-88.
39. Boshku AA, Panova DI, Ivanovska BZ. Adiponectin as a serum marker of adipose tissue dysfunction in women with polycystic ovary syndrome: Correlation with indicators of metabolic disturbances. Acta Endocrinol. 2018;14(3):346-52.

40. Onyegbule OA, Meludu SC, Dioka CE, Okwara JE, Obi-Ezeani CN, NjokuCM. Serum adiponectin and metabolic profile in women with polycystic ovarian syndrome in relation to body mass index. Int J Res Med Sci. 2022;10(3):599-603.
41. Wagh P, Panjwani M, Amrutha S. Early detection of PCOD using machine learning techniques. In: Wagh P, Panjwani M, Amrutha S (Eds). Artificial Intelligence and Speech Technology. Boca Raton, FL, USA: CRC Press; 2021. pp. 9-20.
42. Cook CL, Siow Y, Brenner AG, Fallat ME. Relationship between serum Müllerian-inhibiting substance and other reproductive hormones in untreated women with polycystic ovary syndrome and normal women. Fertil Steril. 2002;77(1):141-6.
43. Dharani B, Angappan S. Targeting obesity in PCOS: a review of current pharmacological interventions and future directions. Medicina Moderna. 2025;32(3):229-48.

CHAPTER 15

Age-related Ovarian Decline and Poor Ovarian Response

Neha Priyadarshini, Shivani Jha

INTRODUCTION

Female fertility is limited by the finite and nonrenewable nature of the ovarian reserve, which forms during fetal development and steadily declines from birth onwards. This loss in both the quantity and quality of oocytes becomes important by a woman's late 30s. This decline is referred to as age-related fertility decline (ARFD). The drop in fertility is not just due to a reduced ovarian reserve; it also involves lower oocyte quality, which raises the chances of chromosomal abnormalities, fertilization failures, poor embryo development, implantation issues, and early pregnancy loss.

Poor ovarian response (POR) occurs during controlled ovarian hyperstimulation (COH) and is usually marked by insufficient follicular recruitment and the recovery of a low number of mature oocytes, even with standard or maximum stimulation protocols.

PATHOPHYSIOLOGY

The reasons behind ARFD and POR are complex. They include structural, molecular, and hormonal changes that collectively damage reproductive potential. While some factors overlap, POR can arise as either an age-related condition or a separate medical issue.

- *Quantitative decline*: Women are born with about one to two million primordial follicles. By the time of menarche, only around 300,000 remain, and fewer than 1,000 last until menopause. Follicular atresia, or the loss of these follicles, happens continuously through cell death. A sharp decline in ovarian reserve occurs around the ages of 37–38 years. As the number of follicles declines, the antral follicle count (AFC) drops, indicating fewer follicles are available for recruitment during COH, leading to POR **(Fig. 1)**.
- *Qualitative decline:*
  - *Spindle instability and chromosomal errors:* Older oocytes are more likely to experience meiotic spindle problems, especially during the long pause at metaphase II. Deterioration of the cohesin complex can lead to improper chromosome separation, increasing the likelihood of chromosomal abnormalities.

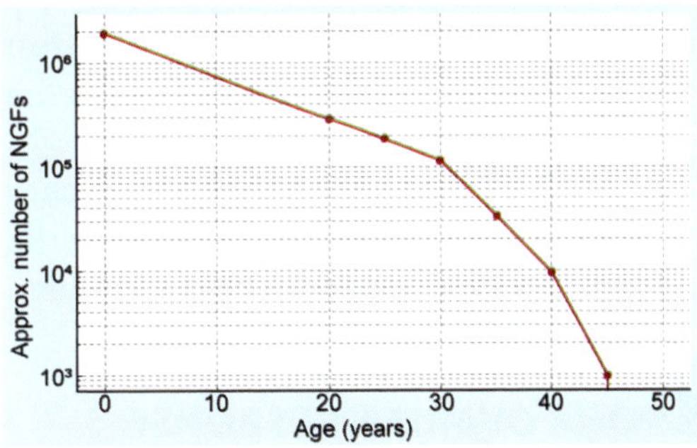

Fig. 1: Decline in nongrowing follicles (NGFs) with age. *Source:* Wallace WH, Thomson AB, Kelsey TW. The radiosensitivity of the human oocyte. Hum Reprod. 2003;18(1):117-21.

    - *Mitochondrial dysfunction:* Mitochondria are inherited from the mother and play a key role in ATP production. As women age, mitochondrial deoxyribonucleic acid (mtDNA) loss and mutations diminish adenosine triphosphate (ATP) levels, which affects oocyte maturation, fertilization, and embryo growth.
    - *Oxidative stress:* Elevated levels of reactive oxygen species (ROS) in the ovarian environment lead to DNA damage, shorter telomeres, and cell death of granulosa and theca cells. This further compromises folliculogenesis and the quality of oocytes.
    - *Epigenetic changes:* Aging impacts histone modifications and DNA methylation patterns, which could disrupt the gene activity important for the development of follicles and early embryos.
- *Epidemiology and clinical impact of ARFD:*
    - *Delayed childbearing and global fertility trends:* Falling fertility rates worldwide partly result from delayed childbearing. Postponing childbirth relates to lower lifetime fertility and a greater dependence on assisted reproductive technology (ART).
    - *Age-related risks:*
        - Miscarriage rates increase (>3% annually), and implantation failures are more common after the age of 40 years.
        - ARFD raises the chances of pregnancy loss, chromosomal issues, stillbirth, and complications during pregnancy.

DEFINING AND DIAGNOSING POOR OVARIAN RESPONSE

- Bologna criteria European Society of Human Reproduction and Embryology (ESHRE), 2011[1]

The ESHRE defines POR as having at least two out of three features:

- Advanced maternal age (40 years or older) or other risk factors.
- History of POR (three or fewer oocytes with standard stimulation).
- Abnormal ovarian reserve test [AFC <7 or anti-Müllerian hormone (AMH) <1.1 ng/mL]
- *POSEIDON stratification (2016)*: POSEIDON classifies "low prognosis" women into four groups based on age, AMH/AFC, and oocyte yield. This classification focuses on the likelihood of producing at least one euploid embryo, not just the quantity of oocytes **(Fig. 2)**.
- *Guidelines from ESHRE 2025 update:*[2]
    - *Ovarian response prediction:* There is a strong recommendation to use AMH or AFC; age, basal FSH, inhibin B, estradiol, and body mass index (BMI) are not recommended for this prediction.
    - *Pregnancy/live birth prediction*: Female age and BMI are useful predictors, while AMH, AFC, and basal hormones do not provide sufficient predictive value.
- *American Society for Reproductive Medicine (ASRM) recommendations:*[3] ASRM recommends that women aged 35 years or older who do not conceive after 6 months should be evaluated for low ovarian reserve; those aged 40 years and up should see reproductive endocrinologists.
    - ASRM clinical guideline (2018) on POR strategies explores mild versus conventional stimulation; mild cycles may lower gonadotropin exposure while having similar live birth rates in expected poor responders **(Table 1)**.

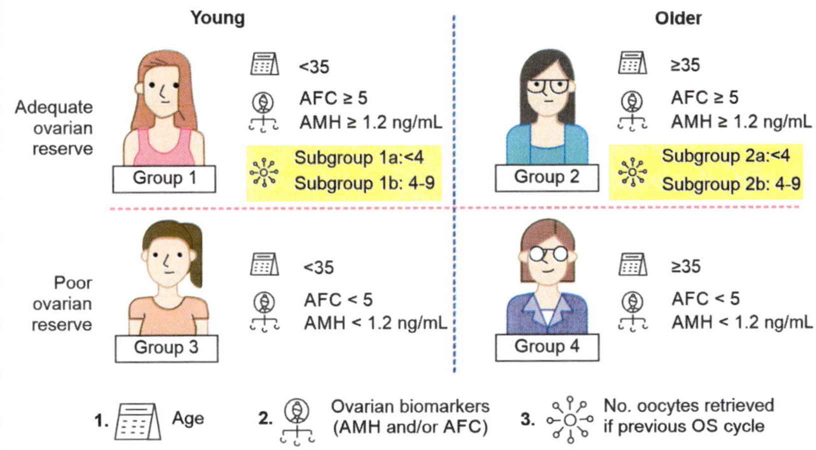

Fig. 2: Low-prognosis groups.
Source: Poseidon Group (Patient-Oriented Strategies Encompassing Individualized Oocyte Number); Alviggi C, Andersen CY, Buehler K, Conforti A, De Placido G, et al. A new, more detailed stratification of low responders to ovarian stimulation: from a poor ovarian response to a low prognosis concept. Fertil Steril. 2016;105(6):1452-3.

TABLE 1: Strength of evidence for intervention in ARFD/POR.[4,5]

Intervention/test	*Recommendation (ESHRE/ ASRM/Evidence reviews)*	*Strength of evidence (practical grading)*	*Key notes/clinical interpretation*
AMH/AFC for predicting ovarian response	Recommended to predict ovarian response (used to counsel on expected oocyte yield)	Moderate—good for response prediction; not a strong predictor of pregnancy/live birth	Use AMH/AFC to estimate ovarian reserve and tailor stimulation. Emphasize limits: They predict oocyte yield, not live birth
Female age (chronological)	Strong predictor of pregnancy/euploidy/live birth (central prognostic marker)	Strong—highest prognostic importance for live birth and embryo euploidy	Always include age in counseling and prognosis calculations (POSEIDON uses age for stratification)
GnRH antagonist vs. GnRH agonist long protocol (choice of COS)	Individualize based on prior response; no universal superiority for POR. Reviews/ guidelines support an individualized approach	Moderate—protocol choice individualized; evidence mixed	Consider prior cycle response, convenience, and patient preference

Contd...

Contd...

Intervention/test	*Recommendation (ESHRE/ ASRM/Evidence reviews)*	*Strength of evidence (practical grading)*	*Key notes/clinical interpretation*
Mild ovarian stimulation (lower gonadotropin dose/ oral agents)	Option for some POR/ predicted poor responders; may reduce medication burden with similar LBR in certain groups (evidence variable)	Weak–moderate—evidence mixed; may be reasonable in selected patients	Use when the goal is fewer injections/cost reduction; discuss potentially lower oocyte yield
DuoStim (double stimulation within the same cycle)	Emerging option to increase oocyte yield in POR; promising cohort data; guideline discussion ongoing	Low–moderate—promising but limited high-quality RCT data	Consider in selected POR patients (e.g., urgent fertility preservation, low oocyte yield history). Counsel on experimental/ limited evidence
LH supplementation/ LH activity (r-LH and hMG)	Evidence is inconsistent; some meta-analyses suggest benefit in specific subgroups (older patients/very low responders), but overall mixed	Weak—mixed results; may benefit select subgroups	Consider individualization—may help when endogenous LH is low or in older poor responders; not universally supported
DHEA (androgen pretreatment)	Some small trials and observational studies suggest improved response in POR; RCT evidence is limited and heterogeneous	Low—insufficient high-quality RCT evidence	If used, discuss experimental nature, heterogeneous dosing/ data, and uncertain benefit. Monitor androgenic adverse effects
Coenzyme Q10/ antioxidants	Some small randomized/ observational studies suggest improvement in oocyte quality/response; evidence is not definitive	Low—promising biologic rationale; clinical evidence limited	Can be offered as an adjunct with counseling about limited evidence
PRP (intraovarian platelet-rich plasma)	Not recommended/ experimental. ESHRE add-ons review does not recommend intraovarian PRP; RCTs show no clear benefit for mature oocyte yield in POR	Insufficient/not recommended—evidence currently negative or inconclusive	Use only in well-designed clinical trials; avoid routine clinical use pending better evidence. Cite ethical/informed-consent concerns
IVA and ovarian fragmentation	Experimental; small case series and early trials only	Insufficient/ experimental	Offer only in research settings with ethics approvals and careful counseling
Mitochondrial transfer/mitochondrial therapies	Experimental; ethically and legally restricted in many jurisdictions; insufficient clinical evidence	Insufficient/ experimental	Not recommended outside approved research programs. Discuss ethical and regulatory constraints

Cont...

Contd...

Intervention/test	*Recommendation (ESHRE/ ASRM/Evidence reviews)*	*Strength of evidence (practical grading)*	*Key notes/clinical interpretation*
Elective oocyte cryopreservation (planned/age-based)	Supported as an effective preventive strategy if performed at younger reproductive ages; many guidelines provide counseling frameworks and outcome data (ASRM evidence summary)	Strong for fertility preservation when performed earlier (e.g., <35 years)	Counsel on age-dependent likelihoods of future live birth, realistic expectations, and return/use rates
Oocyte donation	Most effective option for women with severely diminished reserve or advanced maternal age; high live birth rates	Strong—proven high live birth rates	Discuss as a definitive option when autologous success is unlikely; include psychosocial and legal counseling

(AFC: antral follicle count; AMH: anti-Müllerian hormone; ARFD: age-related fertility decline; ASRM: American Society for Reproductive Medicine; COS: controlled ovarian stimulation; DHEA: dehydroepiandrosterone; GnRH: gonadotropin-releasing hormone; IVA: In vitro activation; LBR: live birth rate; LH: luteinizing hormone; POR: premature ovarian failure; POSEIDON: Patient-Oriented Strategies Encompassing Individualized Oocyte Number; RCT: randomized controlled trial; r-LH: recombinant luteinizing hormone)

MANAGEMENT STRATEGIES FOR POOR OVARIAN RESERVE AND AGE-RELATED DECLINE (FLOWCHARTS 1 AND 2)

- *Ovarian stimulation protocols:*[6]
  - There is no clear advantage to using gonadotropin-releasing hormone (GnRH) antagonist versus long agonist protocols for predicted POR; choices depend on each patient's specific needs.
  - Mild stimulation might offer similar live birth rates with less medication needed, but strong evidence is still lacking.
  - DuoStim (double stimulation in one menstrual cycle) may lead to more oocyte retrieval in POR, but long-term effects are still being studied.
- *Additional drug and nutritional treatments:*
  - Dehydroepiandrosterone (DHEA) and coenzyme Q10 have shown potential in improving ovarian response and pregnancy rates in POR patients, though more extensive randomized trials are needed.

Flowchart 1: Step-by-step diagnostic evaluation of age-related fertility decline and poor ovarian reserve.

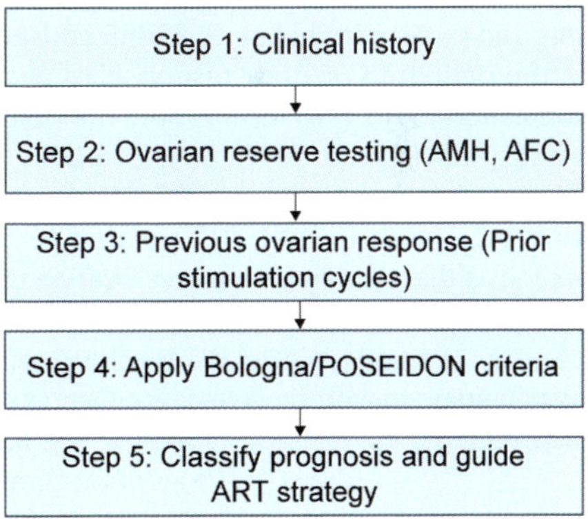

(AMH: anti-Müllerian hormone; AFC: antral follicle count; ART: assisted-reproductive technology; POSEIDON: Patient-Oriented Strategies Encompassing Individualized Oocyte Number)
Source: Broekmans FJ.

Flowchart 2: Management strategies for POR.[10,11]

Ovarian stimulation protocols
- GnRH antagonist
- GnRH agonist (long/short)
- Mild stimulation
- DuoStim

Adjuvant therapies
- DHEA
- Coenzyme Q10
- LH supplementation
- Antioxidants

Emerging approaches
- PRP intraovarian injection
- In vitro activation
- Mitochondrial therapies

Definitive options
- Elective oocyte/embryo cryopreservation
- Oocyte donation

(DHEA: dehydroepiandrosterone; GnRH: gonadotropin-releasing hormone; LH: luteinizing hormone; POR: poor ovarian response; PRP: platelet-rich plasma)

Source:

1. Ferraretti AP, La Marca A, Fauser BC, Tarlatzis B, Nargund G, Gianaroli L; et al. ESHRE consensus on the definition of 'poor response' to ovarian stimulation for in vitro fertilization: the Bologna criteria. Hum Reprod. 2011;26(7):1616-24.
2. Kasaven LS, Saso S, Getreu N, O'Neill H, Bracewell-Milnes T, Shakir F, et al. Age-related fertility decline: is there a role for elective ovarian tissue cryopreservation? Hum Reprod. 2022;37(9):1970-7.
3. Wang X, Wang L, Xiang W. Mechanisms of ovarian aging in women: a review. J Ovarian Res. 2023;16(1):67.

- Supplements such as luteinizing hormone (LH) cotreatment and antioxidants are being explored but require further evidence.

EMERGING AND EXPERIMENTAL APPROACHES

- Autologous intraovarian injection of platelet-rich plasma (PRP) and in vitro activation are being researched to improve follicle development in those with limited reserves.[7]
- Future options may include mitochondrial therapies and epigenetic modulators, based on new insights into ovarian aging. ART choices when oocyte quality is badly impaired.
- Elective cryopreservation of oocytes or embryos at younger ages is a good strategy.[8]
- Oocyte donation remains the best choice for women with significantly reduced reserves or who are older.[9]

COUNSELING AND ETHICAL CONSIDERATIONS

Counseling on Natural Fertility Decline

Clinicians should inform women that fecundity begins to decline in the early to mid-30s, with marked reductions after 38.[12]

Ethics of Elective Fertility Preservation

American Society for Reproductive Medicine Ethics Opinion (2025) emphasizes balancing patient autonomy, realistic expectations, and resource implications when recommending social or elective oocyte cryopreservation.

Decision-making in Poor Prognosis Cases

It is critical to adopt shared decision-making frameworks—discussing chances of success, psychological burden, financial costs, and potential for catastrophic outcomes with advanced age.[13]

CONCLUSION

Age-related fertility declines and POR represent significant, interrelated challenges in reproductive medicine. Advances in understanding ovarian aging mechanisms—including follicular depletion, oocyte quality deterioration, and microenvironmental changes—guide improved diagnosis and personalized management. ESHRE's 2025 updates and ASRM guidance emphasize using AMH and AFC to predict ovarian response; age and BMI are better predictors of live birth outcomes than ovarian reserve markers alone. While strategies to enhance ovarian response (e.g., individualized stimulation protocols, adjuvant treatments, experimental therapies) are emerging, definitive high-level evidence remains limited. Elective fertility preservation and oocyte donation are powerful options to circumvent age-related decline, though they require careful ethical consideration and counseling. Continued research is essential to optimize outcomes and support informed clinical decisions for women across the reproductive age spectrum.

KEY TAKE-HOME MESSAGES FOR CLINICIANS

- Age remains the strongest determinant of fertility potential. Natural fecundity declines after 30 years, accelerates after 35 years, and is marked after 38–40 years.
- Ovarian reserve tests (AMH and AFC) predict ovarian responses but not pregnancy or live birth outcomes; age and BMI remain stronger prognostic markers.
- ESHRE Bologna criteria define poor ovarian response; POSEIDON classification provides better stratification by focusing on the likelihood of achieving a euploid embryo.
- Stimulation protocols (GnRH antagonist, mild stimulation, and DuoStim) should be individualized; no single regimen is universally superior for poor responders.
- Adjuvants (DHEA, CoQ10, LH supplementation, and antioxidants) show promise but require further robust randomized controlled trial (RCT) evidence.
- Experimental therapies (PRP, in vitro activation, mitochondrial transfer) are under investigation and should be used cautiously, ideally within clinical trials.
- Elective oocyte/embryo cryopreservation is the most effective preventive strategy against age-related decline; oocyte donation remains the most successful treatment option for advanced age and severely diminished reserve.
- *Comprehensive counseling is critical*: Realistic expectations, emotional support, and shared decision-making should guide management.

REFERENCES

1. Ferraretti AP, La Marca A, Fauser BCJM, Tarlatzis B, Nargund G, Gianaroli L, et al. ESHRE consensus on the definition of 'poor response' to ovarian stimulation for in vitro fertilization: the Bologna criteria. Hum Reprod. 2011;26(7):1616-24.
2. European Society of Human Reproduction and Embryology. Ovarian stimulation for IVF/ICSI: Guideline update (Stakeholder review draft 2025). [Online] Available from https://www.eshre.eu/Guidelines-and-Legal/Guidelines/Ovarian-Stimulation-in-IVF-ICSI [Last accessed December, 2025].
3. ASRM Ethics Committee. Assisted reproduction with advancing paternal and maternal age: an Ethics Committee opinion. Fertil Steril. 2025;123(6):999-1005.
4. Cedars MI. Managing poor ovarian response in the patient with diminished ovarian reserve. Fertil Steril. 2022;117(1):655-6.
5. Owen A, Carlson K, Sparzak PB. Age-Related Fertility Decline. StatPearls [Internet]. Treasure Island (FL): StatPearls Publishing; 2025.
6. Mauries C, Ranisavljevic N, Mollevi C, Brunet C, Hamamah S, Brouillet S, et al.

"Short agonist stop" protocol, an ovarian stimulation for poor responders in in vitro fertilization (IVF): A pilot study. Front Endocrinol. 2022;13:1056520.
7. Drakopoulos P, Bardhi E, Boudry L, Vaiarelli A, Makrigiannakis A, Esteves SC, et al. Update on the management of poor ovarian response in IVF: the shift from Bologna criteria to the Poseidon concept. Ther Adv Reprod Health. 2020;14:2633494120941480.
8. Kasaven LS, Saso S, Getreu N, O'Neill H, Bracewell-Milnes T, Shakir F, et al. Age-related fertility decline: is there a role for elective ovarian tissue cryopreservation? Hum Reprod. 2022;37(9):1970-7.
9. Wang X, Wang L, Xiang W. Mechanisms of ovarian aging in women: a review. J Ovarian Res. 2023;16(1):67.
10. Wang G, Yang R, Zhang H. Ovarian vascular aging: a hidden driver of mid-age female fertility decline. NPJ Aging. 2025;11(1):24.
11. Conforti A, Carbone L, Di Girolamo R, Iorio GG, Guida M, Campitiello MR, et al. Therapeutic management in women with a diminished ovarian reserve: a systematic review and meta-analysis of randomized controlled trials. Fertil Steril. 2025;123(3):457-76.
12. Carnesi E, Castellano S, Albani E, Busnelli A, Smeraldi A, Bulbul O, et al. Diminished ovarian reserve is associated to euploidy rate: a single center study. Front Endocrinol (Lausanne). 2025;15:1535776.
13. Fauser BCJM, Adamson GD, Boivin J, Chambers GM, de Geyter C, Dyer S, et al. Declining global fertility rates and the implications for family planning and family building: an IFFS consensus |document based on a narrative review of the literature. Hum Reprod Update. 2024;30(2):153-67.

CHAPTER 16

Male Infertility: Emerging Diagnostics and Microsurgical Approaches

Gunupuru Gayatri Swetha, Snigdha Soni, Rekha Ramappa

INTRODUCTION: EPIDEMIOLOGY AND SIGNIFICANCE

Male infertility represents a major contributor to the global infertility burden. Infertility, defined as failure to achieve pregnancy after 12 months of unprotected intercourse (or 6 months if the female partner is >35 years), affects ~15% of couples. A male factor is solely responsible in ~20% and contributory in 30–40%, highlights the importance of comprehensive male evaluation in every infertile couple.[1] Beyond reproduction, infertility often reflects systemic health concerns. Conditions such as hypogonadism may signal broader metabolic, cardiovascular, or skeletal risks. Genetic abnormalities further complicate the picture. Y-chromosome microdeletions and *CFTR* mutations not only impair spermatogenesis or ductal development but also carry heritable consequences, necessitating genetic counseling. Thus, the assessment of male infertility should be approached not merely as reproductive care but as an opportunity for holistic health evaluation.

ADVANCING DIAGNOSTICS

Semen analysis is the cornerstone laboratory test for assessing male fertility. Recognizing discomfort with clinic-based collection, newer systems permit home-based semen testing. Properly obtained home samples may yield higher motility and counts, but accuracy depends on strict protocol adherence. Current home assays remain limited, typically measuring only concentration or motility, and without reliably differentiating progressive motility, a clinically essential parameter. These tests are particularly valuable for post-vasectomy monitoring, where convenience enhances compliance.[2] While they cannot replace comprehensive laboratory analysis, at-home tests may provide a practical first-line screen for fertility concerns.[3]

Conventional semen analysis by manual microscopy is prone to observer variability, and inter-laboratory inconsistencies reduce reliability.[4] Computer-assisted semen analysis (CASA), introduced four decades ago, attempts to standardize results through automated imaging.[5] CASA performs well for sperm count and motility but is less reliable for morphology and still requires manual oversight in severe oligospermia.[6] Future refinements, particularly through AI integration and portable designs, are likely to improve accuracy and promote wider use in clinical practice, while minimizing operator-related variation.[7]

When basic evaluation reveals idiopathic abnormalities or infertility persists despite normal standard tests, *advanced diagnostic tests* can provide deeper insights. These tests assess sperm at the molecular and functional level, evaluate reproductive tract integrity, and identify genetic issues. While not all are indicated in every patient, they are valuable in select clinical scenarios (e.g., recurrent in vitro fertilization (IVF) failure, recurrent pregnancy loss, unexplained infertility).

Sperm DNA Fragmentation Tests (SCSA, TUNEL, and Comet Assays)

Traditional semen analysis does not assess DNA integrity, which is crucial for embryo development and pregnancy. DNA fragmentation tests measure the proportion of sperm with broken DNA strands. Common assays used are described in **Table 1**.

Elevated fragmentation correlates with lower conception rates, poorer assisted reproductive technology (ART) outcomes, and miscarriage. While not part of routine evaluation, testing is valuable in unexplained infertility, recurrent pregnancy loss, or repeated IVF failure.[8] For example, a meta-analysis found that in couples with recurrent miscarriage, the male often had higher sperm DNA damage, and treating that (or using testicular sperm) improved outcomes.[9]

Clinical applications of DNA fragmentation results include:

- *Counseling lifestyle changes and antioxidants:* If fragmentation is high, patients should be advised on measures to reduce oxidative stress (quit smoking, improve diet, etc.), as oxidative damage is a major cause of DNA breaks.
- *Varicocelectomy:* Men with varicocele and high DNA fragmentation may benefit from repair; varicocele repair has been shown to reduce oxidative stress and DNA fragmentation in sperm in some studies.
- *Use of testicular sperm for intracytoplasmic sperm injection (ICSI):* In men with very high ejaculated sperm DNA fragmentation who have failed IVF/ICSI, using sperm retrieved directly from the testis can be beneficial. Testicular sperms often have significantly lower DNA fragmentation than ejaculated sperm in the same men.

TABLE 1: Comparison of commonly used sperm DNA fragmentation assays, their principles, outputs, and clinical interpretation.

Assay	*Principle*	*Output*	*Advantages*	*Limitations*	*Clinical interpretation*
SCSA (sperm chromatin structure assay)	Acridine orange staining + flow cytometry to detect DNA denaturation	DNA fragmentation index (DFI, %)	High-throughput, standardized, reproducible; well-studied cut-offs	Requires flow cytometry; may miss subtle chromatin defects	DFI >25–30% linked to reduced natural conception, poorer ART outcomes, and higher miscarriage risk
TUNEL (terminal dUTP nick end labeling)	Direct labeling of DNA strand breaks with fluorescent dUTP	% TUNEL-positive sperm	Direct measure of DNA breaks; can be done with flow cytometry or microscopy	Time-consuming; variable thresholds; less standardized across labs	>20–25% positive sperm often associated with impaired fertility and IVF failure
Comet assay	Single-cell gel electrophoresis— fragmented DNA migrates as a "comet tail"	Tail length, tail DNA %, intensity	Single-cell resolution; detects single vs. double-strand breaks	Technically demanding; limited reproducibility; no standardized cut-offs	>25–30% DNA in tail considered abnormal; associated with higher miscarriage and lower ART success

This is because sperm DNA damage accumulates during transit/storage in the epididymis. In a study of >100 couples with high fragmentation, using testicular sperm for ICSI resulted in higher live birth rates than using ejaculated sperm.[10] While this approach is somewhat invasive and still debated, it has yielded promising results in select cases.

- *Microfluidics and sperm selection devices:* Microfluidic chips (sometimes called "sperm on a chip") are being developed to improve sperm selection. These devices allow sperm to swim through microscopic channels under conditions mimicking the cervical mucus or tubal environment, essentially performing a gentle "sorting" of sperm. The best sperm (motile, with intact DNA) tend to navigate the channels and can be collected at the outlet, whereas poor sperm do not. One commercially available example is the ZyMot microfluidic device. Studies have shown such devices can significantly reduce DNA fragmentation in the selected sperm population. As microfluidics evolve, they may supplant traditional sperm wash and density gradient techniques, leading to higher quality sperm samples for ART without need for complex lab equipment.

Oxidative Stress Assays (Reactive Oxygen Species Testing)

Oxidative stress is a key contributor to male infertility, arising from an imbalance between reactive oxygen species (ROS) and seminal antioxidants. Excess ROS damages sperm membranes, DNA, and proteins, impairing motility, and fertilization capacity. The MiOXSYS system, which quantifies oxidation-reduction potential (ORP), provides an integrated measure of oxidative stress and has proposed diagnostic cutoffs (~1.34–1.41 mV/10^6 sperm/mL) to differentiate fertile from infertile men.[11] Elevated ORP levels, particularly in conditions such as varicocele, decrease after surgical repair, supporting oxidative stress as a pathogenic mechanism. Additional assays, including chemiluminescence for ROS, total antioxidant capacity (TAC) tests, and measurement of specific ROS species, remain largely research tools but further underscore the relevance of redox imbalance in male infertility.

Sperm Chromatin Maturity Tests (CMA3 Staining, Aniline Blue)

These tests uncover hidden nuclear defects and are especially useful in recurrent ART failure or unexplained infertility. Defective packaging can impair fertility despite normal semen parameters, and cytological stains such as aniline blue (AB) and chromomycin A3 (CMA3) can be used to assess nuclear maturity.[12,13]

ADVANCES IN GENETIC TESTING

- *Y-chromosome microdeletion testing:* It is recommended in men with non-obstructive azoospermia or very low counts (≤1 million/mL) along with evidence of impaired sperm production (high FSH, small testes).[1] Earlier guidelines used a ≤5 million threshold, but newer data show very few deletions when count is 1–5 million, so the cutoff has been lowered to 1 million)
- *Other genetic tests/gene panels:* With advances in genomics, multi-gene including genes such as *KITLG, NR5A1, TEX11, AR,* and others associated with spermatogenic failure in rare cases are developed. As of 2025, broad NGS panels are not standard of care but are

an emerging area for men with persistent infertility with no identifiable cause. They might especially become relevant for counseling in cases of non-obstructive azoospermia (NOA) where microsurgical testicular sperm extraction (micro-TESE) failed.

ADVANCES IN DIAGNOSTIC APPROACH: APHRODITE CRITERIA

The ***APHRODITE*** criteria (short for *Addressing male Patients with Hypogonadism and/or infertility Owing to altereD, Idiopathic TEsticular function*) represent a newly proposed stratification system for men infertility. As an emerging diagnostic framework, APHRODITE helps move beyond "ICSI for everyone" by enabling clinician-patient discussions grounded in a structured, evidence-informed classification. It classifies patients into five groups based on a combination of semen analysis parameters, serum FSH, and total testosterone levels, allowing more precise characterization of their underlying hypogonadism or altered spermatogenesis. The groups range from hypogonadotropic hypogonadism (low FSH + low T) to idiopathic infertility with normal hormone levels but impaired semen parameters, to hypergonadotropic hypogonadism (high FSH). The goal is to identify which men might benefit from hormonal therapy (e.g., FSH, hCG) or more tailored treatments, to improve spermatogenesis, sperm retrieval success, and ultimately fertility outcomes.[14]

ROLE OF PREOPERATIVE IMAGING

Ultrasound is emerging as a valuable adjunct in planning sperm retrieval for men with NOA. *Gray scale ultrasound (GSUS)* can highlight enlarged or oblique seminiferous tubules that correlate with spermatogenic activity, with studies showing good sensitivity and specificity in predicting micro-TESE yield.[15] *Power Doppler ultrasound (PDU)* and *color Doppler* can map areas of increased vascularity, often corresponding to active spermatogenesis, though sensitivity remains modest.[16,17] Contrast-enhanced ultrasound (CEUS) adds perfusion mapping, while MRI-derived parameters (testicular volume, ADC, MTR) show correlation with histology and sperm retrieval outcomes.[18] Given the high cost and the need for further validation, its use should be considered experimental at present.[19-21]

MICROSURGICAL INTERVENTIONS

When specific correctable causes of male infertility are identified, *microsurgical interventions* can dramatically improve a couple's chance of conception—either naturally or in conjunction with assisted reproductive techniques. These surgeries require specialized training and operating microscopes (or magnifying loupes) to deal with small reproductive structures and achieve high success with minimal complications. The key microsurgical approaches in male infertility include *varicocele repair, vas deferens/epididymal reconnections, and sperm retrieval techniques.* Below, we discuss each, focusing on indications, techniques, and outcomes.

Varicocelectomy

Indications

Varicocelectomy is among the most frequently performed surgeries for male infertility, with clear guideline-based indications. It is recommended in infertile men with at least one palpable varicocele and abnormal semen parameters, provided female factors are favorable. Additional indications include adolescents with testicular growth arrest and men with symptomatic varicocele pain. In contrast, subclinical varicoceles detected only on ultrasound should not be treated, as they do not improve fertility outcomes. The role in NOA remains debated, though some evidence suggests improved micro-TESE outcomes after repair.[1]

Technique

The *microsurgical subinguinal approach* (Marmar technique) is now considered the gold standard. Performed under local anesthesia with sedation or general anesthesia, the procedure involves a small (~2–3 cm) incision below the external inguinal ring, avoiding disruption of abdominal muscles. Under magnification (6–25×), dilated internal spermatic, cremasteric, and gubernacular veins are ligated while preserving arteries, lymphatics, and the vas deferens. Delivering the testis through the incision allows treatment of external gubernacular veins, minimizing recurrence.[22,23]

Outcomes

Compared to laparoscopic or open approaches, microsurgical varicocelectomy yields superior results:

- Recurrence <2%, hydrocele <3%, artery injury exceedingly rare (5–15% recurrence and 5–10% hydrocele risk seen with older non-microscopic or laparoscopic approaches).[24,25]
- Improvements in semen parameters in 70% of men within 6 months, with sperm counts rising by 10–20 m/mL, motility, and morphology also improving.
- Spontaneous pregnancy rates of 40–60% within 1–2 years; meta-analyses show a 3-fold higher pregnancy likelihood compared to no repair.
- In NOA, repair increases sperm retrieval rates at micro-TESE (53 vs. 30%).[26]

Vasovasostomy and Vasoepididymostomy

Indications

Microsurgical reconstruction restores continuity of the reproductive tract in obstructive azoospermia. The most common indication is vasectomy reversal, but obstruction from infection, trauma, or congenital anomalies may also be treated.

Vasovasostomy

When vasal obstruction is localized, the cut ends of the vas deferens are reanastomosed under the microscope using ultra-fine sutures (10–0). The presence of sperm in vasal fluid predicts success. Double-layer anastomosis (mucosa of the vas is reapproximated with ultra-fine interrupted sutures 10–0, followed by closure of the muscular layer with slightly larger sutures) achieves patency rates >90% with experienced surgeons.[27] Outcomes decline with time since vasectomy but successful reversals are possible even decades later, although prolonged obstruction increases the likelihood of secondary epididymal blockages, in which case a vasoepididymostomy (VE) may be required.

Vasoepididymostomy

If vasal fluid lacks sperm, epididymal obstruction is suspected. VE bypasses the block by joining the vas directly to an epididymal tubule. The operation involves making a fine incision in an epididymal tubule (only 0.2–0.3 mm wide) and suturing it to the vas lumen. Modern techniques, such as the two-suture intussusception (invagination) method, use 10–0 sutures to draw the tubule edge into the vas, creating a functional bypass. Patency rates of 60–70% and pregnancy rates of 30–40% are reported, though outcomes are lower than

TABLE 2: Comparison of vasovasostomy (VV) and vasoepididymostomy (VE)—indications, techniques, and outcomes.

	Vasovasostomy	*Vasoepididymostomy*
Indication	Obstruction at vas (e.g., vasectomy)	Epididymal obstruction, pasty/aspermic vasal fluid
Technique	End-to-end anastomosis, double-layer suturing	Intussusception (vas to epididymal tubule)
Patency	>90% (expert hands)	50–70%
Pregnancy rate	~50% overall; higher with short obstructive interval	30–40%
Time to sperm return	1–3 months	6–9 months
Predictors of success	Sperm present in vasal fluid; shorter interval	Surgeon expertise; site of obstruction

VV due to epididymal fragility. Often, VE is performed on one side while vasovasostomy (VV) is possible on the other, depending on intraoperative findings.

Outcomes and Considerations

- *Patency:* 70–95% overall, pregnancy ~50% across large series.
- VV achieves up to 97% patency and 76% pregnancy if vasectomy interval <3 years; rates decline with longer intervals.[28,29]
- *Time to sperm return:* 1–3 months post-VV, up to 9 months post-VE.
- *Cost-effectiveness:* Reconstructive surgery is often cheaper than IVF/ICSI and permits multiple pregnancies naturally. However, IVF may be preferable when female age is advanced.
- Comparison between the two techniques is presented in **Table 2**.

Surgical Sperm Retrieval

Microsurgical Testicular Sperm Extraction

Indications: Introduced by Schlegel in 1999, it is the landmark technique for NOA.[26] Any man with NOA who wants biological child and is willing to undergo ICSI can be offered a micro-TESE, after appropriate genetic/hormonal evaluation and possibly medical optimization (e.g., treating hypogonadism with clomiphene or hCG for a few months if needed, to improve intratesticular testosterone, which can aid spermatogenesis.

Technique: Under anesthesia, the testis is widely opened (usually a large equatorial incision in the tunica albuginea), and under high magnification (20–25×) seminiferous tubules are examined. This maximizes sperm yield while sparing tissue. *Dilated, opaque tubules* are preferentially harvested, as they are more likely to contain active spermatogenesis, whereas thin, transparent tubules often indicate Sertoli-cell-only regions.

Outcomes:

- Sperm retrieval rates with micro-TESE are ~50% overall, compared to ~30% with traditional random TESE.[26]
- Less disruption of testicular blood supply and fewer complications such as hematoma
- Despite being an extensive procedure does not significantly drop testosterone levels long-term, likely because it is targeted and tissue-sparing.

Microsurgical Epididymal Sperm Aspiration

Performed by surgically exposing the testis and epididymis and aspirating sperm-rich fluid from dilated epididymal tubules (usually in the caput epididymis) using fine glass micropipettes. Very high sperm retrieval success rate of ~95–100% are seen in cases of obstructive azoospermia.[30]

Compared to percutaneous epididymal sperm aspiration (PESA), which is less invasive but often yields a smaller and blood-tinged sperm sample, microsurgical epididymal sperm aspiration (MESA) provides a more abundant, higher-quality specimen with minimal red blood cell contamination (due to direct visualization and meticulous microsurgical technique).[30]

FUTURE DIRECTIONS

- *Advanced imaging and AI diagnostics:* AI and machine learning algorithms are being applied to automated CASA with morphology, sperm selection techniques, DNA fragmentation recognition.[31] In varicocele patients, AI is being studied to grade varicoceles on ultrasound or predict which patients benefit most from surgery.
- *Robotics and advanced surgical tools:* Tremor-free precision in varicocelectomy and vas reconstruction.[32]
- *Non-invasive biomarkers in seminal plasma:* Proteins, cytokines, and microRNAs may non-invasively reflect spermatogenesis, reducing need for biopsies.

CONCLUSION

Male infertility contributes to nearly half of infertility cases and demands comprehensive evaluation. While semen analysis remains the foundation, advanced diagnostics—fragmentation assays, redox testing, chromatin maturity, genetic analysis, and imaging—offer deeper insights. Among treatments, microsurgical interventions stand out as the most impactful, restoring fertility through varicocelectomy, tract reconstruction, or refined sperm retrieval. The future promises AI, molecular biomarkers, and precision frameworks such as APHRODITE, ushering in an era of individualized male infertility care.

REFERENCES

1. Brannigan RE, Hermanson L, Kaczmarek J, Kim SK, Kirkby E, Tanrikut C. Updates to Male Infertility: AUA/ASRM Guideline (2024). J Urol. 2024;212(6):789-99.
2. Gonzalez D, Narasimman M, Best JC, Ory J, Ramasamy R. Clinical Update on Home Testing for Male Fertility. World J Mens Health. 2021;39(4):615-25.
3. Yu S, Rubin M, Geevarughese S, Pino JS, Rodriguez HF, Asghar W. Emerging technologies for home-based semen analysis. Andrology. 2018;6(1):10-9.
4. Tomlinson MJ. Uncertainty of measurement and clinical value of semen analysis: has standardisation through professional guidelines helped or hindered progress? Andrology. 2016;4(5):763-70.
5. Finelli R, Leisegang K, Tumallapalli S, Henkel R, Agarwal A. The validity and reliability of computer-aided semen analyzers in performing semen analysis: a systematic review. Transl Androl Urol. 2021;10(7):3069-79.
6. Mortimer ST, van der Horst G, Mortimer D. The future of computer-aided sperm analysis. Asian J Androl. 2015;17(4):545-53.
7. Agarwal A, Sharma R, Gupta S, Finelli R, Parekh N, Selvam MKP, et al. Standardized Laboratory Procedures, Quality Control and Quality Assurance Are Key Requirements for Accurate Semen Analysis in the Evaluation of Infertile Male. World J Mens Health. 2022;40(1):52-65.

8. Diaz P, Dullea A, Chu KY, Zizzo J, Loloi J, Reddy R, et al. Future of Male Infertility Evaluation and Treatment: Brief Review of Emerging Technology. Urology. 2022; 169:9-16.
9. McQueen DB, Zhang J, Robins JC. Sperm DNA fragmentation and recurrent pregnancy loss: a systematic review and meta-analysis. Fertil Steril. 2019;112(1):54-60.e3.
10. Esteves SC, Roque M, Bradley CK, Garrido N. Reproductive outcomes of testicular versus ejaculated sperm for intracytoplasmic sperm injection among men with high levels of DNA fragmentation in semen: systematic review and meta-analysis. Fertil Steril. 2017;108(3):456-467.e1.
11. Agarwal A, Panner Selvam MK, Arafa M, Okada H, Homa S, Killeen A, et al. Multi-center evaluation of oxidation-reduction potential by the MiOXSYS in males with abnormal semen. Asian J Androl. 2019;21(6):565-9.
12. Sellami A, Chakroun N, Ben Zarrouk S, Sellami H, Kebaili S, Rebai T, et al. Assessment of Chromatin Maturity in Human Spermatozoa: Useful Aniline Blue Assay for Routine Diagnosis of Male Infertility. Adv Urol. 2013;2013:578631.
13. Iranpour FG. Impact of sperm chromatin evaluation on fertilization rate in intracytoplasmic sperm injection. Adv Biomed Res. 2014;3:229.
14. Najari BB. Ultrasound evaluation of seminiferous tubules: a promising prognostic tool for men with nonobstructive azoospermia undergoing microsurgical testicular sperm extraction. Fertil Steril. 2020;113(1):73-4.
15. Zhang S, Du J, Tian R, Xie S, Li F, Li Z. Assessment of the use of contrast enhanced ultrasound in guiding microdissection testicular sperm extraction in nonobstructive azoospermia. BMC Urol. 2018;18(1):48.
16. Nariyoshi S, Nakano K, Sukegawa G, Sho T, Tsuji Y. Ultrasonographically determined size of seminiferous tubules predicts sperm retrieval by microdissection testicular sperm extraction in men with nonobstructive azoospermia. Fertil Steril. 2020;113(1): 97-104.e2.
17. Xue H, Wang SY, Cui LG, Hong K. Can Contrast-Enhanced Ultrasound Increase or Predict the Success Rate of Testicular Sperm Aspiration in Patients With Azoospermia? AJR Am J Roentgenol. 2019;212(5): 1054-9.
18. Regent B, Skrobisz K, Kozak O, Matuszewski M, Studniarek M. MRI in the evaluation of the azoospermic male. Diagn Interv Radiol. 2020;26(4):271-6.
19. Ntorkou A, Tsili AC, Goussia A, Astrakas LG, Maliakas V, Sofikitis N, et al. Testicular Apparent Diffusion Coefficient and Magnetization Transfer Ratio: Can These MRI Parameters Be Used to Predict Successful Sperm Retrieval in Nonobstructive Azoospermia? AJR Am J Roentgenol. 2019; 213(3):610-8.
20. Ito Y, Unagami M, Yamabe F, Mitsui Y, Nakajima K, Nagao K, et al. A method for utilizing automated machine learning for histopathological classification of testis based on Johnsen scores. Sci Rep. 2021;11(1):9962.
21. Esteves SC, Humaidan P, Ubaldi FM, Alviggi C, Antonio L, Barratt CLR, et al. APHRODITE criteria: addressing male patients with hypogonadism and/or infertility owing to altered idiopathic testicular function. Reprod BioMed Online. 2024;48(4):103647.
22. Kavoussi PK, Gilkey MS, Machen GL, Kavoussi SK, Dorsey C. Varicocele Repair Improves Static Oxidation Reduction Potential as a Measure of Seminal Oxidative Stress Levels in Infertile Men: A Prospective Clinical Trial Using the MiOXSYS System. Urology. 2022;165:193-7.
23. Cho SJ, Kim SC, Kim KS, Park S. Magnification-Assisted Subinguinal Varicocelectomy with Testicular Delivery in Children: A Preliminary Report. The World Journal of Men's Health. 2014;32(2):93-8.
24. Al-Kandari AM, Khudair A, Arafa A, Zanaty F, Ezz A, El-Shazly M. Microscopic subinguinal varicocelectomy in 100 consecutive cases: Spermatic cord vascular anatomy, recurrence and hydrocele outcome analysis. Arab Journal of Urology. 2018;16(1):181-7.

25. Çift A, Yucel MO. Outcomes of microsurgical subinguinal varicocelectomy to treat painful recurrent varicocele. Andrologia. 2018;50(10):e13105.
26. C. Esteves S. What is New in the Clinical Assessment and Treatment of the Infertile Male. TORSJ. 2011;3(1):16-26.
27. Belker AM, Thomas AJ, Fuchs EF, Konnak JW, Sharlip ID. Results of 1,469 Microsurgical Vasectomy Reversals by the Vasovasostomy Study Group. J Urol. 1991;145(3):505-11.
28. Davis NF, Gnanappiragasam S, Nolan WJ, Thornhill JA. Predictors of live birth after vasectomy reversal in a specialist fertility centre. Ir Med J. 2017;110(1):495.
29. Herrel LA, Goodman M, Goldstein M, Hsiao W. Outcomes of microsurgical vasovasostomy for vasectomy reversal: a meta-analysis and systematic review. Urology. 2015;85(4):819-25.
30. Bernie AM, Ramasamy R, Stember DS, Stahl PJ. Microsurgical epididymal sperm aspiration: indications, techniques and outcomes. Asian J Androl. 2013;15(1):40-3.
31. Qaderi K, Sharifipour F, Dabir M, Shams R, Behmanesh A. Artificial intelligence (AI) approaches to male infertility in IVF: a mapping review. Eur J Med Res. 2025;30(1):246.
32. Mohd Hashim MH, Fam XI, Azizi MH, Khoo HC, Shukor S. Microscopic subinguinal varicocelectomy with video telescopic operating microscope (VITOM) telescope: outcome analysis. Transl Androl Urol. 2024;13(4):560-7.

CHAPTER 17

Impact of Cancer Treatment on Fertility and Preservation Strategies

Prachi Singh, Varsha Agrawal

INTRODUCTION

As cancer therapy has improved, and effective treatment has advanced the life span of affected children and reproductive aged people, fertility preservation (FP) has emerged as an essential consideration.

Clinicians should inform and educate patients regarding (1) effect of cancer and the consequences of treatment on reproductive ability, (2) effect of cancer and its treatment on fertility, (3) FP methods available, (4) necessity of cryopreservation of gametes/ tissue after FP, (5) subsequent infertility treatment available, (6) effect of gonadotoxic treatment or underlying condition on subsequent pregnancy, and (7) various childbearing and parenting options.[1]

In the Indian scenario, late diagnosis of cancer is a problem, more so in the rural setting. Cancer screening provision and uptake have to improve in both urban and rural areas in order to make an early diagnosis so as to improve survival rates and quality of life of survivors. FP is only feasible in early-stage cancers with a good prognosis.[2]

Female breast cancer is the most common diagnosed cancer (26.6%), and 8% of women with breast cancer are less than 35 years of age.[3]

Various cancer therapies including chemotherapy, radiation, and surgery have a negative effect on reproductive health, hence the need to address fertility concerns as early as possible in the treatment planning process.

People with cancer should be evaluated and counseled about reproductive risks at diagnosis and during survivorship. FP options should be discussed before cancer treatment is started. In males, sperm cryopreservation or testicular sperm extraction if unable to provide semen samples are valid options. In females, established FP methods comprise embryo, oocyte, ovarian tissue cryopreservation (OTC), ovarian transposition, and conservative gynecological surgery. In vitro maturation (IVM) of oocytes is not widely available but may be offered as an emerging method.[4]

GONADOTOXIC TREATMENTS

Treatments for cancer may cause gonadal damage by directly affecting growing and nongrowing ovarian follicle pool, the ovarian stroma, or the blood supply to the ovary. Treatment-induced gonadotoxicity may lead to premature ovarian insufficiency (POI) defined as the absence of menstrual cycles for ≥4 months and elevated follicle-stimulating hormone (FSH) levels in adult women of 40 years of age or younger.[5]

The type and dose of chemotherapy are the main factors determining the extent of gonadotoxicity **(Table 1)**.

Chemotherapy regimens used for treating young women with gynecological cancers: Platinum agent and taxane for epithelial ovarian cancer and cervical cancer, and BEP

TABLE 1: Cytotoxic agents according to degree of gonadotoxicity.[2]

High risk with alkylating agents	*Intermediate risk with platinum and taxanes*	*Low/no risk with antimetabolites*	*Unknown risk*
• Busulfan • Chlorambucil • Cyclophosphamide • Dacarbazine • Melphalan • Nitrogen mustard • Procarbazine • Ifosfamide • Chlormethine • Mechlorethamine • Carmustine	• Adriamycin • Doxorubicin • Carboplatin • Cisplatin • Dacarbazine • Thiotepa • Gemcitabine • Cytarabine • Daunorubicin	• Actinomycin D • 5-Fluorouracil • Methotrexate • Vincristine • Mitomycin • Dactinomycin • 6-Mercaptopurine • Vinblastine • Azathioprine • Fludarabine	• Bleomycin • Daunorubicin/ anthracycline • Oxaliplatin • Irinotecan • Vinca alkaloids • Monoclonal antibodies • (Trastusumab bevacizumab, cetuximab) • Tyrosine kinase inhibitiors (erlotinib, imatinib)

(bleomycin, etoposide, and cisplatin) or EP (etoposide and cisplatin) chemotherapy for nonepithelial ovarian cancer have a low risk of gonadotoxicity. The risk significantly depends on the type of chemotherapy agent, the dose and length of exposure, and the age of patient at the time of treatment.

The gonadotoxicity of radiotherapy is dependent on the field of radiation, dose, and fractionation. Radiotherapy can directly damage ovarian follicles and other ovarian tissues and may also cause an adverse effect on other reproductive organs, mainly uterus.[6]

Besides the gonadotoxic treatments, the disease itself (e.g., lymphoma) can be associated with gonadal damage and diminished ovarian reserve.[7]

In terms of patient characteristics, age and pretreatment ovarian reserve are the most important factors affecting the risk of gonadotoxicity.

Gonadotoxicity of Treatment of Various Malignancies

Breast Cancer

There is a known gonadotoxic effect of chemotherapy in premenopausal women with early breast cancer as observed in various studies reporting on rates of POI (mostly defined as treatment-induced amenorrhea) as well as an impact on the patient's ovarian reserve [measured by anti-Müllerian hormone (AMH)].

In early breast cancer patients undergoing systemic chemotherapy, the gonadotoxic risk is highest with the use of alkylating agent cyclophosphamide which is commonly given as part of (neo)adjuvant chemotherapy regimens. In chemotherapy regimens using cyclophosphamide, there is significantly higher risk of POI, with more than double the chances of developing treatment-induced amenorrhea as compared to regimens without this drug.[8]

The use of anthracycline and taxane-based regimens has also been shown to significantly increase the risk of subsequent amenorrhea.

After administration of all these chemotherapy agents, AMH becomes undetectable in most women and remains at very low levels after completion of treatment, the extent of recovery being determined by age and pretreatment AMH levels.[9]

Targeted treatments: There is not much data available on the risk of gonadotoxicity subsequent to treatment with targeted agents. Nevertheless, there is evidence of gonadal safety with use of chemotherapy with anthracycline and/or taxane-based regimens plus anti-HER2 agents trastuzumab and/or lapatinib as regards to treatment-induced amenorrhea, as reported in two studies.[10]

Endocrine treatments: Hormone receptor-positive breast cancer patients are treated with endocrine therapy which is standard of care for these patients. The three main approaches available are tamoxifen alone, gonadotropin-releasing hormone (GnRH analogue plus tamoxifen, and GnRH analogue plus an aromatase inhibitor[11] depending on the patient's individual risk of relapse, given for a duration of 5 years (possibly prolonged to 10 years). Although tamoxifen following use of chemotherapy appears to increase the risk of amenorrhea, there is no negative effect of these agents on the ovarian reserve, but since it is used for a long period of time, the patient will slowly have an age-related decrease in ovarian reserve.

Patient-related factors: Age represents the most important factor influencing the risk of treatment-induced gonadotoxicity,[12] high risk (>80% risk of treatment-induced amenorrhea) in patients older than 40 years and low risk (<20% risk of treatment-induced amenorrhea) in patients younger than 30 years.[13]

Baseline ovarian reserve measured by AMH levels predicts the risk of developing treatment-induced amenorrhea.[14]

Hereditary conditions: There is evidence to suggest that there is potential negative effect on baseline ovarian reserve in patients carrying germline *BRCA* mutations.

Hematological Cancers

In premenopausal women with hematological cancers, the use of chemotherapy has been shown to have a gonadotoxic effect as reported in studies assessing POI rates. Most of the available evidence is that for lymphoma.[15]

In Hodgkin's lymphoma, chemotherapy incorporating alkylating agents is most gonadotoxic. When alkylating agent-based chemotherapy was used, the risk of POI was 60% while it was only 3% for women treated with nonalkylating regimens.[16]

When patients with hematological cancers are treated with stem cell transplantation, they are likely to receive pretreatment with high-dose chemotherapy including alkylating agents with or without radiation therapy. Even in the absence of total body irradiation, permanent POI and fertility problems are common.[17] The *age* of the patient at the time of transplantation and *number of chemotherapy cycles* have a large bearing on ovarian function recovery in women undergoing allogenic or autologous stem cell transplantation (risk of POI >80%).

Other than chemotherapy and age at the time of treatment, lymphoma itself has a potential negative effect on baseline ovarian reserve and effectiveness of FP techniques.

Gynecological Cancers

For gynecological cancers, surgical procedures (including hysterectomy and bilateral salpingectomy) have a direct effect on female reproductive potential. Other than surgery, the use of pelvic radiotherapy and/chemotherapy in these patients further accelerates the risk of gonadotoxicity.

Other Cancers

In all women undergoing treatment for cancer, the risk of gonadotoxicity is directly proportional to the use of alkylating agents and older age at time of treatment.

Ovarian Reserve Testing

Cancer negatively affects the fertility potential in premenopausal women. As this population is at higher risk of low ovarian reserve at the time of diagnosis or after treatment/intervention, ovarian reserve testing could be used to guide decisions for FP either at the time of diagnosis or before treatment or intervention.

The ovarian reserve tests recommended for predicting high and low response to ovarian stimulation are either antral follicle count (AFC) or AMH. According to Bologna criteria for the definition of "poor ovarian response" (POR), the cutoff levels for AFC are less than five to seven follicles and AMH levels below 0.5–1.1 ng/mL.

FERTILITY-PRESERVATION INTERVENTIONS

Fertility preservation in males: For a postpubertal male, the primary method of FP is sperm cryopreservation. This should be undertaken prior to any gonadotoxic therapy. In males where a semen sample could not be obtained, testicular sperm aspiration (TESA) and testicular sperm extraction (TESE) can be done. In patients with azoospermia, microdissection (microTESE) is recommended. For prepubertal males, cryopreservation of testicular tissue may be considered under approved clinical trials.

Fertility preservation in females: Since vitrification has a high success rate in postpubertal females, fertility is usually preserved through cryopreservation of oocytes as it gives reproductive autonomy to patients. Embryos can also be preserved and less commonly ovarian tissue, specially in prepubertal girls.

Current Strategies for Fertility Preservation

- *Protective:*
  - *GnRH analogue*
  - *Ovarian transposition*
- *Definitive:*
  - Ovarian stimulation → oocyte/embryo cryopreservation
  - OTC
  - IVM

Patient assessment before FP procedures:

- *Oncological status:* Diagnosis, staging, survival rate
- *Fertility risk assessment:* Disease, treatment protocol, age
- *Ovarian reserve:* FP success depends on OR
- *Estrogen-sensitive tumors:* Tailor OS to reduce estradiol (E2) levels
- *Time available:* Window for FP
- Pubertal status

Protection of Ovaries

GnRH agonists have been used for protection of ovaries against the effects of treatment, especially in breast cancer patients. GnRH agonists reduce uterine-ovarian perfusion so that ovarian exposure to chemotherapy is reduced. FSH and luteinizing hormone (LH) are also reduced so that no follicles will grow and hence will be protected by gonadotoxic agents which affect growing follicles more.

GnRH agonists are started 1 week before CT to avoid the flare effect of agonist and they are given up to 2 weeks after completion of CT. This prolonged use is associated with osteoporosis.

Ovarian transposition is an option in women scheduled for pelvic radiotherapy.

Definitive FP Strategies Currently in Use

Since the development of vitrification, oocyte cryopreservation is a method of choice for FP.

Oocyte vitrification gives reproductive autonomy to the patient but requires a larger number of oocytes as there is loss during thawing, fertilization, and embryogenesis.

Although embryo cryopreservation is commonly available and has been in use in reproductive medicine for a long time, it requires joint legal ownership with the male partner which can have difficult implications later on.

Ovarian Stimulation in Treatments Aimed at FP

Ovarian stimulation for FP is usually an urgent procedure. It may prove difficult to collect a sufficient number of oocytes within a short period of time. The safety of the patient in terms of prevention of complications such as OHSS is paramount while increased risk of an underlying malignant disease and its effect on FP also has to be considered. To circumvent these complications, various approaches such as random-start protocol and use of different drugs to reduce estrogen levels in estrogen-dependent tumors are being practiced.

GnRH Antagonist Protocol

Since there is paucity of time in cancer patients, the antagonist protocol is preferred for ovarian stimulation for FP, since the duration of stimulation is shorter and GnRH agonist for trigger of ovulation can be used which further reduces the risk of OHSS.

For ovarian stimulation in nonurgent situations, the long protocol may be used.

Random-start Protocol

During luteal phase stimulation, if a dominant follicle is 18 mm or more in diameter, ovulation is induced with injection hCG or GnRH agonist, and ovarian stimulation is started 2–3 days later. If the patient has come post ovulation, ovarian stimulation can be started immediately.

Ovarian stimulation initiated in the luteal phase is slightly longer and requires higher gonadotropin doses when compared with stimulation started in the follicular phase.[18]

It has been seen that the number of oocytes obtained and peak serum E2 do not differ between different phases of the cycle at which OS is initiated. Furthermore, it has been observed that oocytes obtained in cycles started in the luteal phase have a better fertilization rate.

Although there is evidence that oocyte quality is probably not adversely affected when ovarian stimulation is initiated in the luteal phase compared to the follicular phase, there are insufficient data on live birth rates. Hence, it is difficult to conclude the role of luteal phase ovarian stimulation for FP, although in urgent situations random-start ovarian stimulation can be done.

Double Stimulation

Double stimulation, also called "dual stimulation", "DuoStim", or the "Shanghai protocol"[19] is useful for poor responders or when urgent FP is required. It involves two stimulations within the same menstrual cycle: The first starting in the follicular phase, and immediately after the oocyte pick up the second stimulation starts in the luteal phase of the same cycle. Hence, two oocyte pickups are performed at approximately 2 weeks' interval, with the potential advantage of recovering more oocytes in a shorter period of time.

Ovarian Stimulation Using Safer Protocols in Estrogen-sensitive Cancer Patients

Fertility preservation in estrogen-sensitive breast cancer patients is challenging since ovarian stimulation results in a supraphysiological serum E2 level. Although the rise of estrogen levels is transient, it could potentially result in the proliferation of malignant cells. There are, however, no data demonstrating any adverse effects of ovarian stimulation for FP in women with breast cancer.

Co-administration of selective estrogen receptor modulators or aromatase inhibitors during ovarian stimulation is commonly used.

Letrozole helps to reduce the E2 levels during OS. It is added in a dose of 2.5–5 mg from the start of gonadotropins and continued for few days after ovum pickup (OPU) till E2 levels fall. In a study by Pereira et al., there was no significant difference in the duration of stimulation and total amount of gonadotropins administered. Peak serum E2 levels were significantly lower in women receiving letrozole. Furthermore, significantly more oocytes were retrieved in women receiving letrozole.[20] The use of an aromatase inhibitor along with GnRH agonist trigger in an antagonist protocol further reduces E2 levels around the time of OPU and progesterone levels during the luteal phase.

In letrozole cycles, antral space is formed earlier, and the trigger criteria should be extended by 2–3 mm to reach the same oocyte maturity seen with standard protocols. Highest maturity rates were obtained at 20.4 mm cutoff.

There is insufficient data on the use of tamoxifen for FP in breast cancer patients.

Ovarian Tissue Cryopreservation

It is recommended to offer OTC in patients undergoing moderate-/high-risk gonadotoxic treatment where oocyte/embryo cryopreservation is not feasible, or at patient preference. OTC should not be recommended in patients with low ovarian reserve (AMH <0.5 ng/mL and AFC <5) or advanced age over 36 years.[21] Slow-freezing protocol is ideal for OTC as it is a well-established and safe procedure.

Ovarian Tissue Transplantation

Ovarian tissue transplantation (OTT) at the orthotopic site, either on the remaining ovaries or in the nearby peritoneal site, is usually performed by laparoscopy and more rarely by minilaparotomy. For OTT, a one-step laparoscopic procedure is commonly performed since it is safe and does not have any additional surgical risk. To restore fertility, OTT at the orthotopic site allows possible natural conception, whereas heterotopic transplantation will require ART. In oncological patients, the decision to perform OTT should be a multidisciplinary decision. It is necessary to exclude the presence of residual neoplastic cells in the ovarian cortex to be transplanted in cancer survivors using appropriate techniques, and patients should be counseled about the theoretical risk of reintroduction of cancer cells. In patients where ovary was involved in the malignancy, the risk of reimplanting cancer seems to outweigh the benefits of the OTT procedure. When oocyte or embryo freezing is not feasible, OTT can be offered in BRCA patients as an alternative, but the implanted ovarian tissue must be completely removed after subsequent pregnancy.

In vitro maturation should be regarded as an innovative FP procedure and is performed when oocyte cryopreservation is required but ovarian stimulation is not feasible.

Before the use of stored tissue, fitness for pregnancy should be thoroughly assessed, taking into account the effects of treatment, the age of the patient, and the interval since treatment.

Pregnancy should only be attempted after 1 year of completion of chemotherapy in order to reduce the risk of pregnancy complications.

CONCLUSION

It is important to emphasize that however promising the emerging technologies, these have to undergo rigorous clinical trials according to internationally accepted standards, before they are implemented in clinical practice. In cancer patients, treatment that is less gonadotoxic is easy to implement, is of low cost, has a lower number of invasive procedures, and maintains both reproductive and endocrine functions. There is need to achieve progress in human folliculogenesis in vitro and enhancing systemic ovarian function, as these technologies may bring revolution in infertility treatment in our modern society.

REFERENCES

1. Goossens J, Delbaere I, Van Lancker A, Beeckman D, Verhaeghe S, Van Hecke A. Cancer patients' and professional caregivers' needs, preferences and factors associated with receiving and providing fertility related information: a mixed-methods systematic review. Int J Nurs Stud. 2014;51:300-19.
2. Mahajan NK, Patil M, Jigre PR. Fertility preservation for patients on gonadotoxic treatment: Recommendations for clinical practice by Fertility Preservation Society (India). Onco Fertility J. 2020;3(2):48-107.
3. Mengxia Fu, Zhiming Peng, Min Wu, Dapeng Lv, Yanping Li, Shuzhen Lyu. Current and future burden of breast cancer in Asia: A GLOBOCAN data analysis for 2022 and 2050. Breast. 2025;79:103835.
4. Su HI, Lacchetti C, Letourneau J, Partridge AH, Qamar R, Quinn GP, et al.. Fertility Preservation in People With Cancer: ASCO Guideline Update. J Clin Oncol. 2025;43(12):1488-515.
5. Webber L, Davies M, Anderson R, Bartlett J, Braat D, Cartwright B, et al. ESHRE Guideline: management of women with premature ovarian insufficiency. Hum Reprod. 2016;31:926-37.
6. Adriaens I, Smitz J, Jacquet P. The current knowledge on radiosensitivity of ovarian follicle development stages. Hum Reprod Update. 2009;15:359-77.
7. Horton J, Sterrenburg M, Lane S, Maheshwari A, Li TC, Cheong Y. Reproductive, obstetric, and perinatal outcomes of women with adenomyosis and endometriosis: a systematic review and meta-analysis. Hum Reprod Update. 2019;25:592-632.
8. Zhao J, Liu J, Chen K, Li S, Wang Y, Yang Y, et al. What lies behind chemotherapy induced amenorrhea for breast cancer patients: a meta-analysis. Breast Cancer Res Treat. 2014;145:113-28.
9. Anderson RA, Themmen AP, Al-Qahtani A, Groome NP, Cameron DA. The effects of chemotherapy and long term gonadotrophin suppression on the ovarian reserve in premenopausal women with breast cancer. Hum Reprod. 2006;21:2583-92.
10. Lambertini M, Martel S, Campbell C, Guillaume S, Hilbers FS, Schuehly U, et al. Pregnancies during and after trastuzumab and/or lapatinib in patients with human epidermal growth factor receptor 2-positive early breast cancer: Analysis from the NeoALTTO (BIG 1-06) and ALTTO (BIG 2-06) trials. Cancer. 2019;125:307-16.
11. Burstein HJ, Lacchetti C, Anderson H, Buchholz TA, Davidson NE, Gelmon KE, et al. Adjuvant Endocrine Therapy for Women With Hormone Receptor-Positive Breast Cancer: American Society of Clinical Oncology Clinical Practice Guideline Update on Ovarian Suppression. J Clin Oncol. 2016;34:1689-701.
12. Silva C, Caramelo O, Almeida-Santos T, Ribeiro Rama AC. Factors associated with ovarian function recovery after chemotherapy for breast cancer: a systematic review and meta-analysis. Hum Reprod. 2016;31:2737-49.
13. Lambertini M, Del Mastro L, Pescio MC, Andersen CY, Azim HA, Jr, Peccatori FA, et al. Cancer and fertility preservation: international recommendations from an expert meeting. BMC Med. 2016;14:1.

14. Anderson RA, Cameron DA. Pretreatment serum anti-mullerian hormone predicts long-term ovarian function and bone mass after chemotherapy for early breast cancer. J Clin Endocrinol Metab. 2011;96:1336-43.
15. Overbeek A, van den Berg MH, van Leeuwen FE, Kaspers GJ, Lambalk CB, van Dulmen-den Broeder E. Chemotherapy-related late adverse effects on ovarian function in female survivors of childhood and young adult cancer: A systematic review. Cancer Treat Rev. 2017;53:10-24.
16. van der Kaaij MA, Heutte N, Meijnders P, Abeilard-Lemoisson E, Spina M, Moser EC, et al. Premature ovarian failure and fertility in long-term survivors of Hodgkin's lymphoma: a European Organisation for Research and Treatment of Cancer Lymphoma Group and Groupe d'Etude des Lymphomes de l'Adulte Cohort Study. J Clin Oncol. 2012;30:291-9.
17. Akhtar S, Youssef I, Soudy H, Elhassan TA, Rauf SM, Maghfoor I. Prevalence of menstrual cycles and outcome of 50 pregnancies after high-dose chemotherapy and auto-SCT in non-Hodgkin and Hodgkin lymphoma patients younger than 40 years. Bone Marrow Transplant. 2015; 50:1551-6.
18. Boots CE, Meister M, Cooper AR, Hardi A, Jungheim ES. Ovarian stimulation in the luteal phase: systematic review and meta-analysis. J Assist Reprod Genet. 2016;33:971-80.
19. Kuang Y, Chen Q, Hong Q, Lyu Q, Ai A, Fu Y, et al. Double stimulations during the follicular and luteal phases of poor responders in IVF/ICSI programmes (Shanghai protocol). Reprod Biomed Online. 2014; 29:684-91.
20. Pereira N, Hancock K, Cordeiro CN, Lekovich JP, Schattman GL, Rosenwaks Z. Comparison of ovarian stimulation response in patients with breast cancer undergoing ovarian stimulation with letrozole and gonadotropins to patients undergoing ovarian stimulation with gonadotropins alone for elective cryopreservation of oocytes dagger. Gynecol Endocrinol. 2016;32:823-6.
21. Gellert SE, Pors SE, Kristensen SG, Bay-Bjorn AM, Ernst E, Yding Andersen C. Transplantation of frozen-thawed ovarian tissue: an update on worldwide activity published in peer-reviewed papers and on the Danish cohort. J Assist Reprod Genet. 2018;35(4):561-70.

SECTION 6

Therapeutics and Adjuncts

18. **Ovulation Induction Protocols and Assisted Reproductive Technology Medications**
Astha Ubeja

19. **Role of Antioxidants and Supplements in Infertility**
Sumavarsha, Veneela Nallani, Jyoti Budi

20. **Growth Factors and Regenerative Medicine: Platelet-rich Plasma in Uterine and Ovarian Applications**
Monisha Singh, Neharika Malhotra

21. **Lifestyle Modifications and Stress Management for Infertility Patients**
Neharika Malhotra, Jaideep Malhotra

CHAPTER 18

Ovulation Induction Protocols and Assisted Reproductive Technology Medications

Astha Ubeja

INTRODUCTION

Ovulation disorders are responsible for 20% of the causes of infertility.[1] Ovulation induction aims to develop a single follicle for anovulation. Ovarian stimulation or controlled ovarian stimulation or superovulation aims at developing multiple follicles and is used in assisted reproductive technology (ART). Patients should be informed about treatment protocols available, the result, and the associated risk. This chapter discusses various ovulation induction and stimulation protocols [clomiphene citrate (CC), gonadotropins, pulsatile gonadotropin-releasing hormone (GnRH) therapy, aromatase inhibitors, and dopamine agonists] and provide approach to the management of patients.[2,3] Classification of anovulatory patients can be performed by using *World Health Organization (WHO) criteria* by Rowe et al.[4]

WORLD HEALTH ORGANIZATION CLASSIFICATION OF OVULATION DISORDERS

- *Group I:* Hypothalamic or pituitary failure, leading to low gonadotropins and estrogen; conditions include hypothalamic amenorrhea (due to stress, low body weight, excessive exercise) and hypogonadotropic hypogonadism.
- *Group II:* Hypothalamic-pituitary-ovarian (HPO) axis dysfunction with normal gonadotropins; this category most commonly includes polycystic ovary syndrome (PCOS) and hyperprolactinemic amenorrhea.
- *Group III:* Primary ovarian insufficiency (POI), characterized by low estrogen and high gonadotropins

Initial evaluation of the patient:

- History and physical examination
- Age of the patient
- Duration of infertility
- Cause of infertility
- Baseline hormonal evaluation thyroid and prolactin levels
- Baseline scan
- Semen analysis

Different regimens used for ovulation protocols:

- CC
- Aromatase inhibitors
- Letrozole
- *Gonadotropins:*
    - hMG (human menopausal gonadotropin)
    - FSH (follicle-stimulating hormone)
    - rFSH (recombinant FSH)
    - LH (luteinizing hormone)
- GnRH analogs
- *Dopamine agonists:*
    - Cabergoline
    - Bromocriptine

Monitoring of ovulation:

- Transvaginal ultrasound (USG)
- Serum estradiol levels

ORAL MEDICATIONS[5]

Clomiphene Citrate

- *Mechanism:* As a selective estrogen receptor modulator (SERM), CC blocks estrogen receptors in the hypothalamus, which tricks the body into producing more FSH and LH.[6] This promotes the growth of ovarian follicles.[7] It is antiestrogenic.
- *Indications:*
  - It can be used in WHO Group 2 women with anovulation; polycystic ovarian disease (PCOD)
  - Unexplained infertility
- *Protocol:* Treatment typically starts on cycle days 2–5 with a dosage of 50 mg for 5 days. If ovulation does not occur, the dose can be increased by 50 mg in subsequent cycles, up to a maximum of 150 mg. Cycles are monitored by USG.
  - *"Stair-step":* This is an alternative approach for women who do not respond to the initial dose. The dose of CC is increased within the same cycle, based on USG monitoring, to induce ovulation.[8]
  - *Results of clomiphene treatment:* Clomiphene will induce ovulation successfully in 70–80% of properly selected women. The overall cycle fecundability is 15%.[9]
- *Side effects:* CC may cause side effects like hot flashes and headaches. It can also have an anti-estrogenic effect on cervical mucus and the uterine lining, potentially affecting implantation.

Chances of multiple pregnancy:

- *Ovarian cancer:* Pooled analysis from eight case-control studies found that infertility drug use among nulliparous, subfertile women was associated with incidence of borderline serous ovarian tumors but not with invasive cancers.[7]
- *Cc resistance:* Failure to ovulate with 3 months of use at 150 mg/day of 5 days; it is mostly encountered in cases of PCOS.
- CC *failure:* Patients who ovulate but do not conceive; they should start some alternative therapy and should be evaluated further.

Aromatase Inhibitors (Letrozole)

Aromatase is the enzyme responsible for the conversion of androgens to estrogens. Aromatase inhibitors block this conversion of androgens to estrogen and result in a relative deficiency of estrogen. This triggers a compensatory release of FSH from the pituitary gland, stimulating follicle growth.[10]

- *Protocol:* A common protocol is 2.5 mg daily for 5 days, starting on cycle days 3–5. The dose can be increased in future cycles if necessary.
- *Extended letrozole regimen:* Studies suggest this low-dose, extended approach can lead to higher ovulation rates, better endometrial thickness, improved clinical pregnancy rates, and potentially better endometrial receptivity than shorter, higher-dose protocol.[11]
- *Dose and duration:* Instead of the typical 5-day regimen (day 2–6 of the cycle), an extended regimen may last for 7–10 days. Letrozole is started at 2.5 mg for 10 days.

Mechanism: The longer stimulation period with a lower daily dose aims to optimize both follicular development and endometrial response, leading to more favorable reproductive outcomes.

In patients with PCOS and women who are resistant to clomiphene, letrozole is associated with higher ovulation and live birth rates than CC and does not have the same negative effects on the uterine lining.[12,13]

- *It should be considered the first-line agent for ovulation induction in anovulatory women with PCOS.*

INJECTABLE MEDICATIONS

Gonadotropins

- Preparations available:
    - hMG
    - Highly purified hMG
    - FSH
    - rFSH and LH

Mechanism: These injectable medications contain FSH, and sometimes LH, to directly stimulate the ovaries and trigger follicle growth. They can be manufactured from the urine of postmenopausal women (hMG) or synthetically (rFSH).

Indications:

- WHO Group 1 (hypogonadotropic hypogonadism, where a combination of FSH and LH stimulation is required).
- Cases of CC resistance or failures or a combination with CC (PCOS, unexplained infertility)[14]
- Controlled ovarian stimulation to induce the development of multiple follicles in in vitro fertilization (IVF)/intracytoplasmic sperm injection (ICSI)
  Before starting stimulation, downregulation should be confirmed.
  Serum estradiol should be <50 pg/m.
  Follicle size should be <10 mm.

Protocols:

- *Fixed dose:* A fixed dose of 75/150 IU is started and serial USG monitoring is done.
    - *Low-dose "step-up"*: It is used to reduce the risk of multiple pregnancies and ovarian hyperstimulation syndrome (OHSS), especially in women with PCOS.[15,16] Low dose of gonadotropin 37.5–75 IU/day is started and dose is increased in small increments if no follicle >10 mm has developed or after 6 days. In subsequent cycles, treatment generally begins at the threshold of response previously determined. Once a mature follicle has developed, exogenous human chorionic gonadotropin (hCG) is administered to stimulate ovulation.[17]
    - *Conventional "step-up"*: A higher starting dose (e.g., 75 IU/day) is used for a shorter duration before a dose increase.
    - *"Step-down"*: This protocol starts with a higher dose that is reduced as the follicles develop. It more closely mimics the natural menstrual cycle starts with 150–225 IU daily and decreases thereafter.

Side effects: This treatment requires close monitoring with serum estradiol levels tests and USG. It has a higher risk of multiple pregnancies and OHSS than oral medications. It is more expensive.

Mild stimulation protocol: This protocol involve clomiphene in combination with hMG, which yields better outcomes compared to HMG alone. These findings were in congruity with another report which showed ovulation and pregnancy rate to be 82% and 21%, respectively, in women who underwent mild ovarian stimulation (MOS) using clomiphene in conjunction with hMG. Moreover, the average cost was much lower (one-third) than the hMG-only protocol.[18] Clomiphene is started at 100 mg daily from day 2 to 6 followed by gonadotropins 75/150 IU. Rest of dose regulation is done by transvaginal USG monitoring[18] **(Fig. 1)**.

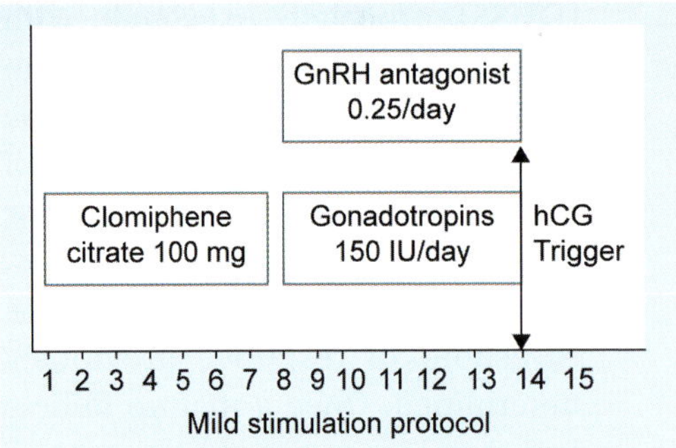

Fig. 1: Single antagonist protocol.

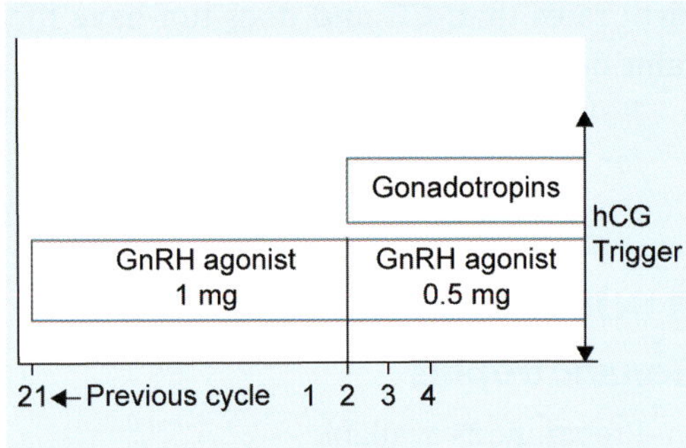

Fig. 2: Long protocol. (GnRH: gonadotropin-releasing hormone; hCG: human chorionic gonadotropin)

Gonadoptropin-releasing Hormone Analogs

Gonadoptropin-releasing hormone agonists downregulate gonadotropin secretion and suppress ovarian function, resulting in a hypoestrogenic state analogous to the hypothalamic hypogonadal state of women with WHO Group I anovulation.[19] Downregulation of the hypothalamic pituitary gonadal axis of women with WHO Group II anovulation with these agonists has been used as an adjunct to the induction of ovulation with exogenous gonadotropins. The GnRH agonist is started in the luteal phase of the previous cycle to suppress the pituitary gland before ovarian stimulation begins. This helps synchronize follicle growth and prevent an untimely LH surge. GnRH agonists or antagonists are used to prevent premature ovulation during the cycle. Addition of GnRh analogs has reduced cycle cancellation rates.

Protocols:

- *Long protocol:* GnRH agonist started in luteal phase (cycle day 21) of the previous cycle until hCG administration **(Fig. 2)**.
- *Short protocol:* GnRH agonist starting on day 1 or 3 of stimulation until hCG administration **(Fig. 3)**
- *Ultrashort protocol:* GnRH agonist is given on day 2 to day 4 **(Fig. 4)**.

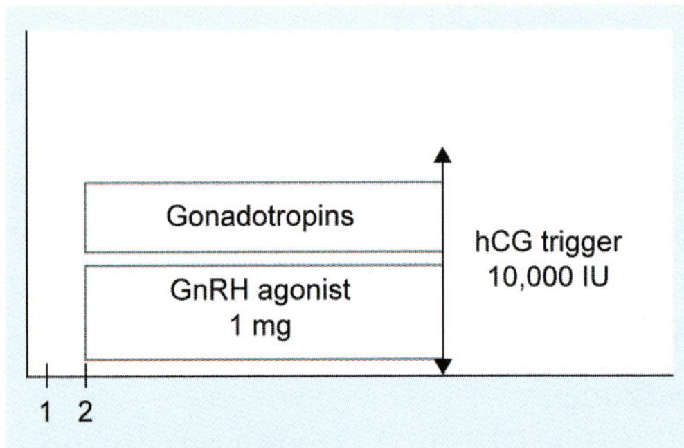

Fig. 3: Short protocol. (GnRH: gonadotropin-releasing hormone; hCG: human chorionic gonadotropin)

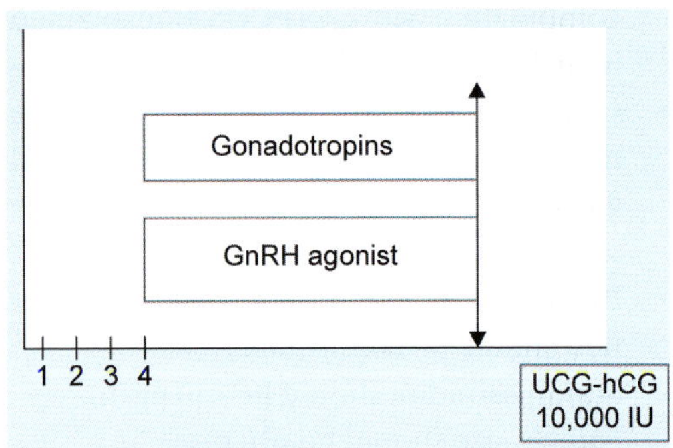

Fig. 4: Ultrashort protocol. (hCG: human chorionic gonadotropin; UCG: urinary chorionic gonadotropin)

- *GnRH antagonist protocol:* The GnRH antagonist binds competitively to the receptors and thereby prevents endogenous GnRH from exerting its stimulatory

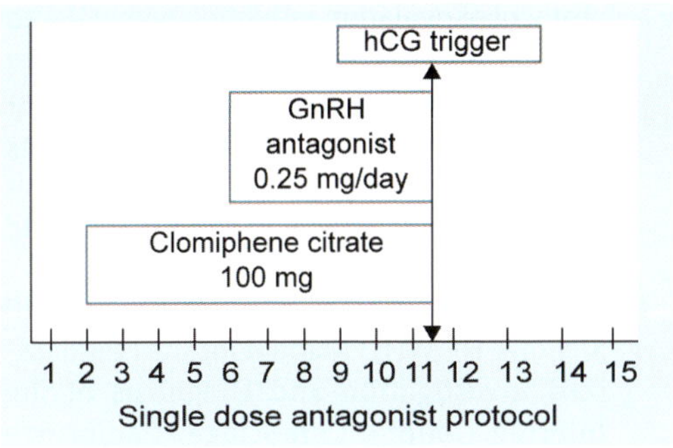

Fig. 5: Multidose antagonist protocol.

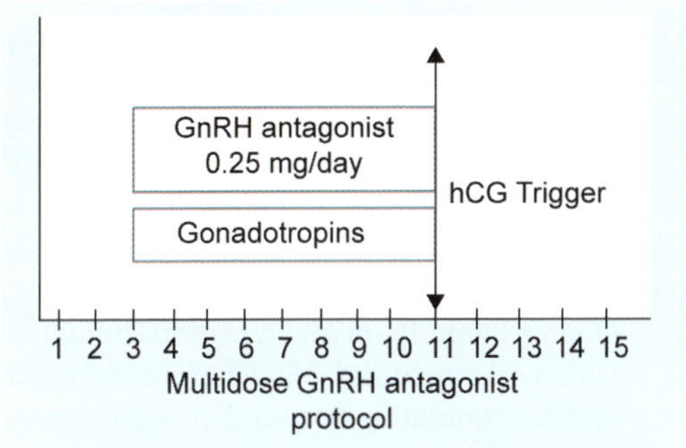

Fig. 6: Mild stimulation protocol.

effect on the pituitary cells. This causes suppression of gonadotrophin secretion which occurs immediately after administration of the antagonist.[20] When using GnRH antagonist in controlled ovarian stimulation, ovulation or maturation of the oocyte can, therefore, be induced by a variety of drugs, e.g., native GnRH, recombinant LH, or short-acting GnRH agonists. Antagonists are started later in the cycle to suppress the LH surge.[21] This protocol is shorter and has a lower risk of OHSS compared to the long agonist protocol **(Figs. 5 and 6)**.

- *hCG "trigger shot":* An injection of hCG of 5,000/10,000 IU is used to trigger the final maturation and release of eggs once the follicles reach the 18–20 mm.

ADJUNCTIVE MEDICATIONS AND PROCEDURES

- *Metformin:* It is an insulin-sensitizing drug that can improve ovulation rates in women with PCOS, especially those with insulin resistance.[22,23] Metformin can be used as an adjunct to clomiphene in PCOS. Dosage is 500 mg daily and can be increased to twice daily. Metformin treatment is beneficial in increasing the clinical pregnancy rates and reducing the OHSS risk in infertile women with PCOS.
    - *Glucocorticoids:* Adjuvant therapy with prednisone in clomiphene-resistant cases can successfully induce ovulation who fail to respond to clomiphene alone.[24] Dose is prednisone (5 mg daily) or dexamethasone (0.5–2 mg daily) from day 5 of the cycle.
    - *Laparoscopic ovarian drilling:* Laparoscopic ovarian drilling is an effective procedure for clomiphene-resistant cases. It helps to restore ovulation, 40% of spontaneous conception within first 6 months of the procedure. The long-term effects on ovarian function may be iatrogenic adhesions and decreased ovarian reserve. Hence, this procedure should be advised in selected CC-resistant cases for the sole purpose of correction of anovulatory infertility.[25]
- *Weight loss:* Lifestyle modification is the first-step treatment for obese anovulatory infertile women with PCOS before switching to pharmacological ovulation induction.[26]
- *Dopamine agonist:* Cabergoline and bromocriptine are primarily used to induce ovulation in anovulation caused by hyperprolactinemia. They have an important role to prevent OHSS

by reducing the effects of vascular endothelial growth factor which increases vascular permeability and leads to fluid leakage during OHSS.

CONCLUSION

Ovulation induction still remains the most common crucial component of fertility treatment. Effective management involves assessing ovarian reserve through tests like antral follicle count and anti-Mullerian hormone to tailor the stimulation protocol to the individual. The goal is to increase the chances of conception either natural cycle or assisted reproductive techniques. Frequent monitoring and strict cancellation criteria can reduce the risks of OHSS.

Lifestyle medication (weight loss and stress management) holds an important role in managing PCOS relation anovulation.

Clomiphene and letrozole if used after proper selection have increased the conceptions rates to 30% and 70%, respectively.

Gonadotropins along with GnRH analogs have revolutionized the approach to ART patients.

By adopting an individualized approach to ovulation induction, more effective, safe, and optimized outcome can be given to patients.

REFERENCES

1. Balen AH, Rutherford AJ. Managing anovulatory infertility and polycystic ovary syndrome. BMJ. 2007;335:663-6.
2. Tan SL, Kingsland C, Campbell S, Mills C, Bradfield J, Alexander N, et al. The long protocol of administration of gonadotropin-releasing hormone agonist is superior to the short protocol for ovarian stimulation for in vitro fertilization. Fertil Steril. 1992;57(4):810-4.
3. D'Amato G, Caroppo E, Pasquadibisceglie A, Carone D, Vitti A, Vizziello GM. A novel protocol of ovulation induction with delayed gonadotropin-releasing hormone antagonist administration combined with high-dose recombinant follicle-stimulating hormone and clomiphene citrate for poor responders and women over 35 years. Fertil Steril. 2004;81(6):1572-7.
4. Rowe PJ, Comhaire FH, Hargreave TB, Mellows HJ. WHO Manual for the Standardized Investigation and Diagnosis of the Infertile Couple. Cambridge: Cambridge University Press; 1993.
5. Amer SA, Li TC, Metwally M, Emarh M, Ledger WL. Randomized controlled trial comparing laparoscopic ovarian diathermy with clomiphene citrate as a first-line method of ovulation induction in women with polycystic ovary syndrome. Hum Reprod. 2009;24(1):219-25.
6. Calaf Alsina J, Ruiz Balda JA, Romeu Sarrió A, Caballero Fernández V, Cano Trigo I, Gómez Parga JL, et al. Ovulation induction with a starting dose of 50 IU of recombinant follicle stimulating hormone in WHO group II anovulatory women: the IO-50 study, a prospective, observational, multicentre, open trial. BJOG. 2003;110:1072-7.
7. Homburg R. Clomiphene citrate—end of an ear? A mini-review. Hum Reprod. 2005;20:2043-51.
8. Agrawal K, Gainder S, Dhaliwal LK, Suri V. Ovulation Induction Using Clomiphene Citrate Using Stair - Step Regimen versus Traditional Regimen in Polycystic Ovary Syndrome Women - A Randomized Control Trial. J Hum Reprod Sci. 2017;10(4):261-4.
9. Balen AH, Rotherford AJ. Managing anovulatory infertility and polycystic ovary syndrome. BMJ. 2007;335:663-6.
10. Plymate SR, Fariss BL, Bassett ML, Matej L. Obesity and its rule in polycystic ovary syndrome. J Clin Endocrinol Metab. 1981;52:1246-8.
11. Zhu X, Fu Y. Extending letrozole treatment duration is effective in inducing ovulation in women with polycystic ovary syndrome and letrozole resistance. Fertil Steril. 2023;119(1):107-13.

12. Mitwally MF, Casper RF. Aromatase inhibition: a novel method of ovulation induction in women with polycystic ovary syndrome. Reprod Technol. 2000;10:244-47.
13. Mitwally MF, Biljan MM, Casper RF. Pregnancy outcome after the use of an aromatase inhibitor for ovarian stimulation. Am J Obstet Gynecol. 2005;192(2):381-6.
14. Mitwally MF, Casper RF. Aromatase inhibitors in ovulation induction. Semin Reprod Med. 2004;22(1):61-78.
15. Donesky BW, Adashi EY, Surgically induced ovulation in the polycystic ovary syndrome: wedge resection revisited in the age of laparoscopy. Fertil Steril. 1995;63:439-63.
16. Homburg R, Levy T, Ben-Rafael Z. A comparative prospective study of conventional regimen with chronic low-dose administration of follicle-stimulating hormone for anovulation associated with polycystic ovary syndrome. Fertil Steril. 1995;63:729-33.
17. Wan JP, Wang ZJ, Sheng Y, Chen W, Guo QQ, Xu J, et al. Effect of HCG-Triggered Ovulation on Pregnancy Outcomes in Intrauterine Insemination: An Analysis of 5,610 First IUI Natural Cycles With Donor Sperm in China. Front Endocrinol (Lausanne). 2020;11:423.
18. Ochin H, Ma X, Wang L, Li X, Song J, Meng Y, et al. Low dose clomiphene citrate as a mild stimulation protocol in women with unsuspected poor in vitro *fertilization* result can generate more oocytes with optimal cumulative pregnancy rate. J Ovarian Res. 2018;11:37.
19. Ho YB, Pride SM. Induction of ovulation with exogenous gonadotropins in anovulatory infertile women. Semin Reprod Med. 1990;8:186-97.
20. Filicori M, Flamigni C, Meriggiola MC, Cognigni G, Valdiserri A, Ferrari P, et al. Ovulation induction with pulsatile gonadotropin-releasing hormone: technical modalities and clinical perspective. Fertil Steril. 1991;56:1-13.
21. Martin K, Santoro N, Hall J, Filicori M, Wierman M, Crowley WF Jr. Clinical review 15: management of ovulatory disorders with pulsatile gonadotropin-releasing hormone. J Clin Endocrinol Metab. 1990;71:1081A-1081G.
22. Cho LW, Jayagopal V, Kilpatrick ES, Atkin SL. The biological variation of C-reactive protein in polycystic ovarian syndrome. Clin Chem. 2005;51:1905-7.
23. Kim LH, Taylor AE, Barbieri RL. Insulin sensitizer and polycystic ovary syndrome: Can a diabetes medication treat infertility ? Fertil Steril. 2000;73(6):1097-8.
24. Lobo RA, Paul W, March CM, Granger L, Kletzy OA. Clomiphene and dexamethasone in women unresponsive to clomiphene alone. Obstet Gynecol. 1982;60:497-501.
25. Bordewijk EM, Ng KYB, Rakic L, Mol BWJ, Brown J, Crawford TJ, et al. Laparoscopic ovarian drilling for ovulation induction in women with anovulatory polycystic ovary syndrome. Cochrane Database Syst Rev. 2020;2(2):CD001122.
26. Lefebvre P, Bringer J, Renard E, Boulet F, Clouet S, Jaffiol C. Influences of weight, body fat patterning and nutrition on the management of PCOS. Hum Reprod. 1997; 12 (Suppl) 1:73-81.

CHAPTER 19

Role of Antioxidants and Supplements in Infertility

Sumavarsha, Veneela Nallani, Jyoti Budi

INTRODUCTION

Infertility affects an estimated 10–15% of couples worldwide and represents a multifactorial condition in which oxidative stress (OS) and micronutrient status often play pivotal roles.[1,2] Reactive oxygen species (ROS) are generated physiologically in gametogenesis, fertilization, and early embryogenesis, but an imbalance between ROS production and antioxidant defenses leads to oxidative damage to lipids, proteins, and nucleic acids, impairing oocyte and sperm function and reducing reproductive outcomes.[3,4] Interest in antioxidant therapies and targeted nutritional supplements has grown over the last two decades as an adjunct to lifestyle measures and assisted reproductive technologies (ARTs).

MECHANISMS: OXIDATIVE STRESS IN MALE AND FEMALE REPRODUCTION

Reactive oxygen species have dual roles: low, regulated ROS concentrations are essential for capacitation, acrosome reaction, and follicular signaling, whereas excessive ROS causes lipid peroxidation, protein oxidation, and deoxyribonucleic acid (DNA) fragmentation.[3,5] Spermatozoa are particularly susceptible to ROS because of their high content of polyunsaturated fatty acids and relatively limited cytoplasmic antioxidant defenses; oxidative damage leads to reduced motility, abnormal morphology, and increased DNA fragmentation that correlate with poor fertility and ART outcomes.[6,7] In the female gamete, OS contributes to mitochondrial dysfunction, chromosomal segregation errors, and impaired granulosa cell function, all of which reduce oocyte quality and embryo developmental competence, particularly in older women and those with diminished ovarian reserve.[8,9] Systemic conditions such as obesity, smoking, environmental toxins, and poor diet increase oxidative burden in both partners and are modifiable contributors to infertility[10] **(Fig. 1)**.

EVIDENCE BASE: METHODOLOGY AND LIMITATIONS

Clinical trials of oral antioxidants and micronutrients vary widely in design, inclusion criteria, endpoints (semen parameters, natural conception, clinical pregnancy, live birth), and supplement formulations. Meta-analyses and systematic reviews often highlight heterogeneity and unclear methodological quality: many randomized controlled trials are small, short-duration, or use composite antioxidant products, making isolation of single-agent effects difficult.[1,11] Cochrane reviews and large systematic analyses report low- to very-low quality

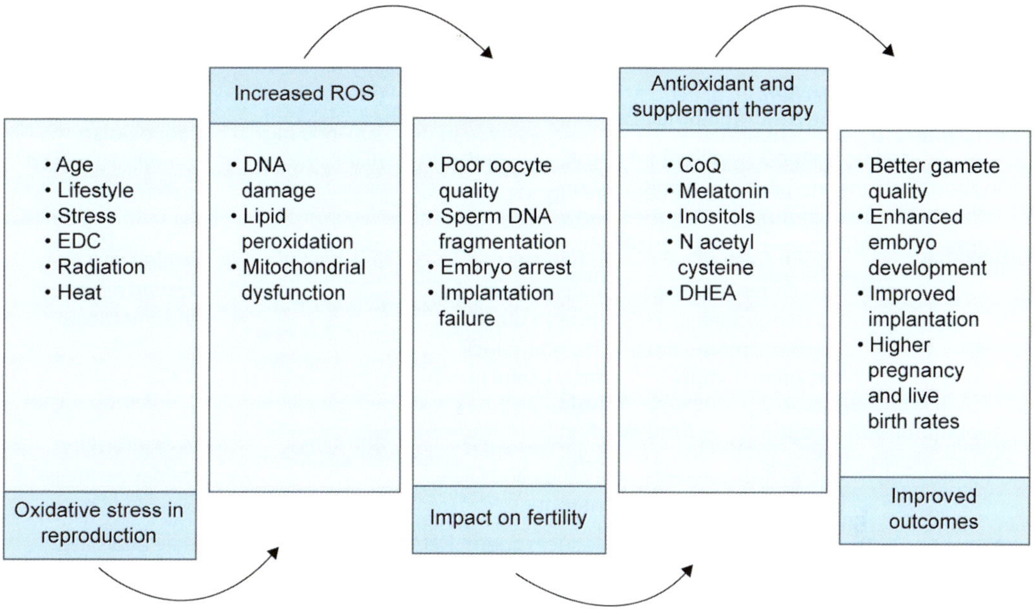

Fig. 1: Mechanism of oxidative stress in reproduction.

evidence for many antioxidant strategies despite promising biological plausibility, and call for larger, adequately powered trials with clinically meaningful endpoints (live birth).[1,12] Nonetheless, moderate-quality evidence exists for certain agents in specific subgroups, such as coenzyme Q10 in older women or men with oxidative stress and omega-3s in male factor infertility.[13,14]

FEMALE INFERTILITY: ANTIOXIDANTS AND SUPPLEMENTS (TABLE 1)

Coenzyme Q10

Coenzyme Q10 (CoQ10) (ubiquinone/ubiquinol) is a mitochondrial electron transport chain component with antioxidant properties. Its levels decline with age, and supplementation has been proposed to improve oocyte mitochondrial function and reduce ROS-mediated damage. Multiple meta-analyses and randomized trials suggest CoQ10 may improve ovarian response, oocyte quality, and clinical pregnancy rates in women with diminished ovarian reserve or advanced maternal age, although heterogeneity and limited sample sizes reduce certainty.[13,15] Typical studied doses range from 100 to 600 mg daily for several weeks before stimulation; safety appears acceptable, but high-dose long-term data are limited.[16]

Myoinositol and Inositol Combinations

Myoinositol (MI) and d-chiro-inositol (DCI) modulate insulin signaling and ovarian steroidogenesis and have been extensively studied in polycystic ovary syndrome (PCOS). MI supplementation improves ovulation rates, reduces gonadotropin requirements during stimulation, and may improve oocyte quality and fertilization rates in PCOS patients undergoing ART.[17,18] Recent large randomized trials and meta-analyses provide supportive evidence for benefits in ovulation induction

TABLE 1: Antioxidants and supplements—summary of mechanisms, evidence, and dosage.

Supplement/ antioxidant	*Mechanism of action*	*Key evidence in reproduction*	*Suggested dose (studied)*	*IVF relevance*
Coenzyme Q10	Mitochondrial cofactor; improves ATP production; ROS scavenger	Improves ovarian response, embryo quality in poor responders	200–600 mg/day	Poor ovarian reserve, advanced maternal age
Melatonin	Potent free radical scavenger; improves mitochondrial function; modulates circadian rhythm	Enhances oocyte quality, embryo quality, and pregnancy rates; useful in endometriosis	3–6 mg/day	Diminished ovarian reserve, endometriosis
Vitamin E (α-tocopherol)	Lipid membrane protection; prevents peroxidation	Improves sperm motility and DNA integrity	400 IU/day	Male infertility (oxidative stress)
Vitamin C (ascorbic acid)	Aqueous-phase ROS scavenger; regenerates oxidized vitamin E	Reduces sperm DNA fragmentation when combined with vitamin E	500–1,000 mg/day	Male infertility, sperm DNA damage
L-carnitine/ Acetyl-L-carnitine	Fatty acid transport enhances mitochondrial function	Improves sperm motility and fertilization	2–3 g/day	Asthenozoospermia, idiopathic male infertility
N-acetyl cysteine (NAC)	Precursor of glutathione; improves insulin sensitivity	Improves ovulation, endometrial thickness in PCOS	600–1,200 mg/day	PCOS, ovulation induction
Omega-3 fatty acids	Anti-inflammatory; membrane fluidity	Improves sperm motility, endometrial receptivity	1–2 g/day	Male infertility, endometrial receptivity
DHEA	Increases IGF-1, reduces ROS, supports folliculogenesis	Improves ovarian response, embryo quality in poor responders	25 mg TDS (75 mg/day)	Poor ovarian reserve
Myo-inositol/d-Chiro-inositol	Insulin sensitizers; antioxidant effect	Improves oocyte quality, fertilization in PCOS	2–4 g/day	PCOS, IVF cycles
Selenium	Cofactor for glutathione peroxidase	Improves sperm motility, DNA integrity	100–200 µg/day	Male infertility
Zinc	Cofactor for SOD; stabilizes sperm DNA	Improves sperm count and motility	30–50 mg/day	Male infertility
Folate	Reduces homocysteine, protects DNA	Improves embryo quality, reduces miscarriage risk	400–800 µg/day	Female infertility, preconception

Contd...

Contd...

Supplement/ antioxidant	*Mechanism of action*	*Key evidence in reproduction*	*Suggested dose (studied)*	*IVF relevance*
Vitamin D	Immunomodulator; implantation support	May improve endometrial receptivity, IVF outcomes	1,000–4,000 IU/day	Recurrent implantation failure, low vitamin D
Resveratrol	Polyphenol; mitochondrial and antiaging effect	Improves ovarian reserve, oocyte competence	200–400 mg/day	Poor ovarian reserve, advanced age
Astaxanthin	Carotenoid antioxidant; membrane stabilization	Improves sperm function, motility	4–12 mg/day	Male infertility
Curcumin	Antioxidant and anti-inflammatory	Preclinical data; limited human IVF evidence	500–1,000 mg/day	Adjunct, experimental

(ATP: adenosine triphosphate; DNA: deoxyribonucleic acid; IVF: in vitro fertilization; IGF-1: insulin-like growth factor 1; IU: international unit; ROS: reactive oxygen species)

and metabolic parameters, though recent pregnancy-outcome trials highlight the need for context-specific recommendations.[11,19] Typical regimens use MI 2–4 g/day, often combined with folic acid.

Melatonin

Melatonin is both an endocrine regulator and a powerful antioxidant that concentrates in follicular fluid. Observational and randomized controlled studies indicate melatonin supplementation may improve oocyte quality, reduce oxidative markers in follicular fluid, and increase fertilization rates in selected groups, particularly women with poor oocyte quality or PCOS undergoing ART. Evidence remains mixed on robust endpoints such as live birth, and dosing in studies varies (commonly 3–6 mg nightly).[18,20]

N-acetylcysteine

N-acetylcysteine (NAC) is a glutathione precursor with antioxidant and insulin-sensitizing actions. Trials in PCOS show NAC can improve ovulation and, in some studies, pregnancy rates when used as an adjunct to clomiphene citrate in resistant PCOS, though results are inconsistent and larger trials are needed.[12,21] Typical NAC doses in fertility studies range from 600 to 1800 mg/day.

Dehydroepiandrosterone

Dehydroepiandrosterone (DHEA) is an adrenal androgen precursor used empirically to improve ovarian response in women with diminished ovarian reserve or poor response to stimulation. Systematic reviews show mixed results: some meta-analyses report improved oocyte yield and embryo numbers, but consistent improvement in live birth remains unproven, and routine use is not universally recommended.[22] Dosing typically ranges from 25 to 75 mg/day; potential androgenic side effects and lack of robust randomized controlled trial (RCT) data mandate caution.

Folic Acid, B Vitamins, and Antioxidants in Pregnancy Planning

Periconceptional folic acid remains standard of care to prevent neural tube defects and may be associated with improved ART outcomes when combined with other B-vitamins.[23] Antioxidant vitamins such as vitamin C and E have biological rationale but inconsistent clinical benefit when given alone; combinations with micronutrients (e.g., selenium and zinc) have shown improvements in some semen or oocyte-related parameters but high-quality evidence for improved live birth is lacking.[24,25]

Male Infertility: Evidence for Antioxidants and Micronutrients

Given the central role of ROS in sperm dysfunction, antioxidant therapy for male infertility has been intensively studied. Trials test single agents (vitamin E, vitamin C, L-carnitine, CoQ10, selenium, and zinc) and combination products; outcomes commonly assessed are semen parameters, seminal oxidative markers, DNA fragmentation, and pregnancy rates.[6,26]

CoQ10, L-carnitine, and Carnitine Esters

Coenzyme Q10 and L-carnitine have demonstrated improvements in sperm motility and concentration in several randomized trials and meta-analyses, with some studies showing higher pregnancy rates after supplementation. Doses studied include CoQ10 100–300 mg/day and L-carnitine 1–3 g/day, often studied for 3–6 months (one spermatogenic cycle).[13,27]

Vitamins C and E, Selenium, and Zinc

Vitamin E (alpha-tocopherol) and vitamin C are classical antioxidants; supplementation trials show mixed impacts on semen parameters and oxidative markers. Selenium (often 100 μg/day) combined with vitamin E improved sperm motility and morphology in some studies, while zinc, essential for spermatogenesis, correlates with seminal quality; supplementation studies report variable outcomes, and optimal dosing remains unclear.[7,24,28]

Omega-3 Fatty Acids

Dietary omega-3 polyunsaturated fatty acids (PUFAs) are structural components of sperm membranes and may improve sperm motility and morphology. Systematic reviews suggest omega-3 supplementation increases certain semen parameters, though evidence linking intake to natural conception or live birth is limited.[14]

Sperm Deoxyribonucleic Acid Fragmentation: Targeted Antioxidant Therapy?

Elevated sperm DNA fragmentation (SDF) is associated with reduced fertility and poor ART outcomes. Antioxidant therapy may reduce SDF in some men, but randomized evidence demonstrating improved live birth after intervention for high SDF is limited; careful patient selection and addressing reversible causes (smoking, varicocele, heat exposure, and infections) remain primary strategies.[6,29]

SAFETY, INTERACTIONS, AND POTENTIAL HARMS

Antioxidants are generally well tolerated, but safety is not guaranteed. Excessive antioxidant supplementation can paradoxically impair ROS-dependent physiological processes, and high doses of certain vitamins (for example, high-dose vitamin E or folic acid) may be associated with adverse outcomes or interactions.[30] Supplements are not tightly regulated, leading to variability in dose and purity; clinicians should recommend third-party tested formulations and be alert to interactions with medications (e.g., anticoagulants with high-dose vitamin E). Women trying to conceive should continue standard periconception folic acid dosing, and any additional supplement should be considered in the context of baseline nutritional status and clinical evidence.[23,30]

CLINICAL APPROACH: PRACTICAL RECOMMENDATIONS

- *Lifestyle first:* Optimize body mass index (BMI), smoking cessation, alcohol moderation, dietary pattern rich in antioxidants (fruits, vegetables, and oily fish), control chronic disease, and minimize environmental exposures before defaulting to supplements.[10]
- *Individualize:* consider targeted supplementation for men with documented oxidative stress, elevated SDF, or idiopathic abnormal semen parameters after ruling out reversible causes.[6]
- *Use evidence-based agents for specific indications:* CoQ10 for older women/ diminished ovarian reserve (100–600 mg/day) and for men with poor motility (100–300 mg/day); myo-inositol for PCOS (2–4 g/day); L-carnitine for male motility (1–3 g/day); NAC as adjunct in CC-resistant PCOS (600–1800 mg/day)[13,17,21,27]
- *Duration and timing:* Allow at least one spermatogenic cycle (approximately 3 months) when treating male factor; in women, a 6–12 weeks preconception window is common for mitochondrial-targeted agents. Consult current guidelines and evidence when planning longer courses.[6,13]
- *Monitor and document:* Baseline nutritional and hormonal assessment as indicated (vitamin D, folate, and selenium), semen analysis, and, when relevant, oxidative or DNA fragmentation testing to guide therapy and measure response.[15]
- *Prioritize high-quality evidence:* Discuss uncertainties with patients, emphasizing that while some supplements may improve intermediate outcomes (semen parameters and oocyte markers), robust evidence for increased live birth is limited for many agents.[1,12]

RESEARCH GAPS AND FUTURE DIRECTIONS

Important gaps include the need for adequately powered randomized controlled trials with live birth as the primary endpoint, head-to-head comparisons of single agents versus combination formulations, and stratification by meaningful subgroups (age, ovarian reserve, PCOS phenotype, and defined male oxidative stress). Biomarker development to identify patients who will benefit from antioxidant therapy (for example, validated measures of seminal oxidative stress or follicular redox status) would permit precision supplementation. Additionally, longer-term safety data and exploration of mechanistic endpoints using modern molecular methods will refine therapeutic choices.[11,15]

CONCLUSION

Antioxidants and nutritional supplements occupy an appealing niche in infertility treatment due to biological plausibility and relative safety. Evidence supports selective use—CoQ10, myoinositol, L-carnitine, and NAC have demonstrated benefits in particular settings—yet many studies are limited by heterogeneity in design and endpoints. Clinicians should prioritize lifestyle optimization, use targeted supplementation based on clinical phenotype and available data, counsel patients transparently about benefits and limitations, and encourage participation in well-designed trials to strengthen the evidence base. Ultimately, supplements can complement but not replace evidence-based fertility care. European Society of Human Reproduction and Embryology (ESHRE) and American Society for Reproductive Medicine (ASRM) do not currently recommend routine antioxidant supplementation for all infertile couples due to insufficient high-quality evidence.[1]

REFERENCES

1. Showell MG, Mackenzie-Proctor R, Brown J, et al. Antioxidants for female subfertility. Cochrane Database Syst Rev. 2020;2020(8): CD007807.
2. Dutta S, Walsh S. Oxidative stress and sperm function: a systematic review. Reprod Biomed Online. 2019;38(4):563-579.
3. Agarwal A, Majzoub A, Esteves SC. Oxidative stress and assisted reproduction. Reprod Biol Endocrinol. 2022;20:100.
4. Begum IA, Khan S. Oxidative stress: oocyte quality and infertility. Hum Reprod Update. 2025;31(2):123-140.
5. Wang Y, Li X. Mechanisms of oxidative stress-induced sperm dysfunction. Front Endocrinol (Lausanne). 2025;16:1520835.
6. Ahmadi S, Kazerouni F. Antioxidant supplementation on male fertility—A review. Clin Exp Reprod Med. 2016;43(4):189-203.
7. Fallah A, Mohammad-Hasani A, Colagar AH. Zinc is an essential element for male fertility: a review. Clin Biochem. 2018;62:34-44.
8. Shang Y, Liu B. Antioxidants and fertility in women with ovarian aging. Clin Med Insights Reprod Health. 2024;18:117955812412 34567.
9. Florou P, Vlahos NF. Does coenzyme Q10 supplementation improve fertility? A systematic review and meta-analysis. Oxid Med Cell Longev. 2020;2020:1234567.
10. World Health Organization. WHO Laboratory Manual for the Examination and Processing of Human Semen, 5th Edition. Geneva: World Health Organization; 2010.
11. Ross C, Morriss A, A review of oral antioxidants for male infertility: systematic review. Hum Reprod. 2010;25(9):e1-e11.
12. Thakker D, Shah H. N-acetylcysteine for polycystic ovary syndrome: systemic review and meta-analysis. J Ovarian Res. 2015;8:52.
13. Lin G, Li X. Clinical evidence of coenzyme Q10 pretreatment for IVF outcomes: a meta-analysis. J Assist Reprod Genet. 2024;41(3):567-80.
14. Falsig AM, Friis M. The influence of omega-3 fatty acids on semen quality: A review. Nutrients. 2019;11(2):311.
15. Pilehvari S, et al. The boosting effects of melatonin on IVF outcomes: clinical trials review. Clin Endocrinol (Oxf). 2023;98(4):301-15.
16. Florou P. Coenzyme Q10: mechanisms, dosing, and safety. J Clin Med. 2020;9(8):2540.
17. Zhang J, Zhang H, Zhou W, Jiang M, Lin X. Effect of myo-inositol supplementation in mixed ovarian response IVF cohort: a systematic review and meta-analysis. Front Endocrinol (Lausanne). 2025;16:1520362. doi:10.3389/fendo.2025.1520362.
18. Hu KL, Ye X, Wang S, Zhang D. Melatonin application in assisted reproductive technology: a systematic review and meta-analysis of randomized trials. Front Endocrinol (Lausanne). 2020;11:160. doi:10.3389/fendo.2020.00160.
19. Aragona C, Russo M, Myers SH, Espinola MSB, Bilotta G, Unfer V. A retrospective study "myo-inositol is a cost-saving strategy for controlled ovarian stimulation in non-polycystic ovary syndrome art patients." Reprod Biomed Online. 2025;50(1):120-8.
20. Pilehvari S. Melatonin clinical trial in PCOS and IVF. J Endocrinol Invest. 2023;46(9):1989-98.
21. Salehpour S, Sene AA, Saharkhiz N, Sohrabi MR, Moghimian F. N-acetylcysteine as an adjuvant to clomiphene citrate for successful induction of ovulation in infertile patients with polycystic ovary syndrome. J Obstet Gynaecol Res. 2012;38(9):1182-6. doi:10.1111/j.1447-0756.2012.01844.x.

22. Zhang J, Wang X. Efficacy of DHEA priming in poor ovarian responders: systematic review. Fertil Steril. 2023;119(6):1234-42.
23. Toivonen KI, Lacroix E, Flynn M, Ronksley PE, Oinonen KA, Metcalfe A, et al. Folic acid supplementation during the preconception period: a systematic review and meta-analysis. Prev Med. 2018;114:1-17. doi:10.1016/j.ypmed.2018.05.023.
24. Ahmadi S, et al. Antioxidant supplements and semen parameters: systematic review. Andrology. 2016;4(6):1020-30.
25. Dimitriadis F, et al. Antioxidant supplementation on male fertility—comprehensive review. Nutrients. 2023;15(4):1012.
26. Xu L, Hu C, Liu Q, Li Y. The effect of dehydroepiandrosterone (DHEA) supplementation on IVF or ICSI: a meta-analysis of randomized controlled trials. Geburtshilfe Frauenheilkd. 2019;79(7):705-712. doi:10.1055/a-0882-3791.
27. Matorras R, Pérez-Sanz J, Corcóstegui B, Pérez-Ruiz I, Malaina I, Quevedo S, et al. Effect of vitamin E administered to men in infertile couples on sperm and assisted reproduction outcomes: a double-blind randomized study. FS Rep. 2020;1(3):219-226. doi:10.1016/j.xfre.2020.09.006.
28. Agarwal A, Parekh N, Panner Selvam MK, Henkel R, Shah R, Homa ST, et al. Male oxidative stress infertility (MOSI): proposed terminology and clinical practice guidelines for management of idiopathic male infertility. World J Mens Health. 2019;37(3):296–312. doi:10.5534/wjmh.190055.
29. Ledowsky C, Scarf V, Sobczyńska-Malefora A, Carter T, Timbrell NE, Steel A. Health effects of excess folic acid use and high blood folate during preconception and pregnancy: a systematic review. Reprod Biomed Online. 2025;105240. doi:10.1016/j.rbmo.2025.105240.
30. World Health Organization. Who should consume high-dose folic acid supplements? BMJ. 2022;377:o67728.

CHAPTER 20

Growth Factors and Regenerative Medicine: Platelet-rich Plasma in Uterine and Ovarian Applications

Monisha Singh, Neharika Malhotra

INTRODUCTION

Regenerative medicine has emerged as one of the most promising frontiers in modern healthcare, offering novel ways to repair or restore damaged tissues and organs. Unlike conventional therapies that focus on symptom management, regenerative medicine aims to harness the body's innate healing potential through biological mediators such as stem cells, growth factors, and bioengineered scaffolds. Within this paradigm, *platelet-rich plasma (PRP)* has attracted growing interest.

Platelet-rich plasma is an autologous concentration of platelets suspended in plasma, prepared from a patient's own blood. Upon activation, platelets release an array of *growth factors*—including platelet-derived growth factor (PDGF), vascular endothelial growth factor (VEGF), transforming growth factor beta (TGF-β), epidermal growth factor (EGF), and insulin-like growth factor-1 (IGF-1). These signaling proteins promote angiogenesis, tissue remodeling, cell proliferation, and anti-apoptotic activity **(Table 1)**.

In gynecology and reproductive medicine, PRP is being explored as a treatment for *thin endometrium, Asherman's syndrome, repeated implantation failure (RIF), premature ovarian insufficiency (POI), poor ovarian reserve, and infertility related to advanced maternal age*. These conditions often have limited conventional treatment options, and PRP—being autologous, minimally invasive, and relatively cost-effective—presents an appealing adjunct or alternative therapy.[1]

This chapter reviews the biological rationale, mechanisms, evidence, and future perspectives of PRP in *uterine and ovarian applications*, while critically analyzing its advantages, limitations, and potential role in regenerative reproductive medicine **(Fig. 1)**.

TABLE 1: Key growth factors in PRP and their functions.

Growth factor	*Main function in regeneration*	*Relevance in uterus/ovary*
PDGF	Fibroblast proliferation, angiogenesis	Endometrial stromal proliferation
VEGF	Angiogenesis, vascular permeability	Improves uterine blood flow
TGF-β	Collagen synthesis, ECM remodeling	Scar reduction in Asherman's
EGF	Epithelial proliferation	Endometrial lining growth
IGF-1	Anti-apoptosis, cell survival	Ovarian follicle activation

(ECM: extracellular matrix; EGF: epidermal growth factor; IGF-1: insulin-like growth factor-1; PDGF: platelet-derived growth factor; TGF-β: transforming growth factor beta; VEGF: vascular endothelial growth factor)

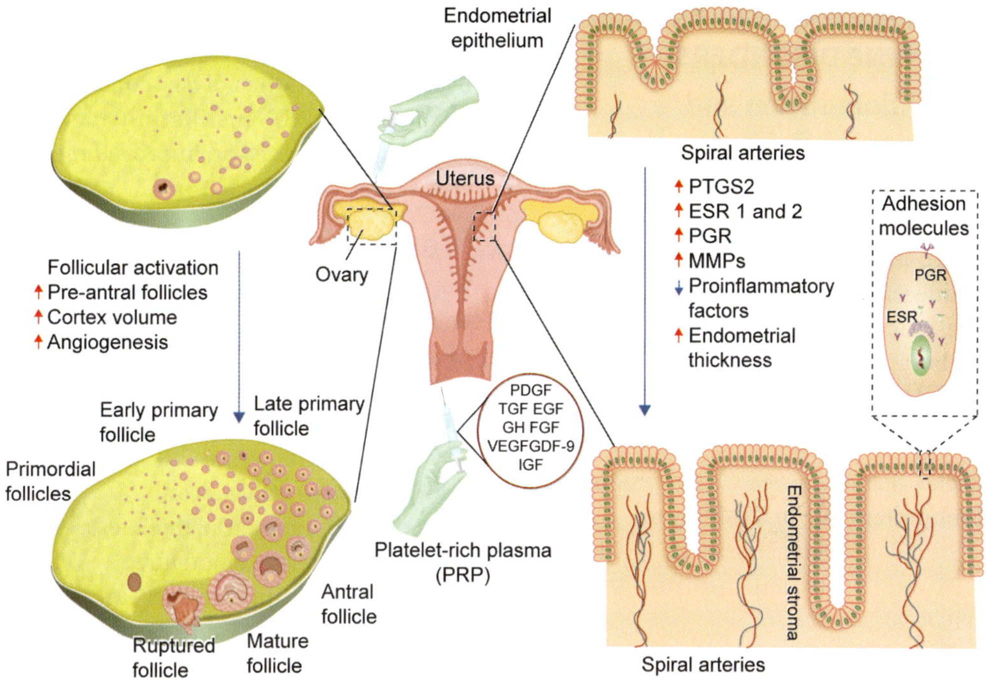

Fig. 1: Use of PRP in uterine and ovarian insufficiency.

BIOLOGICAL BASIS OF PLATELET-RICH PLASMA

Platelet Biology

Platelets, derived from megakaryocytes in the bone marrow, are small, anucleate cell fragments circulating in blood. While traditionally recognized for their role in hemostasis, platelets are also reservoirs of *bioactive proteins* contained within α-granules. Upon activation, they release growth factors and cytokines that orchestrate local healing responses.

Platelet-rich Plasma Preparation Techniques

Platelet-rich plasma is typically obtained through centrifugation of autologous venous blood, which separates red cells, white cells, and platelets into distinct layers. The platelet-rich fraction is then aspirated and prepared for therapeutic use.

- *Single-spin versus double-spin methods*: Double-spin methods generally yield higher platelet concentrations.
- *Leukocyte-rich PRP versus leukocyte-poor PRP:* Controversy exists regarding which is superior; leukocytes may provide additional growth factors but also trigger inflammation.
- *Activation:* PRP can be activated with calcium chloride or thrombin to release growth factors before injection, or injected unactivated, allowing in vivo activation.

Growth Factors in Platelet-rich Plasma

Table 1 provides key growth factors in PRP and their functions.

Together, these mediators create a microenvironment conducive to tissue healing, angiogenesis, and regeneration, which underlies the rationale for PRP use in gynecological disorders.

PLATELET-RICH PLASMA IN UTERINE DISORDERS

Thin Endometrium and Asherman's Syndrome

Thin endometrium (<7 mm) is associated with poor implantation rates and recurrent in vitro fertilization (IVF) failures.[2,3] Causes include chronic endometritis, intrauterine adhesions, or repeated curettage. Conventional therapies such as estrogen supplementation, low-dose aspirin, and sildenafil have limited success **(Fig. 2)**.

Platelet-rich plasma has been proposed as a novel strategy due to its ability to:
- Stimulate angiogenesis (via VEGF).
- Promote stromal proliferation (via PDGF).
- Remodel fibrotic tissue (via TGF-β).
- Enhance epithelialization (via EGF).

In *Asherman's syndrome*, where intrauterine adhesions impair endometrial growth, hysteroscopic adhesiolysis combined with intrauterine PRP instillation has shown reduced recurrence and improved menstrual and fertility outcomes.

Repeated Implantation Failure

Repeated implantation failure refers to failure of embryo implantation after transfer of high-quality embryos across multiple IVF cycles. Endometrial receptivity is often compromised in these cases. Studies have shown that intrauterine PRP administration prior to embryo transfer can:
- Increase endometrial thickness.
- Improve uterine blood flow.
- Enhance implantation and clinical pregnancy rates **(Table 2)**.

Clinical studies of PRP in uterine disorders are mentioned in **Table 2**.

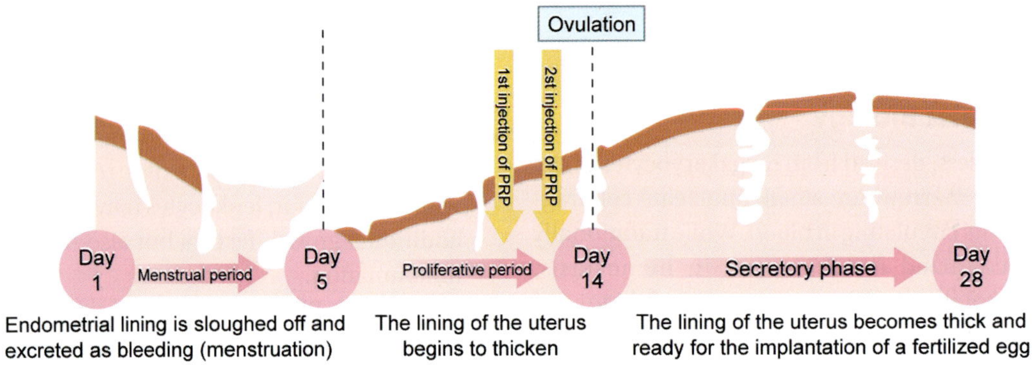

Fig. 2: *Effect and timing of PRP:* PRP infusion → release of growth factor (GF) → angiogenesis, extracellular matrix (ECM) remodeling, epithelial proliferation → thicker, more receptive endometrium → improved implantation.

TABLE 2: Clinical studies of PRP in uterine disorders.

Author, year	*Condition*	*N*	*Intervention*	*Outcome*
Chang et al., 2015	Thin endometrium	5	Intrauterine PRP	Endometrial thickness ↑, pregnancies achieved
Zadehmodarres et al., 2017	RIF	20	Intrauterine PRP	Higher implantation and pregnancy rates
Singh et al., 2019	Asherman's	30	Adhesiolysis + PRP	Reduced adhesion recurrence, restored menstruation

PLATELET-RICH PLASMA IN OVARIAN DISORDERS

Premature Ovarian Insufficiency

Premature ovarian insufficiency affects women under 40 with ovarian follicle depletion or dysfunction. Treatment options are limited, with donor oocytes being the standard in IVF. PRP has been proposed to "rejuvenate" ovarian tissue by:

- Enhancing local angiogenesis
- Supplying anti-apoptotic signals to residual follicles
- Potentially activating dormant primordial follicles

Pilot studies have reported resumption of menstruation, improved serum AMH levels, and even spontaneous pregnancies following intraovarian PRP injections.[4,5]

Poor Ovarian Reserve and Advanced Maternal Age

In women with diminished ovarian reserve or older reproductive age, ovarian response to stimulation is often poor.[6] Intraovarian PRP administration has been studied to improve ovarian performance. Results remain mixed, with some reports showing improved follicular recruitment and live births, while others found no significant benefit **(Table 3)**.

METHODS OF PLATELET-RICH PLASMA ADMINISTRATION IN GYNECOLOGY

Intrauterine Infusion Technique

- Typically it is performed in the mid-proliferative phase or just before embryo transfer.
- A soft catheter is used to instill ~0.5–1 mL PRP into the endometrial cavity.
- Ultrasound guidance ensures proper placement.

Ovarian Injection Technique

- It can be performed laparoscopically or via transvaginal ultrasound-guided injection **(Fig. 3)**.
- Small aliquots of PRP (1–2 mL) are injected into multiple sites within the ovarian cortex.
- Complication rates are minimal, though long-term safety remains under investigation.

ADVANTAGES, LIMITATIONS, AND CHALLENGES

Advantages

- Autologous → low risk of immune reaction
- Simple, outpatient-based procedure

TABLE 3: Clinical studies of PRP in ovarian disorders.

Author, Year	*Condition*	*N*	*Intervention*	*Outcome*
Sills et al., 2018	POI	8	Ovarian PRP injection	2 pregnancies, AMH ↑
Pantos et al., 2019	Poor ovarian reserve	30	Intraovarian PRP	Antral follicle count ↑
Sfakianoudis et al., 2020	Advanced age infertility	60	PRP	Resumed menstruation in some, live births reported

(AMH: anti-Müllerian hormone; POI: premature ovarian insufficiency)

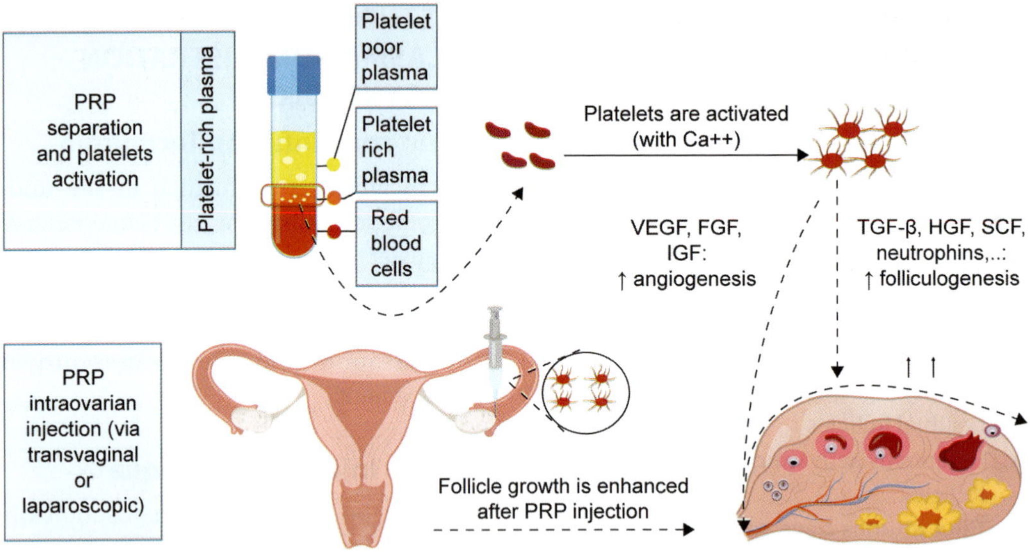

Fig. 3: PRP injection into ovary → release of IGF-1, VEGF, PDGF → angiogenesis + anti-apoptosis → dormant follicle activation → possible oocyte growth.

- Relatively low cost compared to stem cell therapy
- Potential to restore fertility in previously untreatable conditions

Limitations

- Lack of standardized PRP preparation protocols
- Small sample sizes and heterogeneous methodologies in current studies
- Mostly short-term outcomes; limited data on live birth rates
- Placebo effect and natural fluctuations in ovarian/endometrial function may confound results.

Ethical and Safety Concerns

- Premature clinical adoption without large randomized controlled trials (RCTs)
- Unknown long-term risks, especially with intraovarian injections
- Patient counseling must emphasize experimental nature.

FUTURE PERSPECTIVES

- *Combination therapies:* PRP with stem cells or granulocyte colony-stimulating factor (G-CSF)
- *Controlled delivery systems:* Hydrogels, scaffolds, or nanotechnology to sustain growth factor release
- *Personalized PRP:* Tailoring PRP formulations (platelet concentration, leukocyte inclusion) to specific conditions
- *Larger randomized trials:* Needed to define efficacy, standardize protocols, and evaluate long-term reproductive outcomes

CONCLUSION

Platelet-rich plasma represents an exciting intersection of regenerative medicine and reproductive biology. Its ability to deliver autologous growth factors directly to uterine or ovarian tissue provides a biologically plausible means of enhancing regeneration and improving fertility.

Evidence to date suggests potential benefits in *thin endometrium, Asherman's syndrome, RIF, POI, and poor ovarian reserve,* but current studies are limited by small sample sizes, heterogeneity, and lack of long-term follow-up.

As research evolves, PRP may establish itself as a valuable adjunct in fertility treatment, potentially transforming the management of previously refractory gynecological conditions. However, until robust randomized trials confirm its efficacy and safety, clinicians must approach PRP as an *experimental therapy,* offering it with appropriate patient counseling and within ethical frameworks.

REFERENCES

1. Chang Y, Li J, Chen Y, Wei L, Yang X, Shi Y. Autologous platelet-rich plasma promotes endometrial growth and improves pregnancy outcome during in vitro fertilization. Int J Clin Exp Med. 2015;8(1):1286-90.
2. Zadehmodarres S, Salehpour S, Saharkhiz N, Nazari L. Treatment of thin endometrium with autologous platelet-rich plasma: a pilot study. JBRA Assist Reprod. 2017;21(1):54-6.
3. Singh N, Mohanty S, Seth T, Shankar M, Bhaskaran S, Dharmendra S. Autologous platelet-rich plasma for treatment of thin endometrium in infertility patients: A pilot study. J Hum Reprod Sci. 2019;12(3):208-14.
4. Sills ES, Rickers NS, Li X, Palermo GD. First data on safety and efficacy of autologous platelet-rich plasma for ovarian rejuvenation. Hum Reprod Open. 2018;2018(3):hoy006.
5. Pantos K, Simopoulou M, Pantou A, Rapani A, Tsioulou P, Nitsos N, et al. A case series on platelet-rich plasma revolutionary management of poor responders. Front Endocrinol (Lausanne). 2019;10:806.
6. Sfakianoudis K, Simopoulou M, Grigoriadis S, Pantou A, Rapani A, Nitsos N, et al. Autologous platelet-rich plasma treatment enables resumption of menses in patients with premature menopause. Hum Fertil. 2020;23(1):1-8.

CHAPTER 21

Lifestyle Modifications and Stress Management for Infertility Patients

Neharika Malhotra, Jaideep Malhotra

INTRODUCTION

Infertility affects nearly 10–15% of couples worldwide, representing a complex interplay between biological, environmental, and psychosocial factors **(Fig. 1)**. While advances in assisted reproductive technology (ART) have improved outcomes, nonmedical determinants such as lifestyle choices and stress profoundly influence both natural conception and ART success rates **(Fig. 2)**. Addressing these modifiable factors forms an essential component of comprehensive infertility management.[1]

LIFESTYLE FACTORS INFLUENCING FERTILITY

Body Weight and Nutrition

Both undernutrition and obesity adversely affect fertility **(Table 1)**. Adipose tissue influences the hypothalamic-pituitary-gonadal (HPG) axis through leptin and insulin pathways.[1] In women, obesity is associated with anovulation, PCOS, and reduced ART success. In men, obesity leads to altered testosterone and estrogen balance, decreased sperm count, and motility.[2]

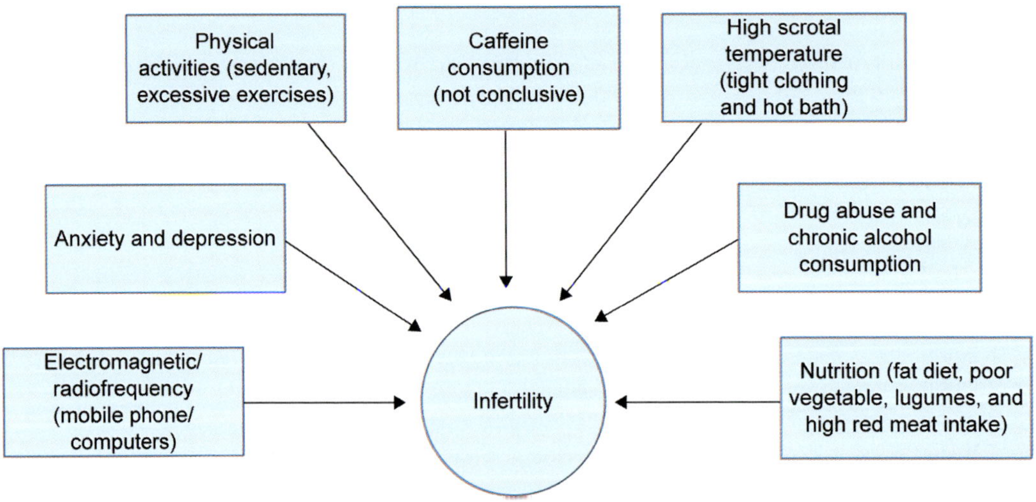

Fig. 1: Causes of infertility.

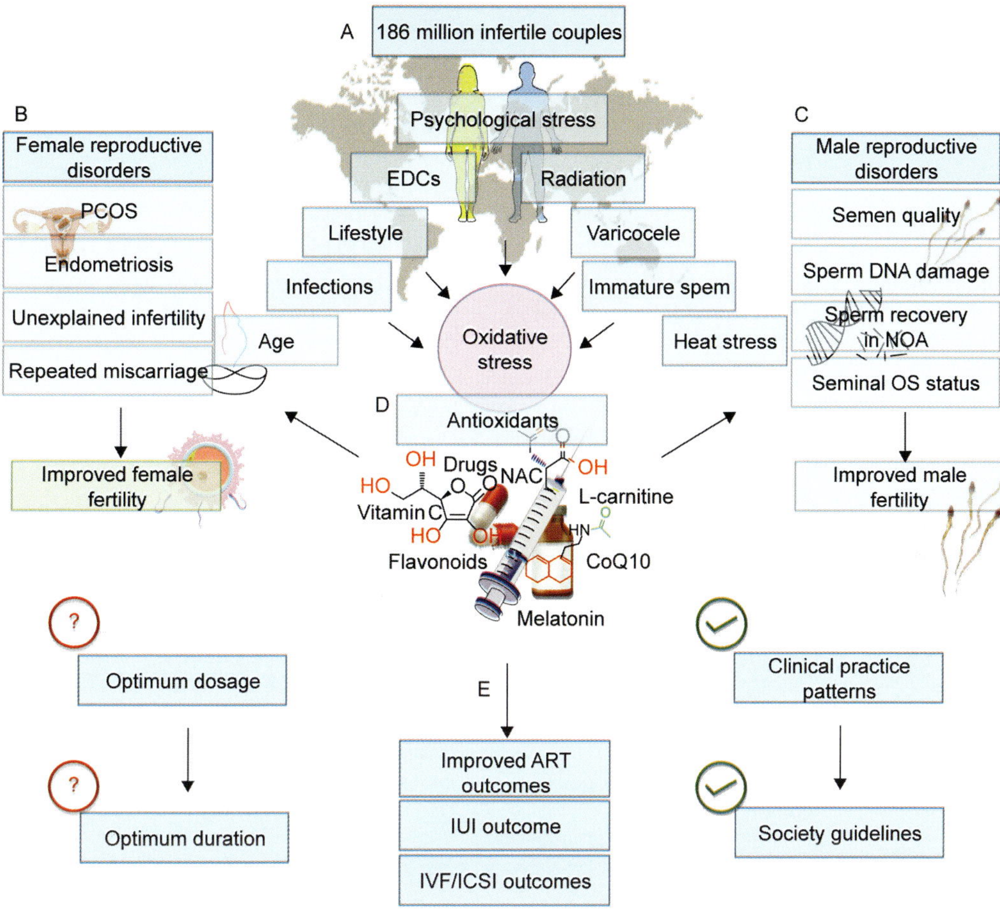

Fig. 2: Impact of oxidative stress on infertility and the role of antioxidants in improving reproductive outcomes. Oxidative stress, influenced by factors such as psychological stress, endocrine-disrupting chemicals (EDCs), radiation, varicocele, infections, age, and lifestyle, affects both male and female fertility (A). In females (B), oxidative stress contributes to conditions like polycystic ovary syndrome (PCOS), endometriosis, unexplained infertility, and recurrent miscarriage, while in males (C), it impacts semen quality, sperm DNA integrity, nonobstructive azoospermia (NOA), and seminal oxidative stress status. Antioxidant therapy, including vitamins, flavonoids, N-acetylcysteine (NAC), L-carnitine, and coenzyme Q10 (CoQ10), plays a crucial role in mitigating oxidative stress and improving both male and female fertility (D). However, determining the optimum dosage and duration of antioxidant therapy remains a challenge. Antioxidants have also been shown to enhance outcomes in assisted reproductive technologies (ART), such as intrauterine insemination (IUI) and *in vitro* fertilization/intracytoplasmic sperm injection (IVF/ICSI), contributing to the development of clinical guidelines for infertility management (E).

Dietary interventions such as the Mediterranean diet rich in whole grains, fruits, vegetables, fish, and olive oil are linked to improved fertility outcomes. Reducing trans fats and refined carbohydrates while increasing omega-3 fatty acids and antioxidants (vitamin C, E, selenium, zinc) supports gamete quality **(Table 2)**.

TABLE 1: The effect of several nutritional factors and dietary patterns on female reproductive health.

Nutrients	*Study type/population*	*Findings*	*Evidence*
Proteins	• Cohort study/women reporting ovulatory infertility[10] • Animal study/mice[11] • Cross-sectional study/women cohort	• Animal proteins increased the risk of ovulatory disorders[10] • Low dietary protein improves fertility rate[11] • High soy intake decreases likelihood of pregnancy	+ ± +
Carbohydrates	*Sugars*: • Cohort study/premenopausal women • Animal study/lactating cattle	• High sugar intake is associated with infertility and low rate of pregnancy development	++
	Fibers: • Cohort study/couples attempting to conceive • Cohort study/women (18–44 years)	• Increased chance of conception • Decreased concentration of reproductive hormones and increased risk of anovulation	±
Fats	*PUFA*: • Animal study/female mice • Cohort study/women undergoing IVF/ICSI • Cohort study/women (18–44 years)	• Intake improves oocyte quality and embryo implantation rates • Sea-food ω-3 PUFA associated with increased progesterone concentration; DHA associated with decreased risk of anovulation	++
	Trans fatty acids: • Cohort study/premenopausal women • RCTs/overweight women, healthy men	• Increased intake associated with increased risk of infertility • Negative impact on ovarian function due to insulin resistance and increased inflammation	++
Vitamins	*Multivitamins*: Cohort study/ premenopausal women	• Supplementation inversely correlates with ovulatory dysfunction	+
	Folate: Cohort study/ premenopausal women	• Increased luteal progesterone levels and reduced risk of sporadic anovulation	++
	Vitamin D: • Animal study/rats • RCT/women with history of pregnancy loss • Cohort study/healthy women	• Deficiency associated with reduced fertility rates • No association found between vitamin D and female fertility	±
Minerals	*Iron*: Cohort study/women with history of infertility	• Supplementation associated with decreased risk of ovulatory infertility	+
	Zinc: • Animal studies/rats, rhesus monkey • Cohort study/nulliparous women	• Deficiency causes abnormal menstrual cycles, longer time to pregnancy, and reduced pregnancy rates	++

Contd...

Contd...

Nutrients	Study type/population	Findings	Evidence
	Selenium: Cohort study/nulliparous women	• Low serum concentration associated with increased risk of subfertility and longer time to pregnancy	+
Dietary pattern	*Mediterranean diet*: • Cohort study/healthy women • Cross-sectional study/healthy women[33]	• Reduced risk of ovulatory disorders (66%) and other infertility (27%) • Improved ovarian morphology and ovarian function	++
	Western-like diet: Animal study/macaques	• Low follicle survival rate and reduced androstenedione and estradiol levels	+

(PUFA: polyunsaturated fatty acids; RCT: randomized controlled trial)

TABLE 2: The role of nutrigenomics, nutri-epigenetics and diet–gut microbiome axis in influencing ART outcomes.

Nutrients	Study type/population	Nutrigenomics and nutrigenetics	Nutri-epigenetics	Diet–gut microbiome
Fats	PUFA: • Animal study/mice SFA: • Animal study/mice	• PUFA intake is associated with upregulation of genes involved in folliculogenesis (*BMPER, FLT4, BDNF, CKR1, AGT*), ovulation (*CCR3, PTX3, AGT*), and steroidogenesis (*CRHR1, AGT, BDNF*) • SFA intake is associated with downregulation of the embryonic gene *TWIST1* and differential expression of ovulation genes (*EDN2, TNFAIP6, ERRFIL, PRKG2, NFIL6, EDN2*, and *NR4A1*)	No evidence available	No evidence available
Carbo-hydrates	• Animal study/*Drosophila melanogaster* • Cell model/Bovine fibroblast cell line	High sucrose diet is associated with decreased expression of antioxidant and mitochondrial genes, impairing oocyte maturation	Low carbohydrate intake increases levels of BOHB, which is associated with elevated H3K9ac levels, leading to enhanced *FOXO3A* expression in the blastocyst	No evidence available

Contd...

Contd...

Nutrients	*Study type/ population*	*Nutrigenomics and nutrigenetics*	*Nutri-epigenetics*	*Diet–gut microbiome*
Protein	Cross-sectional study/women undergoing IVF	No evidence available	No evidence available	Animal protein-derived TMAO is decreased in follicular fluid of oocytes developing high-quality embryos
Fibers	RCT/infertile women undergoing IVF	No evidence available	No evidence available	Fiber intake is associated with increased abundance of *Bifidobacterium*, decreased abundance of *Paraprevotella* and *Blautia*, and increased ART success rate
Micro-nutrients	*Vitamin D*: • RCT/infertile women candidates for IVF; women undergoing ART with vitamin D deficiency *Vitamin B:* • Animal study/D. melanogaster • Animal study/ Black × Holstein F1 cows *Folate:* RCT/women with history of miscarriage *Selenium and zinc:* • RCT/women with PCOS candidates for IVF • Animal study/mice	• Vitamin D supplementation improves glycemic profile via upregulation of *PPAR-γ, GLUT-1, LDLR, VDR, GSTA3,* and *IL-21R*; and downregulation of *PTGS2, AGER*, and *RXRB* • Folate supplementation reduces homocysteine concentration in women homozygous for the *MTHFR* gene *(677C>T)* • *Selenium supplementation:* Upregulation of *VEGF, PPAR-γ*, and *GLUT-1;* downregulation of *IL-1, TNF-α*, and *LDLR*	• Biotin deficiency is associated with decreased biotinylated histones and reduced fertility rates • Vitamin B mixture increases methylation level of H3K27 • Reduced DNA methylation variance in *KCNQ1OT1, SNRPN,* and *PEG1;* increased global DNA methylation levels in both embryonic and placental tissues • Zinc deficiency is associated with decreased histone H3K4 and global DNA methylation in oocytes	No evidence available

(GLUT-1: glucose transporter type 1; IL-21R: interleukin-21 receptor; IVF: in vitro fertilization; LDLR: low-density lipoprotein receptor; PCOS: polycystic ovary syndrome; PPARγ: peroxisome proliferator-activated receptor gamma; RCT: randomized controlled trial; VEGF: vascular endothelial growth factor; VDR: vitamin D receptor)

Source: Kohil A, Chouliaras S, Alabduljabbar S, Lakshmanan AP, Ahmed SH, Awwad J, et al. Female infertility and diet, is there a role for a personalized nutritional approach in assisted reproductive technologies? A Narrative Review. Front Nutr. 2022;9:927972.

Physical Activity

Moderate physical activity enhances insulin sensitivity, reduces inflammation, and optimizes reproductive function. Excessive exercise, however, may disrupt the HPG axis leading to amenorrhea and anovulation. For men, a sedentary lifestyle and prolonged sitting increase scrotal temperature and oxidative stress, impairing spermatogenesis. Recommended: 150 minutes/week of moderate-intensity aerobic activity (WHO guidelines).[3,4]

Smoking, Alcohol, and Substance Use

Nicotine and cadmium from tobacco are gonadotoxins that impair ovarian reserve, sperm DNA integrity, and IVF outcomes. Alcohol alters gonadal steroids and increases miscarriage risk. Illicit drugs such as marijuana and cocaine are associated with oligozoospermia and anovulation.[5] Cessation is advised for both partners at least 3 months before conception.

Caffeine and Environmental Exposures

High caffeine intake (>300 mg/day) may delay conception. Exposure to endocrine-disrupting chemicals [bisphenol A (BPA), phthalates, pesticides] affects gametogenesis and embryo quality. Encourage use of glass or steel containers and organic foods.[5,6]

Sleep and Circadian Rhythms

Sleep deprivation disrupts melatonin secretion and gonadotropin release. Night shift workers have higher infertility prevalence. Recommend 7–8 hours of regular nocturnal sleep with reduced screen time before bed.[7]

PSYCHOLOGICAL STRESS AND INFERTILITY

Infertility is a potent psychological stressor leading to anxiety and depression. Chronic stress activates the hypothalamic-pituitary-adrenal (HPA) axis, increasing cortisol which suppresses GnRH pulsatility and impairs reproduction.

Stress Management Strategies

Mind-body interventions such as cognitive behavioral therapy (CBT), mindfulness-based stress reduction (MBSR), and yoga improve psychological resilience and ART outcomes. Group therapy and relaxation techniques (guided imagery, breathing exercises) reduce stress hormones. Integrating daily mindfulness routines creates a holistic fertility approach.[8,10]

Clinical Implementation

Lifestyle and stress management should be part of preconception counseling **(Fig. 3)**. Use validated stress scales (Fertility Problem Inventory, Perceived Stress Scale). Offer multidisciplinary support from nutritionists, psychologists, and yoga therapists.[8,9]

CONCLUSION

- Lifestyle and stress significantly influence reproductive health **(Fig. 4)**.
- Balanced diet, moderate exercise, and elimination of harmful substances enhance fertility.
- Stress reduction improves conception and ART outcomes.
- Holistic, patient-centered approaches are vital.[11]

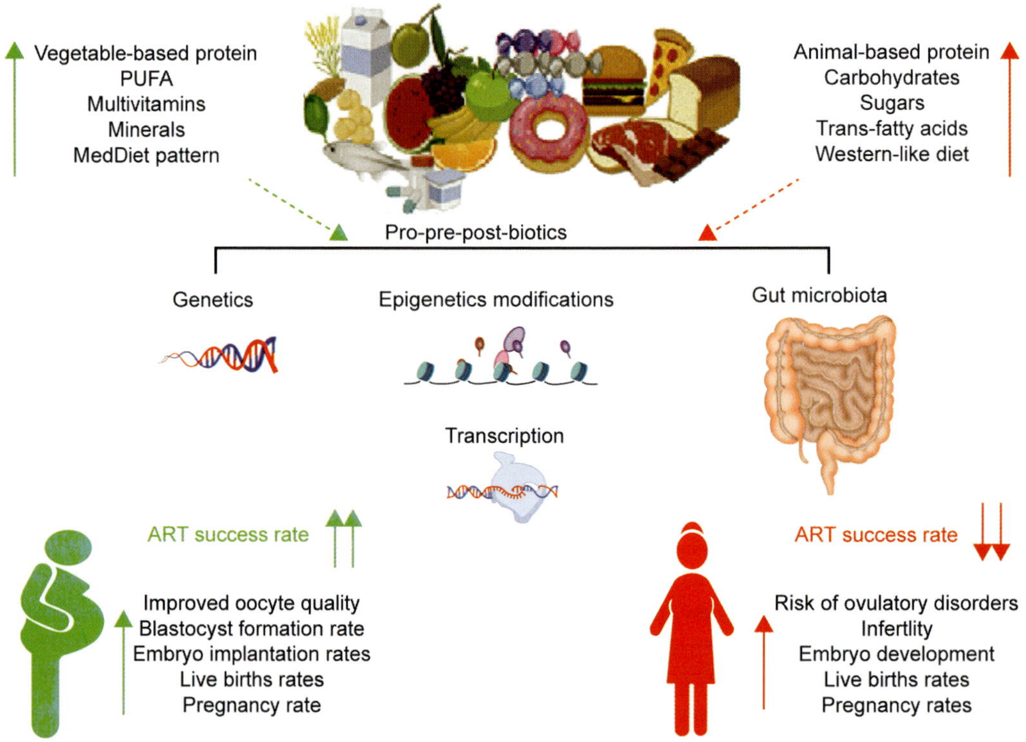

Fig. 3: Graphical summary of the impact of nutrition on female fertility.
Source: Created with BioRender.com.

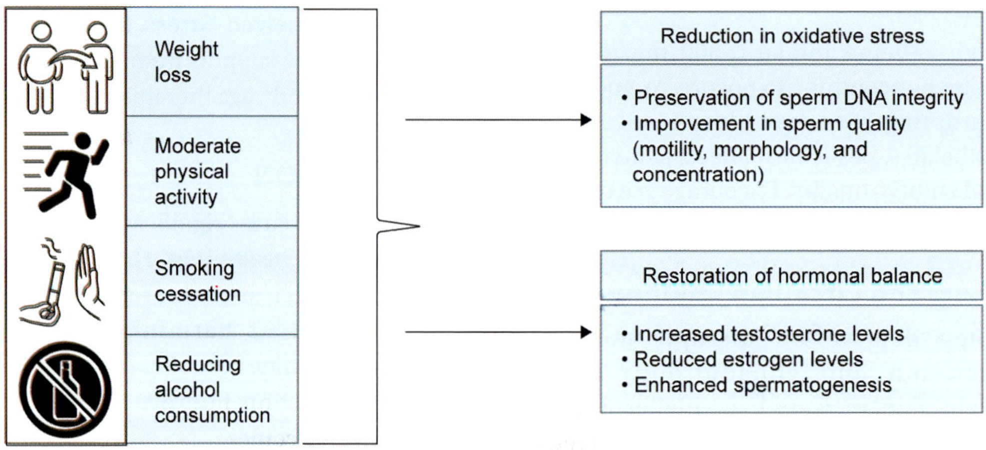

Fig. 4: Lifestyle modifications to reduce oxidative stress, restore hormonal balance, and enhance male fertility.

REFERENCES

1. Chavarro JE, Rich-Edwards JW, Rosner BA, Willett WC. Diet and lifestyle in the prevention of ovulatory disorder infertility. Obstet Gynecol. 2007;110(5):1050-8.
2. Lynch CD, Sundaram R, Maisog JM, Sweeney AM, Buck Louis GM. Preconception stress increases the risk of infertility: results from a couple-based prospective cohort study—the LIFE study. Hum Reprod. 2014;29(5):1067-75.
3. Domar AD, Rooney KL, Wiegand B, Orav EJ, Alper MM, Berger BM, et al. Impact of a group mind/body intervention on pregnancy rates in IVF patients. Fertil Steril. 2011;95(7):2269-73.
4. Palomba S, Falbo A, Valli B, Morini D, Villani MT, Nicoli A, et al. Physical activity before IVF and ICSI cycles in infertile obese women: an observational cohort study. Reprod Biomed Online. 2014;29(2):138-46.
5. Sharma R, Biedenharn KR, Fedor JM, Agarwal A. Lifestyle factors and reproductive health: taking control of your fertility. Reprod Biol Endocrinol. 2013;11:66.
6. Rooney KL, Domar AD. The relationship between stress and infertility. Dialogues Clin Neurosci. 2018;20(1):41-7.
7. Eskew AM, Gurumurthy S. The impact of dietary patterns on fertility treatment outcome. Hum Reprod Update. 2011;17(2): 197-207.
8. World Health Organization. Global Recommendations on Physical Activity for Health. Geneva: WHO; 2020.
9. Vessa B, Perlman B, McGovern PG, Morelli SS. Endocrine disruptors and female fertility: a review of pesticide and plasticizer effects. F S Rep. 2022;3(2):86-90.
10. Kalra S, Baruah MP. Stress and reproductive endocrinology. Indian J Endocrinol Metab. 2018;22(3):258-62.
11. Torkel S, Moran L, Wang R, Villani A, Mantzioris E, Norman RJ, et al. Barriers and enablers to a healthy lifestyle in people with infertility: a qualitative descriptive study. Reprod Biol Endocrinol. 2025;23(1):52.

SECTION 7

Clinical Challenges and Controversies

22. **Managing Unexplained and Idiopathic Infertility**
Aditi Nadkarni

23. **In Vitro Fertilization in Low-resource Settings: Challenges, Innovations, and Global Lessons**
Rutuja R Athawale

CHAPTER 22

Managing Unexplained and Idiopathic Infertility

Aditi Nadkarni

INTRODUCTION

Unexplained and idiopathic infertility remains one of the most debated entities in reproductive medicine. Despite advances in diagnostics, 10–30% of couples are still classified as having "unexplained infertility" after a standard work-up.[1,2] This uncertainty often leads to dilemmas: Should clinicians recommend expectant management, ovulation induction with intrauterine insemination (IUI), or move directly to in vitro fertilization (IVF)?[3,4]

From 2019 to 2024, several high-quality randomized controlled trials (RCTs), systematic reviews, and guideline updates [American Society for Reproductive Medicine (ASRM), European Society of Human Reproduction and Embryology (ESHRE), and National Institute for Health and Care Excellence (NICE) have redefined how we approach these cases. This chapter synthesizes recent evidence, explores controversies [endometrial receptivity analysis (ERA), immunology, artificial intelligence (AI), sperm deoxyribonucleic acid (DNA) fragmentation], compares international guidelines, and illustrates clinical decision-making through practical scenarios.[4-8]

DEFINITIONS AND EPIDEMIOLOGY

- *Unexplained infertility:* Failure to conceive after 12 months (6 months if age >35 years) of unprotected intercourse, despite normal ovulation, tubal patency, and semen parameters.
- *Idiopathic infertility:* Often used interchangeably but may suggest subtle abnormalities undetected by standard tests (e.g., gamete dysfunction and endometrial receptivity defects).

Globally, unexplained infertility accounts for *15–25% of infertility cases*, with prevalence slightly higher in high-income countries. *Idiopathic infertility contributes an additional ~10%.* Together, unexplained and idiopathic infertility may represent up to one-third of infertility cases. Reporting prevalence alongside *fertility percentages* provides a clearer clinical picture for prognosis and counseling.

PATHOPHYSIOLOGICAL HYPOTHESES AND POSSIBLE CAUSES

- *Gamete quality defects:* Subtle oocyte dysfunction, sperm DNA fragmentation index (DFI).[1,2]
- *Fertilization and embryo development:* Defective zona binding, mitochondrial DNA deletions.[3,4]
- *Endometrial receptivity:* Window of implantation shifts, homeobox A10 (HOXA-10) dysregulation, microbiome dysbiosis.[5-7]

- *Immunological factors*: Altered uNK activity, Th1/Th2 imbalance, antibodies.[8-10]

Expanded possible causes include:

- Ovarian factors
- Endocrine factors
- Immunological factors
- Tubal and peritoneal factors
- Cervical factors
- Male factors
- Embryo-related factors

DIAGNOSTIC APPROACH (FLOWCHART 1)

- *Step 1:* Basic work-up
  - *Ovulation assessment* → midluteal progesterone levels or ultrasound monitoring.[36]
  - *Semen analysis* → performed according to World Health Organization (*WHO) 2021 criteria.*[37]

Flowchart 1: Diagnostic algorithm.

• Start

↓

Couple presents with infertility (>12 months; >6 months if female >35 years)

↓

Basic work-up:

Ovulation: Mid-luteal progesterone/ultrasound
• *Semen analysis:* WHO 2021
• *Tubal patency:* HSG/saline sonohysterography/hysterolaparoscopy (gold standard)
If abnormal → manage specific abnormality

↓

If normal → diagnose as unexplained infertility

↓

Extended testing (optional):
- Sperm DNA fragmentation
- ERA/receptivaDx (CBCL-6, CD138; for RPL, progesterone resistance)
- Immunological/thrombophilia screen
- Antisperm antibodies
- Microbiome profiling

↓

Choose management:
1. Expectant management
2. Ovulation induction + IUI
3. IVF/ICSI

↓

Continuous counseling and psychological support

- No → manage specific abnormality

[CBCL-6: child behavior checklist 6-18 (referring to the age range of 6 to 18 years); CD138: cluster of differentiation 138; DNA: deoxyribonucleic acid; ICSI: intracytoplasmic sperm injection; IUI: intrauterine insemination; IVF: in vitro fertilization; HSG: hysterosalpingogram; RPL: recurrent pregnancy loss; WHO: World Health Organization]

- *Tubal patency assessment* →
  - Hysterosalpingography (HSG)
  - *Saline sonohysterography* (minimally invasive option),
  - *Hysterolaparoscopy* (considered the *gold standard*).[38]
- *Step 2:* Extended evaluation (selective, controversial)
  - *Sperm DNA fragmentation (SDF) testing.*
  - *Endometrial receptivity assays (ERA, ReceptivaDx)* → include markers such as B-cell lymphoma 6 (*BCL-6*) and Cluster of differentiation 138 (*CD138*), which may be useful in:
    - Implantation failure,
    - *Recurrent pregnancy loss (RPL)*
    - *Progesterone resistance*
  - *Immunological testing* → includes screening for *antisperm antibodies.*
  - *Thrombophilia screening.*
  - *Microbiome profiling* → emerging tool to evaluate uterine and vaginal flora balance.

MANAGEMENT STRATEGIES AND EVIDENCE (TABLES 1 AND 2)

- Expectant management: 1–4% per cycle, 20–30% in 12 months (Smith 2021).[2]
  - *Pregnancy rates: 1–4% per cycle, 20–30% at 12 months.*
  - Best suited for *young couples with a short duration of infertility.*
- Ovulation induction + IUI: LIVE trial (Lancet 2022) shows significant benefit.[3]
  - LIVE (Liraglutide's Effect on Left Ventricular Function) trial (Lancet 2022): Significant benefit in unexplained infertility.
  - *Pregnancy rates: 7–12% per cycle, 30–40% cumulative at 12 months.*

TABLE 1: Comparative pregnancy rates in unexplained infertility.

Strategy	*Pregnancy rate per cycle (%)*	*Cumulative 12-month pregnancy (%)*	*Notes*
Expectant management	1–4	20–30	Best for young couples, short infertility[2]
IUI + stimulation	7–12	30–40	Modest benefit; cost-effective first line[3]
IVF/ICSI	30–40	50–60	Highest efficacy; invasive and costl[4-6]

(ICSI: intracytoplasmic sperm injection; IUI: intrauterine insemination; IVF: in vitro fertilization)

TABLE 2: Comparison between unexplained infertility and idiopathic infertility.

Parameter definition	• Unexplained infertility[7] • Infertility despite normal standard evaluation[9]	• Idiopathic Infertility[8] • Subtle undetected defects (gamete, endometrium, immune, etc.)[10]
Prevalence	15–25% of infertility cases	10 of infertility cases[11]
Causes Prognosis (natural)	• Diagnostic exclusion • Fair, better in younger couples	• Possible underlying factors (oocyte, sperm, endometrium, and immune) • Slightly poorer if underlying subtle causes exist
Management[24]	Stepwise: Expectant → IUI → IVF[12]	Similarly, but IVF may be considered earlier in poor responders[13]

(ICSI: intracytoplasmic sperm injection; IUI: intrauterine insemination; IVF: in vitro fertilization)

- Represents a *modest but cost-effective first-line treatment.*[39]
- *In vitro fertilization (IVF)/intracytoplasmic sperm injection (ICSI):* 50–60% cumulative pregnancy in 12 months, especially in patients >35 years.[5]
  - Highest efficacy among available treatments.
  - *Pregnancy rates*: *30–40% per cycle, 50–60% cumulative at 12 months,* especially for women >35 years or those with failed IUI.
  - However, it is *invasive and costly*.

EMERGING INTERVENTIONS

- Time-lapse embryo monitoring—benefit unproven.
- AI-based embryo selection—promising, Nat Med 2023.
- Microbiome modulation—under study.
- Immunomodulation [intravenous immunoglobulin (IVIG) and intralipids]—inconsistent evidence.

CONTROVERSIES IN DEPTH

- *ERA testing:* No live birth benefit, ASRM against routine use.
- *SDF:* Associated with miscarriage, but not recommended routinely.
- *Immunology:* Not recommended outside trials.
- *AI in embryology:* Promising but costly.

GUIDELINE COMPARISONS (AMERICAN SOCIETY FOR REPRODUCTIVE MEDICINE, EUROPEAN SOCIETY OF HUMAN REPRODUCTION AND EMBRYOLOGY, AND NATIONAL INSTITUTE FOR HEALTH AND CARE EXCELLENCE)[25]

- *ASRM 2023:* Avoid ERA/SDF, starting with IUI.
  - Does not recommend routine use of ERA, immunological testing, or SDF in unexplained infertility.[14]
  - Suggests superovulation with IUI as a first-line therapy in younger women.[15]
  - IVF should be considered after 3–4 failed IUIs or in women >38 years.[16]
- *ESHRE 2023:* ERA/SDF optional in select cases, IVF earlier >38 years.
  - Emphasizes individualized treatment, discourages routine use of advanced diagnostics, but allows selective use in poor-prognosis patients.[17]
  - IVF may be considered earlier in older women or when the duration exceeds 2 years.[18]
- *NICE 2022:* IVF after 2 yrs, discourages immunology/thrombophilia testing.[40]
  - Recommends IVF after 2 years of unexplained infertility in women <40 years.[19,26]
  - Does not support ERA, immunological testing, or thrombophilia screening in routine practice.[20]

CLINICAL SCENARIOS AND DECISION-MAKING

- Case 1: 29 years, 1 year infertility → Expectant/IUI.
  Management: Expectant management or up to three to four cycles of ovulation induction with IUI is reasonable.[21]
- *Case 2:* 36 years, 2 years of infertility → IUI then IVF.
  Management: Initial trial of three cycles of ovulation induction with IUI, followed by IVF if unsuccessful.[22]
- *Case 3*: 40 years, 1 year of infertility → Direct IVF.
  Management: Proceed directly to IVF, as success rates with expectant management or IUI are very low in this age group.[23]

BOX 1: Clinical pearls.[27-35]

- Confirm true *unexplained infertility* only after thorough evaluation
- Expectant management remains a valid option in *younger couples* with a good prognosis
- *IUI* is a cost-effective first-line therapy
- *IVF* is most effective, particularly in women >35 years or following failed IUI
- Use advanced diagnostics *selectively* (avoid unnecessary investigations)
- Always address *psychological support and counseling* as part of care

CONCLUSION

Unexplained infertility remains one of the most perplexing diagnoses in reproductive medicine, accounting for up to one-third of infertility cases worldwide.[1,2] It is fundamentally a diagnosis of exclusion, reflecting the limitations of conventional diagnostics rather than the absence of pathology.[3] Subtle defects in gametes, fertilization, implantation, or early embryogenesis are likely responsible in many cases but remain undetectable with current testing.[4]

From a clinical perspective, UI requires a pragmatic, stepwise approach. In couples with a good prognosis (younger age, short infertility duration), expectant management may be appropriate.[5] Lifestyle modification and psychological support are universal recommendations.[6] OI combined with IUI is widely accepted as a cost-effective first-line therapy, particularly in North America and Europe.[7] IVF remains the most effective treatment when the prognosis is poor, when IUI has failed, or in older women.[8] ICSI should be reserved for couples with failed fertilization in IVF or proven subtle sperm dysfunction and not used empirically in UI[9] **(Box 1)**.

Guideline consensus highlights three essential principles:

- Personalization of care based on prognosis.
- Cost-effectiveness in selecting interventions.
- Evidence-based practice, avoiding unproven therapies, such as immunological interventions.[10-12]

Beyond the biological aspects, clinicians must recognize that UI carries a disproportionate psychological and emotional burden. Counseling and holistic support should be integrated into care alongside medical treatments.[13] Looking forward, advances in genomics, proteomics, endometrial receptivity testing, and AI-driven predictive models are expected to improve diagnostics and shift the paradigm from unexplained infertility to better-classified, personalized subgroups.[14,15] In summary, while UI is frustrating for patients and clinicians alike, adherence to guideline-based, stepwise management combined with emerging technologies and empathetic care offers the best chance of improving reproductive outcomes and patient well-being.[16]

REFERENCES

1. WHO. Infertility definitions and terminology. Geneva: World Health Organization; 2020.
2. Practice Committee of the American Society for Reproductive Medicine. Definition and evaluation of unexplained infertility. Fertil Steril. 2020;113(2):305-9.
3. Ray A, Shah A, Gudi A, Homburg R. Unexplained infertility: an update and review. Reprod Biomed Online. 2012;24(6): 591-602.
4. Gurunath S, Pandian Z, Anderson RA, Bhattacharya S. Defining infertility: a systematic review of prevalence studies. Hum Reprod Update. 2011;17(5):575-88.

5. ESHRE Guideline Group on Unexplained Infertility. ESHRE guideline: unexplained infertility. Hum Reprod Open. 2023;2023(1):hoad002.
6. Bhattacharya S, Johnson NP. Should 'unexplained infertility' be explained? BMJ. 2015;351:h5877.
7. ICMR Task Force on Infertility. Epidemiology of infertility in India. Indian J Med Res. 2019;150(6):586-95.
8. Snick HK, Snick TS, Evers JL, Collins JA. The spontaneous pregnancy prognosis in untreated subfertile couples: the Walcheren primary care study. Hum Reprod. 1997;12(7):1582-8.
9. van der Steeg JW, Steures P, Eijkemans MJ, Habbema JD, Hompes PG, Broekmans FJ, et al. Predictive value of pregnancy history in subfertile couples: results from a nationwide cohort study in the Netherlands. BMJ. 2008;337:a716.
10. Cousineau TM, Domar AD. Psychological impact of infertility. Best Pract Res Clin Obstet Gynaecol. 2007;21(2):293-308.
11. Greil AL, Slauson-Blevins K, McQuillan J. The experience of infertility: a review of recent literature. Sociol Health Illn. 2010;32(1):140-62.
12. Collins JA, Burrows EA, Wilan AR. The prognosis for live birth among untreated infertile couples. Fertil Steril. 1995;64(1):22-28.
13. Broekmans FJ, Soules MR, Fauser BC. Ovarian aging: mechanisms and clinical consequences. Endocr Rev. 2009;30(5):465-93.
14. Lessey BA. Assessment of endometrial receptivity. Fertil Steril. 2011;96(3):522-29.
15. Marcoux S, Maheux R, Bérubé S. Laparoscopic surgery in infertile women with minimal or mild endometriosis. N Engl J Med. 1997;337(4):217-22.
16. Horne AW, Saunders PT. Inflammation and infertility: the role of the fallopian tube. Reproduction. 2019;158(5):R189-99.
17. Moreno I, Franasiak JM. Endometrial microbiota—new player in town. Fertil Steril. 2017;108(1):32-9.
18. Zini A, Boman JM, Belzile E, Ciampi A. Sperm DNA damage and pregnancy loss: systematic review and meta-analysis. Hum Reprod. 2008;23(12):2663-8.
19. Agarwal A, Virk G, Ong C, du Plessis SS. Effect of oxidative stress on male reproduction. World J Mens Health. 2014;32(1):1-17.
20. Aitken RJ. Sperm function tests and fertility. Asian J Androl. 2021;23(1):16-22.
21. Palermo G, Joris H, Devroey P, Van Steirteghem AC. Pregnancies after ICSI of a single spermatozoon. Lancet. 1992;340(8810):17-18.
22. Huntriss J, Elder K, Dale B. Epigenetics and Human Assisted Reproduction. In: In-Vitro Fertilization. Cambridge University Press; 2020:331-57.
23. Practice Committee of the ASRM. Immunological factors in unexplained infertility. Fertil Steril. 2018;110(3):387-95.
24. ASRM Practice Committee. Evidence-based management of unexplained infertility. Fertil Steril. 2020;113(2):305-22.
25. ESHRE Guideline Group on UI. ESHRE guideline: unexplained infertility. Hum Reprod Open. 2023;2023(1):hoad002.
26. Dewailly D, Andersen CY, Balen A, Broekmans F, Dilaver N, Fanchin R, et al. Physiology and utility of AMH in women. Hum Reprod Update. 2014;20(3):370-85.
27. Crosignani PG, Collins J, Cooke ID, Diczfalusy E, Rubin BL. Recommendations for infertility investigation. Hum Reprod. 1993;8(5):953-60.
28. WHO. WHO laboratory manual for human semen. 6th ed. Geneva: WHO; 2021.
29. Evers JL. Female subfertility. Lancet. 2002;360(9327):151-9.
30. Showell MG, Mackenzie-Proctor R, Jordan V, Hodgson R, Farquhar C. Antioxidants for male subfertility. Cochrane Database Syst Rev. 2014;12:CD007411.
31. Guzick DS, Sullivan MW, Adamson GD, Cedars MI, Falk RJ, Peterson EP, et al. Efficacy of clomiphene citrate in unexplained infertility. N Engl J Med. 1998;339(8):517-22.
32. Pandian Z, Bhattacharya S, Ozturk O, Serour G, Templeton A. IUI for unexplained subfertility. Cochrane Database Syst Rev. 2020;4(2):CD003357.

33. Steures P, van der Steeg JW, Mol BW, Eijkemans MJ, van der Veen F, Habbema JD, et al. Cumulative pregnancy rates in UI. Hum Reprod. 2004;19(11):2683-7.
34. Bhattacharya S, Harrild K, Mollison J, Wordsworth S, Tay C, Harrold A, et al. CC, IUI, and IVF for unexplained infertility: randomized trial. Lancet. 2008;371(9613):1703-12.
35. Foong SC, Fleetham JA, O'Keane JA, Scott SG, Tough SC, Greene CA. IVF vs ICSI in UI couples: prospective RCT. Fertil Steril. 2006; 86(3):715-719.
36. Collins JA, Burrows EA, Wilan AR. Prognosis for live birth in untreated infertile couples. Fertil Steril. 1995;64(1):22-8.
37. Hunault CC, Habbema JD, Eijkemans MJ, Collins JA, Evers JL, Te Velde ER. Prediction rules for spontaneous pregnancy. Hum Reprod. 2004;19(9):2019-26.
38. Simon C, Gómez C, Cabanillas S, Vladimirov I, Bernal A, Vilella F, et al. ERA-guided embryo transfer vs standard. Fertil Steril. 2020;114(1):238-46.
39. McLernon DJ, Maheshwari A, Lee AJ, Bhattacharya S. IVF live birth prediction model. BMJ. 2016;355:i5735.
40. National Institute for Health and Care Excellence. Fertility problems: assessment and treatment. Clinical guideline [CG156]. London: National Institute for Health and Care Excellence; 2021.

CHAPTER 23

In Vitro Fertilization in Low-resource Settings: Challenges, Innovations, and Global Lessons

Rutuja R Athawale

INTRODUCTION

Infertility has emerged as a significant global health issue with profound social, cultural, and economic consequences. The World Health Organization (WHO) estimates that approximately 17.5% of the global adult population will experience infertility at some point during their reproductive life, making it a major component of reproductive health worldwide.[1] In high-income countries (HICs), advances in assisted reproductive technology (ART), especially in vitro fertilization (IVF), have transformed the prospects for infertile couples. However, in low- and middle-income countries (LMICs), in vitro fertilization (IVF) remains largely aspirational, constrained by financial, infrastructural, and sociocultural barriers.

The paradox of infertility in LMICs lies in the coexistence of growing demand for ART and the stark inequities in access. Unlike in HICs, where IVF has been integrated into health systems or subsidized by governments, most LMIC couples must pay out-of-pocket for treatment, often at catastrophic costs relative to household incomes.[2] The cultural burden is equally significant: in many societies, parenthood is central to marital and social identity, and childlessness is associated with stigma, psychological stress, and gender discrimination.[3]

This chapter examines the epidemiology and burden of infertility in low-resource settings, the sociocultural context, barriers to IVF access, and the innovative strategies being developed to address these challenges. Drawing from global and regional experiences, it explores policy developments, ethical debates, and future directions that can help bridge the divide between cutting-edge IVF science and equitable access.

EPIDEMIOLOGY AND BURDEN OF INFERTILITY IN LOW-RESOURCE SETTINGS

The prevalence of infertility shows considerable global variation. The WHO estimates that infertility affects between 8% and 15% of couples worldwide, with higher rates reported in South Asia, Sub-Saharan Africa, and parts of the Middle East.[1,4] Data from the International Committee for Monitoring Assisted Reproductive Technologies (ICMART) confirm wide disparities in ART utilization, with over 80% of all IVF cycles performed in HICs, while LMICs collectively contribute <10%.[2]

Primary versus Secondary Infertility

Primary infertility, defined as the inability to conceive after one year of unprotected intercourse without any prior pregnancy, is relatively less common in LMICs compared to secondary infertility. Secondary infertility is prevalent due to factors such as untreated reproductive tract infections (RTIs), unsafe abortions, and complications from poor obstetric care.[5] In Sub-Saharan Africa, for instance, up to 85% of infertility cases are secondary.[6]

Male Infertility

Although male factors contribute to nearly half of infertility cases globally, they remain underdiagnosed in LMICs due to stigma and the lack of routine semen analysis facilities.[7] In many societies, infertility is considered a woman's problem, leading to misdirected blame and care-seeking practices.[8]

Demographic and Lifestyle Shifts

Changing demographics and lifestyle patterns in urban LMIC populations are increasing infertility prevalence. Rising obesity, higher prevalence of polycystic ovary syndrome (PCOS), delayed marriage and childbearing, and lifestyle stressors are well-recognized risk factors.[9] In India, PCOS prevalence is estimated at 20–30% among women of reproductive age, significantly contributing to infertility.[10]

Social and Economic Burden

Infertility has severe social and economic implications in LMICs. In many cultures, childlessness leads to marital instability, domestic violence, social exclusion, and mental health issues.[11] Economically, households incur catastrophic expenditures when seeking IVF, often exceeding annual incomes, thereby reinforcing cycles of poverty.[12]

SOCIOCULTURAL DIMENSIONS OF INFERTILITY

The cultural meaning of infertility in LMICs is profound, often shaping treatment-seeking behavior and psychosocial outcomes.

Stigma and Gender Bias

Women disproportionately bear the blame for infertility, even in cases where male factors are responsible. Studies in India, Nigeria, and Egypt show that infertile women are more likely to experience abandonment, verbal and physical abuse, and marital instability.[13,14] The emphasis on motherhood as central to female identity intensifies this stigma.

Value of Children and Son Preference

In many cultures, children are considered essential for social continuity, old-age support, and spiritual fulfillment. In rural South Asia and parts of Africa, son preference remains a strong determinant of reproductive pressure.[15] This influences ART demand, sometimes leading to misuse of technologies for sex selection despite legal prohibitions.[16]

Treatment-seeking Pathways

Couples in LMICs often exhaust informal or traditional remedies before seeking medical interventions. Faith healers, herbalists, and alternative medicine are commonly consulted, delaying timely access to effective care.[17] This delay contributes to a worsened prognosis by the time ART is pursued.

BARRIERS TO IN VITRO FERTILIZATION IN LOW-RESOURCE SETTINGS

Multiple systemic and individual barriers constrain access to IVF in LMICs.

Economic Cost

The most formidable barrier is cost. In India, a single IVF cycle costs between USD 1,800–3,000, equivalent to three to five times the monthly income of an average urban family, and catastrophic for rural households.[18] In sub-Saharan Africa, IVF costs range from USD 2,000–6,000 per cycle, while average annual per capita income is <USD 1,500.[19] Unlike HICs, where insurance or government subsidies are available, <10% of IVF cycles in LMICs are covered by insurance.[20]

Geographic Disparities

In vitro fertilization clinics are concentrated in metropolitan areas. For example, over 80% of India's IVF clinics are in tier-1 cities, leaving vast rural populations underserved. Travel expenses, accommodation, and wage loss exacerbate inequity.

Infrastructure Challenges

IVF requires specialized laboratory infrastructure, including sterile clean rooms, uninterrupted electricity, CO_2 incubators, and high-cost consumables. In rural LMIC hospitals, these resources are often unavailable.[21] Dependence on imported consumables further inflates costs.

Human Resources

A shortage of trained embryologists, reproductive endocrinologists, and ART nurses limits service delivery. The migration of skilled professionals from public to private or urban clinics exacerbates inequities.[22]

Policy and Regulation

While countries like India have enacted ART and Surrogacy Regulation Acts (2021), implementation remains uneven, particularly outside urban centers. In many LMICs, ART practices remain unregulated, raising concerns about safety, quality, and ethics.[23]

Patient-side Barriers

Low awareness, misconceptions about IVF success rates, cultural hesitancy regarding donor gametes, and limited counseling capacity also restrict uptake.

ADAPTATIONS AND INNOVATIONS

Despite barriers, several innovations are helping to adapt IVF for low-resource contexts.

Low-Cost In Vitro Fertilization Models

The Walking Egg Project, pioneered in Belgium and extended to India and Africa, developed simplified IVF culture systems using affordable incubators and basic laboratory infrastructure. These models reduced cycle costs by up to 80% while maintaining success rates of 20–30%.[24] Indian clinics have piloted portable incubators and mild stimulation regimens to lower costs.[25]

Mild Stimulation and Minimal Monitoring

Protocols using clomiphene or letrozole with low-dose gonadotropins minimize drug costs. Limited ultrasound monitoring (two to three scans instead of daily tracking) further reduces expenditure without compromising safety.[26]

Government and Nongovernmental Organization Initiatives

Public hospitals such as AIIMS Delhi and PGIMER Chandigarh offer subsidized ART services.[27,28] Nongovernmental organizations (NGOs) have collaborated with Indian and African clinics to pilot simplified IVF approaches, improving access.[24]

Financing Innovations

Some IVF chains in India and Africa now provide installment-based payment plans, microfinance-linked packages, or insurance-linked models. This has improved affordability for middle- and lower-income families.

Digital and Telehealth Solutions

Telemedicine platforms are increasingly used to reduce travel burdens, enabling consultations, follow-ups, and counseling in remote areas.[29] AI-based embryo and sperm assessment tools are also being adopted in leading LMIC clinics, potentially reducing failed cycles and cumulative costs.[30]

Local Manufacturing and Renewable Energy

Encouraging local production of culture media, consumables, and incubators can reduce dependency on imports. Experimental solar-powered incubators are being tested for rural IVF laboratories in Africa and South Asia.[31]

OUTCOMES AND EFFECTIVENESS

Low-cost IVF models have shown pregnancy rates of 25–35% per cycle, comparable to global averages for mild stimulation protocols.[24,25] Importantly, complication rates such as ovarian hyperstimulation syndrome (OHSS) and multiple pregnancies are lower in these settings, reflecting safer practice.

However, success rates vary significantly with age, ovarian reserve, and severity of male infertility. Proper patient selection remains critical for cost-effectiveness and safety.[32]

POLICY, ETHICS, AND EQUITY

Policy Frameworks

India's ART Regulation Act (2021) mandates clinic registration, regulates donor gametes, and restricts commercial surrogacy. While it has improved transparency, critics argue that restrictions such as bans on donor surrogacy may limit options for poor couples. Other LMICs lack comprehensive ART laws, creating risks of exploitation and inconsistent standards.[23]

Ethical Concerns

Persistent ethical issues include multiple embryo transfers, misuse of sex selection, commercialization of gametes, and exploitation in surrogacy arrangements.[16,33] Ethical oversight is limited in rural and unregulated clinics.

Equity and Gender Justice

Access to IVF is skewed toward urban, wealthy couples, while rural and low-income populations remain excluded. Women bear the disproportionate physical and psychological burden of infertility and ART treatments.[13,34] Equity-oriented policies are necessary to avoid reinforcing gender and socioeconomic disparities.

FUTURE DIRECTIONS AND RECOMMENDATIONS

To make IVF more accessible and equitable in low-resource settings, a multipronged strategy is needed:

- Scale low-cost IVF models across public hospitals, especially state medical colleges.
- Incorporate IVF under universal health coverage (UHC) frameworks like India's Ayushman Bharat or similar schemes in LMICs.
- Develop regional ART hubs with centralized laboratories and satellite clinics supported by telehealth.
- Invest in training embryologists, reproductive endocrinologists, and ART nurses.

- Promote local manufacturing of consumables and affordable incubators.
- Leverage digital technologies and AI for embryo selection, counseling, and cost reduction.
- Encourage renewable energy integration, e.g., solar-powered IVF laboratories in rural settings.
- Strengthening community awareness and counselling to reduce stigma and misinformation.

CONCLUSION

Infertility represents a significant yet often neglected component of global reproductive health. IVF has revolutionized treatment in HICs but remains inaccessible to the vast majority in LMICs due to economic, infrastructural, and sociocultural barriers. Nevertheless, low-cost IVF models, financing innovations, digital health, and supportive policies offer promising pathways.

India and other LMICs have demonstrated that through innovation, public-private partnerships, and ethical regulation, IVF can be made accessible without compromising quality. Equity must remain at the heart of this expansion, ensuring that reproductive technologies empower rather than exclude. If these innovations are scaled and integrated into national health frameworks, LMICs could emerge as global leaders in democratizing IVF.

REFERENCES

1. World Health Organization. Infertility prevalence estimates, 1990–2021. Geneva: World Health Organization; 2023.
2. Zegers-Hochschild F, Adamson GD, de Mouzon J, Ishihara O, Mansour R, Nygren K, et al. International Committee for Monitoring Assisted Reproductive Technologies (ICMART): world report on ART. Hum Reprod. 2022;37(9):1853-70.
3. Inhorn MC, Patrizio P. Infertility around the globe: new thinking on gender, reproductive technologies, and global movements in the 21st century. Hum Reprod Update. 2015;21(4):411-26.
4. ESHRE Capri Workshop Group. Developing countries and infertility: WHO meeting's outcome. Hum Reprod. 2010;25(12):2833-47.
5. Hammarberg K, Kirkman M. Infertility in resource-poor settings: challenges and strategies. Best Pract Res Clin Obstet Gynaecol. 2013;27(6):891-901.
6. Dyer SJ, Patel M. Infertility in low-resource countries: prevalence, consequences and access to care. Hum Reprod Update. 2012;18(5):603-12.
7. Agarwal A, Mulgund A, Hamada A, Chyatte MR. A unique view on male infertility around the globe. Reprod Biol Endocrinol. 2015;13:37.
8. Ombelet W. Is global access to infertility care realistic? The Walking Egg Project. Reprod Biomed Online. 2014;28(2):267-72.
9. Chambers GM, Sullivan EA, Ishihara O, Chapman MG, Adamson GD. The economic impact of assisted reproductive technology: a review of selected developed countries. Fertil Steril. 2009 Jun;91(6):2281-94.
10. Kaur R, Prasad S. PCOS prevalence and infertility in Indian women. Int J Reprod Contracept Obstet Gynecol. 2020;9(2):760-5.
11. Singh M, Sharma A. Social stigma of infertility in Indian women: a qualitative analysis. Indian J Psychol Med. 2020;42(1):46-52.
12. Raj A, et al. Financial burden of ART in Indian households. Reprod Health Matters. 2023;31(1):1-12.
13. Baveja R, Arora P. Infertility in India: dimensions and care-seeking practices. Indian J Public Health. 2018;62(4):331-6.
14. Dyer SJ, Abrahams N, Hoffman M, van der Spuy ZM. Infertility in South Africa: women's reproductive health knowledge and treatment-seeking behaviour for involuntary childlessness. Hum Reprod. 2002;17(6):1657-62.

15. Inhorn MC. Global infertility and the globalization of new reproductive technologies: illustrations from Egypt. Soc Sci Med. 2003;56(9):1837-51.
16. Shetty P. IVF in India: Growth and inequity. Lancet. 2015;385(9985):1479-80.
17. Patel A, Sharma PSVN. Coping strategies of infertile couples in India. Indian J Community Med. 2018;43(3):220-4.
18. Pandey S, McLernon DJ, Scotland G, Mollison J, Wordsworth S, Bhattacharya S. Cost of fertility treatment and live birth outcome in women of different ages and BMI. Hum Reprod. 2014;29(10):2199-211.
19. Dyer S, Archary P, de Mouzon J, Fiadjoe M, Ashiru O; African Network and Registry for Assisted Reproductive Technology. Assisted reproductive technologies in Africa: first results from the African Network and Registry for Assisted Reproductive Technology, 2013. Reprod Biomed Online. 2019;38(2):216-24.
20. Arora P, Reddy M. Insurance coverage for ART in India: current status and way forward. Indian J Health Econ. 2022;7(1):33-9.
21. Desai N, Nadkarni S. IVF lab management challenges in small cities in India. J Hum Reprod Sci. 2016;9(4):259-64.
22. Saxena P, Mishra A. ART outcomes and challenges in low-resource India. Fertil Sci Res. 2021;8(2):89-96.
23. Springer Medizin. (2020). Infertility policy analysis in LMICs. [Online] Available from https://www.springermedizin.de/infertility-policy-analysis-a-comparative-study-of-selected-lowe/18516178 [Last accessed December, 2025].
24. Ombelet W, Van Blerkom J. Simplified IVF culture systems: a global perspective. Reprod Biomed Online. 2016;32(6):499-502.
25. Gunasheela D. Low-cost IVF approaches in Indian practice. Fertil Steril. 2017;107(5):1042-6.
26. Malhotra N, Singh N, Bahadur A. Low-cost IVF in India: the way forward. J Hum Reprod Sci. 2020;13(3):173-80.
27. All India Institute Of Medical Sciences Delhi. Annual Report on ART services. New Delhi: All India Institute Of Medical Sciences Delhi; 2022.
28. Post Graduate Institute of Medical Education & Research. Annual report on infertility services. Chandigarh: Post Graduate Institute of Medical Education & Research; 2021.
29. Bhat P, Rao K. Role of telemedicine in infertility care during COVID-19 in India. J Hum Reprod Sci. 2021;14(3):215-20.
30. Business Standard. IVF chains in India turn to AI to cut costs and boost accuracy. 2025.
31. Ombelet W. Walking Egg Project outcomes in Africa and Asia. Reprod Biomed Online. 2015;30(3):225-30.
32. Vladimirov IK, Vladimirov M. Introductory chapter: IVF Technology and perspectives. In: Vladimirov IK (Ed). IVF Technologies and Infertility—Current Practices and New Perspectives. London: IntechOpen;2023.
33. Banerjee S, Choudhary N. Economics of infertility treatment in India. Indian J Med Ethics. 2017;2(4):220-5.
34. Talwar P, Sandeep K. Challenges of infertility care in low-resource Indian settings. J Obstet Gynaecol India. 2019;69.

SECTION 8

Support, Ethics, and Broader Outcomes

24. **Counseling Strategies and Supporting Diverse Family Structures**
Shivani Sachdev Gour, Shubhda Gupta

25. **Ethical, Religious, and Legal Considerations in Assisted Reproductive Technology**
Pratibha Singh

26. **Long-term Health of ART: Conceived Children and Reproductive Outcomes**
Rekha Ramappa, Gunupuru Gayatri Swetha

27. **Endometriosis and Assisted Reproductive Technology**
Rekha Rajendra Kumar

CHAPTER 24

Counseling Strategies and Supporting Diverse Family Structures

Shivani Sachdev Gour, Shubhda Gupta

INTRODUCTION

Assisted reproductive technology or ART has revolutionized parenthood, offering hope to individuals and couples facing infertility and reproductive challenges. Techniques like in vitro fertilization (IVF), intracytoplasmic sperm injection (ICSI), gamete/embryo donation, and surrogacy have expanded possibilities for diverse social, cultural, and personal contexts. Alongside medical advancements, ART brings complex psychological, ethical, and social considerations, making counseling an essential part of the process. It helps patients stay informed, emotionally prepared, and supported while balancing clinical outcomes with personal expectations.

EVOLUTION OF ASSISTED REPRODUCTIVE TECHNOLOGY

Since the birth of the first "test-tube baby" Louise Brown, in 1978, ART has advanced from limited procedures to widely accessible technologies like cryopreservation, genetic testing, donor programs, and surrogacy. Beyond infertility treatment, ART now supports family planning, fertility preservation, and gender-affirming care. Increasingly, single parents, same-sex couples, and transgender individuals are seeking ART, reflecting broader societal shifts in the definition of family.

NEED FOR COUNSELING IN ASSISTED REPRODUCTIVE TECHNOLOGY

Assisted reproductive technology involves emotional, ethical, and financial challenges alongside uncertain outcomes. Patients often face anxiety, depression, social stigma, and relationship stress. Counseling offers:

- Clear understanding of treatment and risks
- Guidance on realistic expectations
- Emotional support during failures or repeated cycles
- Preparation for alternative options like adoption or donor programs

Effective counseling empowers patients, improving decision-making, psychological well-being, and treatment outcomes.

IMPORTANCE OF ADDRESSING DIVERSE FAMILY STRUCTURES

Modern families seeking ART include single parents by choice, same-sex couples, transgender individuals, and blended families. Each group faces unique emotional, legal, and societal challenges:

Single parents: Concerns about readiness and long-term planning

Same-sex couples: Donor selection, legal parentage and societal biases

Transgender individuals: Preserving fertility and ensuring identity-respecting care

Cultural, religious, and socioeconomic factors also influence decisions. Counseling must be inclusive, patient-centered, and sensitive to diverse values and aspirations, ensuring equitable and ethical reproductive care.

OVERVIEW OF ASSISTED REPRODUCTIVE TECHNOLOGY

Historical Perspective and Milestones

Assisted reproductive technology has its roots in mid-20th-century animal research, notably the successful birth of rabbits conceived via in vitro fertilization in the 1950s, which validated the feasibility of fertilization outside a living organism.[1] The first human birth resulting from IVF occurred in 1978, when Louise Brown was born in Oldham, England, a monumental milestone in reproductive medicine.[2] This breakthrough earned Dr Robert Edwards, who collaborated with Patrick Steptoe and Jean Purdy, the Nobel Prize in Physiology or Medicine in 2010.[3]

Following these achievements, ART rapidly evolved. In India, Dr Indira Hinduja and Dr T C Anand Kumar played pivotal roles in pioneering IVF and gamete intrafallopian transfer (GIFT), leading to the first recorded IVF and GIFT births in India during the 1980s.[4] Since then, millions of children have been born worldwide through ART, reflecting its transition from experimental to mainstream clinical practice.[5]

TYPES OF ASSISTED REPRODUCTIVE TECHNOLOGY PROCEDURES[6-9]

Assisted reproductive technology encompasses a range of sophisticated interventions designed to assist individuals or couples with infertility. The principal modalities are given in **Flowchart 1**.

Increasing Demand and Changing Societal Trends

Demand for ART has grown substantially in recent decades, propelled by shifts in social

Flowchart 1: Types of assisted reproductive technology (ART) procedures.

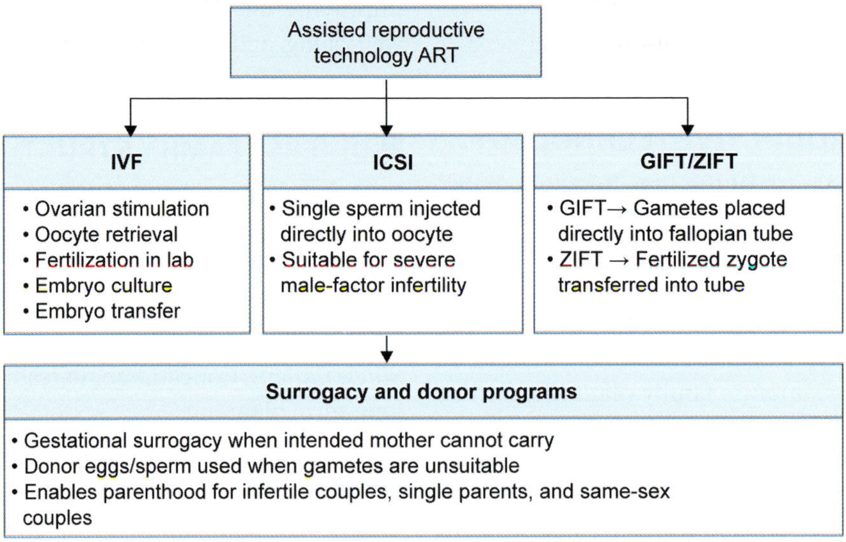

(ICSI: intracytoplasmic sperm injection; IVF: in vitro fertilization)

norms, delayed childbearing, and evolving family structures. It is estimated that while 85–90% of infertility cases resolve with low-tech interventions (e.g., medication, surgery, lifestyle changes), fewer than 5% require ART.[10] Nevertheless, ART remains a critical avenue for achieving parenthood across diverse populations.

Social acceptance has also expanded significantly. Initially controversial, ART including IVF and surrogacy has become more widely embraced over time, with media portrayals (such as the Netflix film *"Joy"* spotlighting Jean Purdy's role) contributing to broader public understanding.[11] As reproductive technologies evolve, they now serve not only infertile heterosexual couples but also single individuals, same-sex couples, and transgender persons seeking parenthood.

Diversity in Family Structures Seeking Assisted Reproductive Technology

Advances in ART have transformed pathways to parenthood, enabling a wide range of family structures to achieve conception and childbirth. Modern ART practices address diverse social, cultural, and biological needs, extending beyond traditional heterosexual couples to include same-sex partners, single parents, transgender individuals, and blended families. Understanding these variations is essential for ensuring inclusive counseling, ethical treatment planning, and culturally sensitive practices.

Heterosexual Couples with Infertility

Heterosexual couples remain the largest group seeking ART services globally. Causes of infertility may be female factors (e.g., anovulation, tubal block), male factors (e.g., low sperm count), combined factors, or unexplained infertility. ART modalities such as IVF and ICSI provide effective solutions when conventional treatments fail. In India, this group forms nearly *70–80%* of ART users, while worldwide, similar trends are reported.[12]

Same-sex Couples

Assisted reproductive technology has enabled same-sex couples to become parents through donor sperm, donor oocytes, surrogacy, and reciprocal IVF.

Female couples often choose donor sperm, with one partner carrying the pregnancy.

Male couples typically require donor eggs and gestational surrogacy.

The European Society of Human Reproduction and Embryology (ESHRE) and American Society for Reproductive Medicine (ASRM) emphasize nondiscriminatory access to ART for same-sex partners, though legal frameworks differ globally. In India, the Surrogacy (Regulation) Act currently restricts commercial surrogacy but permits altruistic arrangements under specific conditions.[13]

Single Parents by Choice

Single men and women are increasingly opting for ART to achieve biological parenthood.

Single women frequently utilize donor sperm with IVF or intrauterine insemination (IUI).

Single men may seek donor oocytes and gestational surrogacy.

Legal accessibility varies significantly. In India, the ART (Regulation) Act, 2021 permits single women to use ART but imposes restrictions on single men seeking surrogacy, highlighting ongoing policy debates.[14]

Transgender and Nonbinary Individuals

Transgender and gender-diverse individuals increasingly utilize ART to preserve fertility or achieve biological parenthood:

Transgender men (assigned female at birth) may choose to freeze oocytes or carry pregnancies if the uterus is intact.

Transgender women (assigned male at birth) may freeze sperm before gender-affirming treatments.

Ethical guidelines from ASRM and ESHRE advocate equitable access, fertility preservation counseling, and psychological support for gender-diverse patients.[15]

Blended and Extended Families

Blended families where one or both partners bring children from previous relationships are increasingly common among ART users. Many couples seek ART to have a genetically related child together. Extended family involvement in ART decision-making is particularly prominent in South Asian contexts, where cultural norms and joint-family systems influence treatment choices.[16]

CULTURAL AND RELIGIOUS INFLUENCES ON FAMILY FORMATION

Cultural, social, and religious beliefs significantly shape ART accessibility and decision-making:

In India, traditional family expectations often influence couples' treatment preferences, including stigma around donor gametes.

Islamic countries frequently prohibit third-party gamete donation but may allow ART using the couple's own gametes.

Catholic doctrine generally discourages IVF but permits natural fertility enhancement techniques.[17]

Importance of Counseling in Assisted Reproductive Technology

Counseling forms a cornerstone of modern ART practices, ensuring that patients are informed, emotionally supported, and guided through complex medical, psychological, ethical, and legal decisions. The diversity of ART users including heterosexual couples, single parents, same-sex partners, and transgender individuals makes a structured counseling approach essential to deliver holistic and patient-centered care.

Role of Counseling in Reproductive Medicine

Counseling in ART focuses on three primary domains:

1. *Informative counseling*: Educates patients about ART options, procedures, risks, outcomes and success rates, empowering them to make informed decisions
2. *Supportive counseling*: Helps individuals and couples cope with the emotional, psychological, and relational stresses of infertility and ART treatments.
3. *Decision-making counseling*: Assists patients in navigating sensitive topics such as donor gametes, surrogacy and embryo storage, considering personal, ethical and cultural factors.

Studies have shown that structured pretreatment counseling *improves treatment adherence and psychological well-being* in ART patients.[18]

Infertility and ART treatments can have significant emotional and relational impacts **(Table 1)**.[19]

Counseling ensures that patients feel supported, reducing treatment dropouts and improving mental health outcomes.[20]

LEGAL AND ETHICAL CONSIDERATIONS IN COUNSELING

Assisted reproductive technology raises complex legal and ethical challenges that require clear guidance during counseling sessions.

TABLE 1: Psychosocial challenges faced by patients.

Psychosocial challenge	*Impact on patients*	*Role of counseling*
Emotional distress	Anxiety, depression, and uncertainty due to repeated failures or financial burden	Provides coping strategies, relaxation techniques, and psychological support
Relationship conflicts	Stress within marital or family relationships due to infertility or donor involvement	Couple counseling fosters communication, understanding, and shared decision-making
Social stigma	Cultural shame, family pressure, and societal judgment, especially in India and conservative regions	Encourages emotional resilience and provides tools to handle societal pressures

Surrogacy Laws

India: The *Surrogacy (Regulation) Act, 2021* permits only altruistic surrogacy; commercial surrogacy is banned.

Counseling ensures that patients understand eligibility, surrogate rights, and legal obligations.[21]

Donor Anonymity versus Transparency

India: The *ART (Regulation) Act, 2021* mandates donor anonymity; clinics maintain records but do not reveal identities.

ESHRE and ASRM: Some regions allow children born via ART to access donor information upon adulthood.

Counseling prepares parents for potential identity disclosure challenges in the future.[13]

Parental Rights

Clarifies legal parentage in cases of surrogacy, donor gametes, and embryo adoption.
Educates patients on required consent forms (e.g., Forms 6–15 under Indian ART Rules).
Ensures ethical and legal compliance before treatment initiation.[22]

COUNSELING STRATEGIES IN ASSISTED REPRODUCTIVE TECHNOLOGY

Effective counseling in ART involves a multidimensional approach that addresses

Flowchart 2: Counseling workflow in assisted reproductive technology (ART).

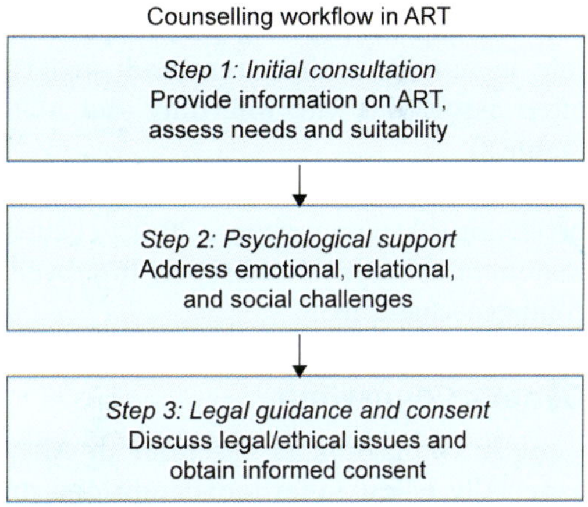

medical, psychological, ethical, and family-related concerns. It ensures that patients are fully informed, emotionally prepared and supported throughout their treatment journey, improving adherence, satisfaction, and overall outcomes **(Flowchart 2)**.

Pretreatment Counseling

Pretreatment counseling serves as the foundation of ART planning, focusing on preparing patients both medically and emotionally. It involves educating individuals and couples about ART procedures, success rates, possible complications, and available treatment options. Counselors also discuss emotional readiness, financial implications, and lifestyle adjustments, ensuring that patients have realistic expectations regarding treatment outcomes and the possibility of multiple cycles.

Additionally, legal obligations, including consent forms and donor agreements, are reviewed. For example, before initiating IVF, patients should be informed about potential risks such as ovarian hyperstimulation, chances of multiple pregnancies, and associated financial considerations.[20]

Psychological Counseling

Psychological counseling plays a critical role in managing the stress and anxiety often associated with infertility and ART **(Table 2)**.

Studies suggest that patients receiving psychological support show a 20–30% better treatment adherence and report improved coping mechanisms.[13]

Genetic Counseling

Genetic counseling is essential in ART, especially when inherited conditions or chromosomal abnormalities are suspected.

Indications:
- Advanced maternal age
- History of recurrent miscarriages
- Positive family history of genetic disorders
- Preimplantation genetic testing (PGT) considerations

Key benefits:
- Explains risks of passing on heritable diseases
- Guides informed decision-making regarding donor gametes
- Helps couples evaluate options for PGT and embryo selection
- ESHRE and ASRM guidelines recommend mandatory genetic counseling before donor egg/sperm use and when PGT is planned[23]

Couple and Family Counseling

Assisted reproductive technology decisions often affect relationships and family dynamics, making couple and family counseling essential. It helps strengthen marital bonds by encouraging open communication between partners and reducing conflicts. In the Indian context, where extended families often influence ART-related choices, involving them can improve understanding and acceptance. Counseling also prepares families for the emotional, legal, and social implications of using donor gametes or surrogacy. Additionally, it promotes participation in support networks and peer groups, helping patients share experiences and cope with the psychological challenges of ART.[24]

TABLE 2: Psychological impact of infertility and appropriate counseling approaches.

Psychological concern	*Impact on patients*	*Counseling approach*
Anxiety and depression	Fear of failure, emotional instability	Cognitive behavioral therapy, relaxation techniques
Repeated ART failures	Hopelessness, treatment fatigue	Resilience-building sessions, coping strategies
Financial burden	Stress due to high treatment costs	Emotional support, financial planning
Social stigma	Shame or pressure from family/ society	Counseling on self-esteem, group therapy

SUPPORTING DIVERSE FAMILY STRUCTURES IN ASSISTED REPRODUCTIVE TECHNOLOGY (TABLE 3)

Assisted reproductive technology is increasingly sought by individuals and couples from diverse family structures. Counseling in this context must be inclusive, nonjudgmental, and tailored to address specific psychosocial, cultural, and legal challenges.

Inclusive Counseling Approaches

Counselors must adopt strategies that respect cultural diversity, gender inclusivity, and individual choices:

Culturally sensitive practices: Different communities have varying attitudes toward infertility, donor gametes, and surrogacy. Counselors must adapt approaches based on patients' social and religious contexts.

Addressing stigma and biases: In conservative societies, infertility and nontraditional families face discrimination. Counseling provides emotional support, coping strategies, and community resources.

Empathetic, neutral communication: Using inclusive language fosters trust, particularly for LGBTQ individuals and single parents.[25]

Tailored Strategies for Same-sex Couples

ART options: Reciprocal IVF, donor sperm, donor eggs, and gestational surrogacy are common pathways for same-sex couples.

Legal Considerations

India: Under the *Surrogacy Regulation Act, 2021*, surrogacy for same-sex couples remains restricted.

International perspective: Countries like the US and Canada allow ART for same-sex couples with legal recognition of parental rights.

Psychosocial support: Counseling addresses discrimination, family rejection, and relationship concerns.[13,20]

Addressing Needs of Single Parents

Single mothers by choice: They often use donor sperm with IUI or IVF. Counseling includes emotional preparation, financial planning, and family readiness.

Single fathers by choice: They require donor oocytes and gestational surrogacy, which faces legal limitations in India.[14]

TABLE 3: Counseling focus across diverse family structures.[25]

Family type	*Key challenges*	*Counseling strategies*
Heterosexual couples	Infertility distress, family pressures	Pretreatment counseling, emotional support
Same-sex couples	Legal restrictions, social stigma	Tailored ART pathways, advocacy support
Single parents	Financial stress, social judgment	Peer networking, legal counseling
Transgender and nonbinary	Fertility preservation, disclosure issues	Identity-affirming counseling, reproductive planning
Children born via ART	Identity and belonging concerns	Gradual disclosure, emotional integration

(ART: assisted reproductive technology)

Counseling for Transgender and Nonbinary Individuals

Fertility preservation: Gamete or embryo freezing before starting hormone therapy or gender-affirming surgeries.

- *Parenthood pathways:* Use of partner gametes, donor gametes, or gestational carriers depending on reproductive capacity
- Counselors explain legal and medical limitations based on jurisdiction.

Psychological support: Focuses on identity affirmation, disclosure decisions, and emotional well-being.[15]

CHILDREN BORN THROUGH ART: PSYCHOLOGICAL CONSIDERATIONS

Identity formation: Children conceived through donor gametes or surrogacy may have questions about genetic heritage and family origins.

Disclosure strategies: The ASRM and ESHRE guidelines recommend age-appropriate disclosure to promote trust and emotional stability.[25]

Counselors guide parents in planning open and supportive communication.

Social adaptation: Families receive tools to address external stigma and ensure a positive self-identity for the child.

ETHICAL, LEGAL, AND POLICY PERSPECTIVES IN ASSISTED REPRODUCTIVE TECHNOLOGY

Assisted reproductive technology operates within a complex ethical, legal, and policy framework that balances patient autonomy, donor rights, child welfare, and societal norms. Given the diversity of family structures and cross-border treatments, clinicians must remain updated on national laws and international guidelines to ensure compliance and patient safety **(Table 4)**.

NATIONAL AND INTERNATIONAL GUIDELINES[20]

Comparison of ART guidelines are shown in **Table 4**.

INFORMED CONSENT AND AUTONOMY

In ART, informed consent is not just procedural but ethical:

- Patients must fully understand treatment options, risks, success rates, and legal implications before consenting.
- In India, Forms 6–15 under the ART Rules ensure legal documentation of consent for IVF, gamete donation, embryo freezing, and surrogacy.
- The ESHRE and ASRM recommend shared decision-making, where clinicians

TABLE 4: Comparison of ART guidelines.

Aspect	*India (ICMR, ART Act 2021)*	*ASRM (USA)*	*ESHRE (EU)*
Clinic registration	Mandatory	State-dependent	Varies by country
Surrogacy	Altruistic only	Allowed, regulated	Often prohibited
Donor age (egg)	23–35 years	21–34 years	18–35 years
Donor age (sperm)	21–55 years	21–45 years	18–40 years
Embryo storage	Max 10 years	Program-defined	5–10 years (country-specific)
Access	Married couples, some single women	Inclusive, LGBTQ+ friendly	Country-dependent

and patients collaboratively determine the best pathway based on medical, ethical, and psychosocial factors.[13,25]

DONOR RIGHTS, SURROGACY REGULATIONS, AND PARENTAGE LAWS

Donor Rights

In India, donor identity remains confidential; recipients cannot access identifying information.

The ESHRE promotes anonymous or identity-release donation based on country-specific laws.

The ASRM supports voluntary disclosure, depending on mutual agreement between donor and intended parents.

Surrogacy Regulations

India: Altruistic surrogacy is permitted; commercial surrogacy is prohibited.

Europe: Countries like France, Germany, and Italy prohibit surrogacy; others (e.g., Greece) allow regulated surrogacy.

USA: Most states permit both altruistic and commercial surrogacy under legally binding contracts.[13,24,25]

Parentage Laws

Indian law automatically grants legal parentage to the intending couple under the ART and Surrogacy Acts.

In the US, parentage laws are state-specific and often require prebirth or post-birth orders.

In the EU, parentage recognition varies, especially in cross-border surrogacy arrangements.[26]

Confidentiality and Data Protection

India: ART clinics must maintain detailed donor and patient records through the National ART Registry. Data sharing without consent is prohibited.

ESHRE (EU): Enforces GDPR (General Data Protection Regulation) compliance, ensuring strict control over genetic and personal data.

ASRM (USA): Promotes HIPAA (Health Insurance Portability and Accountability Act) regulations to protect patient privacy.

ROLE OF MULTIDISCIPLINARY TEAMS IN ASSISTED REPRODUCTIVE TECHNOLOGY

Assisted reproductive technology requires collaboration among medical, psychological, genetic, and social care professionals to provide holistic patient support. A multidisciplinary approach ensures personalized treatment, informed decision-making, and optimal clinical outcomes[24] **(Table 5)**.

TABLE 5: Role of multidisciplinary teams in ART.

Team member	*Primary role*	*Key contributions*
Psychologist	Emotional and mental health support	Reduces stress, enhances coping skills
Genetic counselor	Risk assessment and genetic testing guidance	Assists in PGT, donor selection
Social worker	Navigates legal, financial, and social aspects	Links to resources and support systems
Physician	Designs treatment plans and supervises care	Guides ART protocols, coordinates team
Embryologist	Handles gametes and embryos in the laboratory	Ensures laboratory safety and embryo quality

Collaborative Decision-making for Optimal Care

A well-coordinated multidisciplinary team improves ART outcomes through:

- *Shared decision-making:* Aligning medical advice, patient preferences, and psychosocial needs
- *Integrated care pathways:* Regular interdepartmental case discussions to ensure unified treatment goals
- *Holistic patient support:* Addressing emotional, financial, legal, and medical concerns together[20]

FUTURE DIRECTIONS IN COUNSELING FOR ART

As ART technologies evolve, counseling practices are rapidly adapting to digital health tools, artificial intelligence (AI) integration, and inclusive care models. Future counseling will focus on enhanced personalization, accessibility, and inclusivity ensuring that all individuals and families receive comprehensive support.

Integration of Digital Counseling Platforms

Online counseling platforms enable remote sessions, improving access for patients in rural and underserved areas.

Video-based consultations help provide psychological support and educational resources before, during, and after ART cycles.

Patient Portals and E-Learning Tools

Mobile applications and digital platforms provide procedure information, consent forms, emotional health resources, and progress tracking. Indian Council of Medical Research (ICMR) and international bodies are exploring standardized digital counseling modules to ensure uniformity in patient education. Digital counseling improves treatment compliance, reduces travel costs, and helps patients engage in informed decision-making.[27]

ARTIFICIAL INTELLIGENCE IN ASSISTED REPRODUCTIVE TECHNOLOGY COUNSELING

Artificial intelligence tools analyze patient history, ovarian reserve, sperm quality, and embryo grading to predict ART outcomes more accurately. Algorithms can help physicians and counselors guide patients on realistic expectations, reducing emotional distress.

Applications

- Predicting IVF success rates
- Optimizing personalized treatment protocols
- Offering risk-based counseling on multiple cycles

The ESHRE and ASRM are exploring frameworks to ethically integrate AI into ART counseling while maintaining patient autonomy and confidentiality.

INCREASING ACCESSIBILITY FOR MARGINALIZED FAMILIES

Rural populations, LGBTQ individuals, single parents, and economically disadvantaged groups face limited access to ART counseling. Policies must encourage subsidized counseling and simplified procedures to reduce disparities.

CULTURALLY INCLUSIVE COUNSELING

Counseling should respect religious beliefs, gender identities, and community norms, adapting information to patient contexts.

The World Health Organization (WHO) and ESHRE emphasize removing financial, legal, and social barriers that restrict ART access. Digital tools and hybrid counseling models are increasingly being adopted for equity in reproductive care.[25,28]

CONCLUSION

Assisted reproductive technology counseling today provides holistic support by integrating psychological, genetic, ethical, and legal guidance, enabling patients to make informed decisions. Emphasizing inclusivity and empathy ensures care for diverse family structures while reducing stigma. Moving forward, simplified regulations, stronger patient rights on consent and privacy, and broader awareness campaigns are vital for making ART more accessible, transparent, and socially acceptable.

REFERENCES

1. Wikipedia. History of in vitro fertilisation. Nature. First non-human IVF birth in mammals (1959) and first human IVF baby (1978). [online] Available from https://en.wikipedia.org/wiki/In_vitro_fertilisation [Last accessed December, 2025].
2. TIME Magazine. Robert Edwards awarded 2010 Nobel Prize for pioneering IVF in humans. [online] Available from https://time.com [Last accessed December, 2025].
3. Pacific Fertility Center; Chang MC, et al. Early animal IVF research successes in the 1950s. [online] Available from https://www.pacificfertilitycenter.com [Last accessed December, 2025].
4. Wikipedia. Indira Hinduja and T.C. Anand Kumar: India's pioneer IVF and GIFT achievements. [online] Available from https://en.wikipedia.org/wiki/In_vitro_fertilisation [Last accessed December, 2025].
5. NCBI. Overview of IVF steps: controlled ovarian stimulation to embryo transfer. [online] Available from https://www.ncbi.nlm.nih.gov [Last accessed December, 2025].
6. Pacific Fertility Center. Definition and process of IVF ("in glass" fertilisation). [online] Available from https://www.pacificfertilitycenter.com [Last accessed December, 2025].
7. Wikipedia. Intracytoplasmic sperm injection (ICSI): Method description and applications. [online] Available from https://en.wikipedia.org/wiki/Intracytoplasmic_sperm_injection [Last accessed December, 2025].
8. EBSCO Reproductive Facts. GIFT and ZIFT techniques explained. [online] Available from https://www.reproductivefacts.org [Last accessed December, 2025].
9. Wagner K. What is in vitro fertilization (IVF)? Verywell Health [Internet]. Updated 2023 Nov 30 [cited 2025 Jan 10]. [online] Available from https://www.verywellhealth.com/ivf-5119348. [Last accessed January, 2026].
10. Madormo C. What's the difference between IUI vs. IVF for fertility treatment? Verywell Health [Internet]. Published 2025 Feb 26 [cited 2025 Jan 10]. [online] Available from: https://www.verywellhealth.com/iui-vs-ivf-8779517. [Last accessed January, 2026].
11. Decider. Media portrayal of IVF pioneers 'Joy' film. [online] Available from https://decider.com [Last accessed December, 2025].
12. Vander Borght M, Wyns C. Fertility and infertility: Definition and epidemiology. Clin Biochem. 2018;62:2-10.
13. Ethics Committee of the ASRM. Access to ART for same-sex couples: Updated guidelines. Fertil Steril. 2021;116(4):887-93.
14. Kashyap S, Tripathi P. The Surrogacy (Regulation) Act, 2021: A critique. Asian Bioeth Rev. 2022;15(1):5-18.
15. Schwartz AR, Moravek MB. Reproductive potential and fertility preservation in transgender and nonbinary individuals. Curr Opin Obstet Gynecol. 2021;33(4):327-34.
16. Skarbek K, Kierzkowska M. Family relationships and parenting dynamics in blended families. Studia Paedagogica Ignatiana. 2024;27:19-41.
17. Ardakani Z, Navabakhsh M, Tremayne S, Akhondi M, Ranjbar F, Tabrizi A. The impact of third-party reproduction on family and kinship. J Reprod Infertil. 2020;22(1):1-9.

18. Kaur KK. Editorial: Reviews in assisted reproduction: 2022. Front Reprod Health. 2023;5:1174047.
19. Verhaak CM, Smeenk JMJ, Evers AWM, Kremer JAM, Kraaimaat FW, Braat DDM. Emotional impact of unsuccessful ART: A systematic review. Hum Reprod Update. 2020;26(5):584-603.
20. Gameiro S, Verhaak CM, Kremer JA, Boivin J. Why we should talk about compliance with assisted reproductive technologies (ART): a systematic review and meta-analysis of ART compliance rates. Hum Reprod Update. 2013;19(2):124-35.
21. Kashyap S, Tripathi P. The Surrogacy (Regulation) Act, 2021: a critique. Asian Bioeth Rev. 2022;15(1):5-18.
22. European Society of Human Reproduction and Embryology (ESHRE). Guidelines, consensus documents and recommendations [Internet]. Brussels: ESHRE. [online] Available from https://www.eshre.eu/Guidelines-and-Legal [Last accessed December, 2025].
23. Boivin J, Gameiro S. Evolution of psychology and counseling in infertility. Fertil Steril. 2015;104(2):251-9.
24. Gameiro S, Boivin J, Dancet E, de Klerk C, Emery M, Lewis-Jones C, et al. ESHRE guideline: routine psychosocial care in infertility and medically assisted reproduction a guide for fertility staff. Hum Reprod. 2015;30(11):2476-85.
25. European Society of Human Reproduction and Embryology. (2023). ESHRE Guidelines. Ethical, social and legal perspectives in ART. [online] Available from https://www.eshre.eu [Last accessed December, 2025].
26. International Bar Association (IBA). Surrogacy abroad: Legal pathways for Indian couples. London: IBA. [online] Available from https://www.ibanet.org/surrogacy-abroad-legal-pathways-for-Indian-couples [Last accessed December, 2025].
27. Wu YC, Su ECY, Hou JS, Lin CJ, Lin KB, Chen CH. Artificial intelligence and assisted reproductive technology: a comprehensive systematic review. Taiwan J Obstet Gynecol. 2025;64(1):11-26.
28. World Health Organization (WHO). Recommendations on digital interventions for health system strengthening. Geneva: WHO; 2019. [online] Available from https://apps.who.int/iris/handle/10665/311941 [Last accessed December, 2025].

CHAPTER 25

Ethical, Religious, and Legal Considerations in Assisted Reproductive Technology

Pratibha Singh

INTRODUCTION

Assisted reproductive technology (ART) has revolutionized infertility management, offering hope to millions of couples who previously faced permanent childlessness. Techniques such as in vitro fertilization (IVF), intracytoplasmic sperm injection (ICSI), surrogacy, and gamete donation have expanded the scope of reproductive options. However, the rapid growth of ART raises *profound ethical, religious, and legal dilemmas*. These issues surpass clinical practice, impacting patients, healthcare providers, lawmakers, and society at large.[1]

Questions surrounding embryo status, gamete ownership, third-party reproduction, surrogacy, genetic selection, and equitable access highlight the delicate balance between technological advancement and societal values. Diverse religious perspectives and evolving legal frameworks add complexity.

ETHICAL CONSIDERATIONS IN ASSISTED REPRODUCTIVE TECHNOLOGY (BOX 1)

- *Core bioethical principles:* The application of ART must align with fundamental principles of bioethics:[2]
    - *Autonomy:* Respecting patients' reproductive choices, informed consent, and decision-making
    - *Beneficence:* Acting in the best interests of the couple and the child-to-be
    - *Nonmaleficence:* Minimizing risks to the woman, gamete donors, and offspring
    - *Justice:* Ensuring equitable access and fair distribution of resources
- *Ethical issues in gamete donation:*[4]
    - *Anonymity versus transparency:* Debate over whether donor identity should remain confidential or be disclosed to offspring
    - *Exploitation concerns:* Commercialization of egg donation may exploit economically vulnerable women.
    - *Consent:* Donors must receive full disclosure of medical risks and long-term implications.
- *Embryo-related ethical questions:*
    - *Status of the embryo:* Differing views on moral and legal status of preimplantation embryos[5]

BOX 1: Ethical principles in ART.[3]

- *Autonomy:* Right to choose or refuse treatment
- *Beneficence:* Acting for the welfare of patient and child
- *Nonmaleficence:* Avoiding harm (medical, psychological, social)
- *Justice:* Fairness in access and treatment distribution

TABLE 1: Ethical issues in surrogacy.

Concern	*Ethical dilemma*	*Possible safeguard*
Exploitation	Poor women as surrogates for affluent couples	Strong regulation, fair compensation
Autonomy	Pressure from family or brokers	Independent counseling and consent
Child's rights	Multiple claims of parenthood	Clear prebirth legal contracts

- *Cryopreservation:* Ethical dilemmas in storage, ownership, and disposal of surplus embryos
- *Preimplantation genetic testing (PGT):* Balancing prevention of genetic disease versus concerns about "designer babies"

- *Surrogacy ethics **(Table 1)**:*[6]
  - *Altruistic versus commercial surrogacy:* Many countries ban commercial surrogacy due to exploitation risks.
  - Gestational versus traditional surrogacy*:* In gestational surrogacy, the surrogate has no genetic link to the child, while in traditional surrogacy she does
  - *Exploitation and coercion:* Safeguards needed to ensure voluntary participation
  - *Parentage rights:* Ethical dilemmas when intended parents or surrogates change their minds
  - *PGT and sex selection:*
    - PGT allows detection of genetic disorders before embryo transfer.
    - Ethical concerns:
      - *Discrimination* against embryos with disabilities.
      - *Slippery slope* toward "designer babies"

Sex selection is legally prohibited in India under the *PCPNDT Act (1994)* due to the risk of skewed sex ratios

  - *Embryo creation, freezing, and disposal*
    - ART often results in surplus embryos.
    - Ethical dilemmas:
      - Is discarding embryos equivalent to destruction of potential life?
      - Should couples be allowed to donate embryos for research?
      - Duration of embryo storage and decisions in case of divorce/death
- *Access and equity in ART:* ART is expensive and often inaccessible to low-income couples. Ethical responsibility lies in balancing advanced technology with equitable healthcare distribution. There is always debate over state funding of ART in resource-limited countries.

RELIGIOUS CONSIDERATIONS IN ASSISTED REPRODUCTIVE TECHNOLOGY (TABLE 2)

Religious beliefs significantly shape attitudes toward ART. Positions vary across traditions:

- *Hinduism* is generally supportive of procreation as they feel it is a sacred duty. Use of ART is acceptable if marital fidelity is preserved, although donor gametes may raise ethical doubts regarding lineage (*gotra* and *varna* purity).[7]
- *Islam:* ART is permitted between husband and wife only. Usually, third-party reproduction (donor sperm, donor egg, surrogacy) is strictly prohibited. Embryo cryopreservation is allowed if used within the marital bond.
- *Christianity:*
  - *Catholic Church* has strong opposition to ART involving third-party gametes,

surrogacy, or embryo destruction. IVF itself is discouraged due to separation of conception from marital act.
- *Protestant denominations:* They are more permissive but concerned about embryo handling and commercialization.

- *Judaism:* It is supportive of ART, as they fulfil the commandment "Be fruitful & multiply." Donor gametes and surrogacy are acceptable under rabbinical guidance. Lineage and identity of the child must be clarified within Jewish law.[8,9]
- *Buddhism:* Generally, this accepts ART as long as it does not cause harm. Embryo destruction (e.g., in selective reduction) may conflict with *ahimsa* (nonviolence).[10]

LEGAL CONSIDERATIONS IN ASSISTED REPRODUCTIVE TECHNOLOGY[11-13]

- *Global legal landscape* **(Box 2)**:[14,15]
  - *International legal perspectives:* Laws vary globally, reflecting cultural and ethical diversity.
    - *UK* Human Fertilisation and Embryology Authority (HFEA): Regulates IVF, embryo research, and surrogacy; allows donor anonymity to be removed at 18 years[16]
    - *USA*: Regulation is state-specific, leading to variation in surrogacy and donor gamete practices[17]
    - *France and Germany:* Restrictive policies, banning commercial surrogacy and embryo research[18,19]

TABLE 2: Religious views on ART.

Religion	*Acceptable practices*	*Prohibited/discouraged practices*
Hinduism	IVF within marriage	Donor gametes (controversial)
Islam	IVF with couple's gametes	Third-party gametes, surrogacy
Catholicism	Natural conception only	IVF, donor gametes, embryo destruction
Protestantism	IVF with restrictions	Commercial surrogacy, embryo misuse
Judaism	IVF, surrogacy with guidance	Ambiguity around lineage without rabbi
Buddhism	IVF, donor gametes acceptable	Embryo destruction, selective reduction

(ART: assisted reproductive technology; IVF: in vitro fertilization)

BOX 2: Landmark case laws in ART and surrogacy (global).[21-23]

- *Johnson v. Calvert (1993, USA)*: Established the "intent test"—legal parentage rests with intended parents, not surrogate
- *Buzzanca v. Buzzanca (1998, USA)*: Commissioning couple declared legal parents even without genetic ties, shaping ART parentage law
- *Mennesson v. France (2014, ECtHR)*: France's refusal to recognize surrogacy-born children violated child's right to identity and family life[24]
- *Paradiso and Campanelli v. Italy (2017, ECtHR)*: Upheld Italy's right to remove a child born via surrogacy abroad with no genetic link, stressing state authority[25]
- *Baby Gammy Case (2014, Thailand)*: Abandoned twin with Down syndrome by commissioning parents triggered ban on commercial surrogacy in Thailand

- *Middle East:* Strict adherence to Islamic law, banning third-party reproduction[20]

- *Local legal landscape* **(Boxes 3 and 4)**:
  - *Indian Legal Framework*: India has undergone significant reforms in ART legislation **(Box 3; Flowchart 1)**:
    - ART (Regulation) Act, 2021
      - Governs clinics and banks offering ART
      - Prohibits sex selection
      - Restricts ART to married couples and certain categories of women
    - Surrogacy (Regulation) Act, 2021[26]
      - Allows only altruistic surrogacy for Indian couples
      - Bans commercial surrogacy
      - Requires surrogate to be a close relative, married, with a child of her own

BOX 3: Key provisions of ART and Surrogacy (Regulation) Acts, 2021.

- Ban on commercial surrogacy
- Only altruistic surrogacy allowed
- Donor gametes regulated through ART banks
- Strict penalties for violations

(ART: assisted reproductive technology)

- *Consent and confidentiality:* Informed consent must cover risks, success rates, alternatives, and legal parentage. Confidentiality of donor and recipient identity is critical, unless disclosure is mandated by law.
- *Legal challenges and gaps:*[27]
  - Exclusion of single parents and LGBTQ+ couples from accessing ART under current laws.
  - Lack of clarity on rights of cryopreserved embryos in divorce or death cases.
  - International surrogacy tourism and cross-border legal disputes

Flowchart 1: ART legal pathways in India.

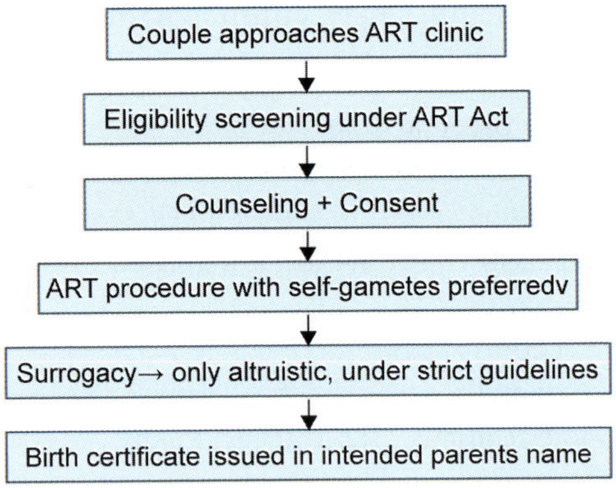

BOX 4: Landmark case laws in ART and surrogacy (India).

- *Baby Manji Yamada vs Union of India (2008, Supreme Court)*
  First major case on surrogacy in India. Led to Surrogacy Regulation Bill debates, pushed lawmakers to create ART Act 2021 and Surrogacy (Regulation) Act 2021
  - Japanese parents had a surrogate child in Gujarat; after divorce, the intended mother refused custody. The child was left in legal limbo until the grandmother was allowed to take custody
  - Court upheld surrogacy but emphasized need for regulation
- *Jan Balaz vs Anand Municipality (2009, Gujarat High Court)*
  - German couple had twins via Indian surrogate. German government refused citizenship; Gujarat HC granted Indian passports
  - Highlighted *citizenship and parentage disputes* in cross-border surrogacy
- *Suchita Srivastava vs Chandigarh Administration (2009, Supreme Court)*
  - Though not ART-specific, upheld a woman's reproductive autonomy as part of Article 21 (Right to Privacy and Dignity)
  - Important precedent for autonomy in ART decisions

(ART: assisted reproductive technology)

- *Emerging issues and future directions:*
  - *Cross-border ART:* Legal parentage conflicts when couples travel abroad for ART services
  - *Artificial gametes and uterine transplants:* Will challenge existing laws
  - *Genomic editing (CRISPR):* Raises profound ethical and legal implications
  - *Balancing regulation with accessibility:* Over-regulation may limit availability of ART services to deserving couples.
- *Surrogacy laws:*[28]
  - *India (2021 Act):* Only altruistic surrogacy permitted; no commercial arrangements
  - *USA:* Surrogacy contracts legally binding in some states; banned in others
  - *UK:* Surrogacy contracts unenforceable; parental orders required
- *Embryo storage and disposal:* Embryos can be stored for limited years (varies by jurisdiction). Consent of both partners is mandatory for use/disposal. Should be careful as legal battles often arise in cases of divorce or separation.
- *ART and child's rights:*
  - *Right to identity:* Many countries now allow donor-conceived children to access donor details upon maturity. Citizenship and parentage disputes arise in cross-border surrogacy cases.

CONCLUSION

Assisted reproductive technology represents a fusion of science, ethics, faith, and law which has provided hope to millions, yet its practice is intertwined with *ethical debates, religious values, and legal challenges.* A balanced approach requires respecting patient autonomy, ensuring justice, and safeguarding against exploitation while remaining sensitive to cultural and religious beliefs. Clinicians must navigate sensibly adhering to legal frameworks.

India's ART and Surrogacy Regulation Acts of 2021 mark a major step toward safeguarding patients, donors, and children. Yet, challenges persist—particularly regarding donor identity, surrogacy exploitation, and affordability.[29] However, further reforms are needed protecting vulnerable populations (as they exclude single men, LGBTQ+ individuals), cross-border issues, and emerging technologies.[30]

Ultimately, ART must be guided not only by technological possibilities but also by a framework that respects human dignity, social justice, and cultural diversity. ART must not only create life but also honor the dignity of all parties involved.

Assisted reproductive technology is a powerful tool in infertility management but is inseparable from *ethical, religious, and legal complexities*. Clinicians must respect patient autonomy, cultural values, and adhere to national laws to ensure *safe, ethical, and socially acceptable practice.* Going forward, a *nuanced, inclusive, and ethically sensitive approach* is essential to ensure that ART is practiced with respect for human dignity, reproductive rights, and cultural diversity.[31-35]

REFERENCES

1. Ethics Committee of the American Society for Reproductive Medicine. Ethical considerations of assisted reproductive technologies. Fertil Steril. 2018;110(6):1022-38.
2. Savulescu J. Procreative beneficence: why we should select the best children. Bioethics. 2001;15(5-6):413-26.
3. Pennings G. Ethical issues of infertility treatment in developing countries. Hum Reprod. 2008;23(8):1608-11.
4. Daar J, Klipstein S. Ethical issues in fertility treatment. Clin Obstet Gynecol. 2019;62(2):215-27.

5. Baylis F, McLeod C. The ethics of creating and selecting embryos. J Med Ethics. 2017;43(1):1-5.
6. Choudhury S, Singh S. Assisted reproductive technologies in India: ethics, economy, and agency. Asian Bioeth Rev. 2012;4(4):303-15.
7. Gurmukh S, Dhillon BS. Hindu religious perspectives on assisted reproductive technologies. Indian J Med Ethics. 2019;4(2):111-5.
8. Zoloth L. Jewish perspectives on assisted reproductive technologies. Camb Q Healthc Ethics. 2015;24(3):303-12.
9. Dorff EN. A Jewish approach to assisted reproduction. Fertil Steril. 2010;94(7):2790-3.
10. Keown D. Buddhism, bioethics and society. J Med Ethics. 2005;31(6):341-5.
11. Indian Council of Medical Research. National Guidelines for Accreditation, Supervision, and Regulation of ART Clinics in India. New Delhi: ICMR; 2021.
12. The Assisted Reproductive Technology (Regulation) Act, 2021. Government of India Gazette.
13. The Surrogacy (Regulation) Act, 2021. Government of India Gazette.
14. Jones HW, Cohen J. IFFS Surveillance 2019. Global trends in reproductive medicine. Fertil Steril. 2019;112(4):667-81.
15. Dickens BM, Cook RJ. Legal regulation of assisted reproduction. Int J Gynaecol Obstet. 2017;138(3):287-94.
16. Human Fertilisation and Embryology Authority (HFEA). Code of Practice. London: HFEA; 2021.
17. Vayena E, Rowe PJ, Griffin PD (Eds). Current practices and controversies in assisted reproduction. Geneva: WHO; 2002.18. Vatican Congregation for the Doctrine of the Faith. Instruction on respect for human life in its origin and the dignity of procreation (Donum Vitae). Rome: Holy See; 1987.
19. Vatican Congregation for the Doctrine of the Faith. Instruction Dignitas Personae on certain bioethical questions. Rome: Holy See; 2008.
20. Qureshi Z, Alkhamees A, Sattar S. Islamic perspectives on assisted reproductive technology. J Reprod Infertil. 2018;19(2):71-6.
21. Inhorn MC, Patrizio P. Infertility around the globe: new thinking on gender, reproductive technologies and global movements in the 21st century. Hum Reprod Update. 2015;21(4):411-26.
22. Blyth E, Frith L. Donor-conceived people's access to genetic and biographical history: an analysis of provisions in different jurisdictions permitting disclosure of donor identity. Int J Law Policy Family. 2009;23(2):174-91.
23. Smajdor A. Ethics of surrogacy: a global review. Bioethics. 2020;34(4):333-40.
24. Robertson JA. Children of Choice: Freedom and the New Reproductive Technologies. Princeton: Princeton University Press; 1994.
25. Maheshwari A, Bhattacharya S. Surrogacy: a reproductive justice perspective. BJOG. 2013;120(13):1633-6.
26. Majumdar A, Inamdar D. The new ART and Surrogacy Acts in India: promises and challenges. Indian J Med Ethics. 2022;7(3):204-10.
27. Hammarberg K, Kirkman M. Infertility in resource-constrained settings: ethical challenges. Reprod Biomed Online. 2013;26(2):162-70.
28. Shenfield F, Pennings G, De Mouzon J, Ferraretti AP, Nygren KG, Tarlatzis B, et al. Cross-border reproductive care in six European countries. Hum Reprod. 2010;25(6):1361-8.
29. Sarojini NB, Sharma A. The political economy of surrogacy in India: understanding exploitation. Dev World Bioeth. 2018;18(1):36-44.
30. Franklin S, Inhorn MC. Introduction to the anthropology of reproductive technologies. Reprod Biomed Soc Online. 2016;2:1-7.
31. Cook RJ, Dickens BM. Human rights and assisted reproductive technologies. Int J Gynaecol Obstet. 2009;104(2):102-6.
32. Harris J. Enhancing Evolution: The Ethical Case for Making Better People. Princeton: Princeton University Press; 2007.
33. Lindheim SR, Sauer MV. Genetic parenthood, donor anonymity, and obligations to children born from assisted reproduction. Fertil Steril. 2013;100(1):36-8.
34. FIGO Committee for the Ethical Aspects of Human Reproduction. Ethical guidelines on assisted reproductive technologies. Int J Gynaecol Obstet. 2019;146(1):1-7.
35. Warnock M. A Question of Life: The Warnock Report on Human Fertilisation and Embryology. Oxford: Oxford University Press; 1985.

CHAPTER 26

Long-term Health of ART: Conceived Children and Reproductive Outcomes

Rekha Ramappa, Gunupuru Gayatri Swetha

INTRODUCTION

Over 10 million assisted reproductive technology (ART) births have occurred worldwide since its debut in 1978 with many of the offsprings being in their adulthood now.[1] Short-term adverse perinatal outcomes of ART like preterm birth, low birth weight, intrauterine growth restriction, perinatal mortality, congenital anomalies associated with multiple and singleton pregnancies alike, large for gestational age (LGA) in frozen embryo transfer (FET) conceptions, preeclampsia, placental dysfunction, and caesarean delivery in ART mothers have been extensively studied.[2,3]

Studies on long-term health outcomes of ART are scarce and controversial. This chapter throws light on the evidence from the available literature, scope for future research, and cautious use of ART practice.

It is difficult to attribute the adverse outcomes to infertility factors or to ART itself.[4] It is ethically not right to randomize fertile group to ART arm to study the effect of ART on long-term outcome. It is equally not right to allow the infertile group to try for natural conception to study the effect of infertility factors.

Most of the ART children are in their young adulthood and need long-term follow-up before we arrive at a conclusion.

Nonuniformity in stimulation protocols, infertility factors, FET protocols, and laboratory and culture conditions make comparison difficult.

Recent popularity of the vitrification technique calls for newer prospective studies and cannot be compared with the older slow-freeze methods.

Animal studies cannot be extrapolated to humans in all contexts.

BASIS FOR POSSIBLE LONG-TERM ADVERSE OUTCOMES OF ART

Epigenetic Aberrations

The Developmental Origins of Health and Diseases (DOHaD) paradigm indicates that there are critical periods of development, including the periconception period where epigenetic reprograming is taking place, which when perturbed predispose an adult to cardiovascular and metabolic disorders.[5] ART alters the environment of both male and female gametes and embryos when epigenetic imprints are being established via ovarian stimulation/ovulation; exposures of gametes and embryos to the in vitro environment in which they mature with changes in temperature, pH, and oxygen tension; intracytoplasmic sperm injection (ICSI); and freeze thaw embryo manipulations.[6]

Parental Infertility

Parents seeking ART are older and have age-associated chromosomal aberrations and obstetric and metabolic complications. Suboptimal intrauterine and perinatal environment can have far-reaching impact on later health in accordance with Barker's hypothesis.[7]

Placental Dysfunction

Placental dysfunction is common in ART pregnancies leading to adverse perinatal and long-term health outcomes.

Nonphysiologic Steroid Hormone Environment

- Maternal hyperestrogenism due to ovarian stimulation persisting into early pregnancy can lead to dyslipidemia, insulin resistance, and placental dysfunction.
- Hyperandrogenism in women with polycystic ovarian syndrome

Nonphysiologic sex steroids can affect epigenetic reprogramming making ART offsprings susceptible to metabolic dysfunction.[7]

Paternal Genome Integrity

Severe oligoasthenoteratozoospermia (OATS) and azoospermia are associated with chromosomal aberrations that are carried to their male offsprings, e.g., Y chromosome deletion, Robertsonian and unbalanced translocations, inversions, deletions, etc.

Effect of Vitrification

Vitrification leads to LGA, epigenetic alteration, mitochondrial dysfunction, oxidative stress, etc., further leading to long-term metabolic effects.[8,9]

There are a number of large databases currently working on long-term outcomes of ART of which the following are noteworthy:[10]

- *CoNARTaS* (The Committee of Nordic ART and Safety) database includes approximately 8 million deliveries from the years 1985 through 2015.
- *Human Fertilization and Embryology Authority (HFEA) register* as being born after ART between 1992 and 2009, their spontaneous conception (SC) siblings, and matched SC population controls linked to the Office for National Statistics birth registration dataset.
- *MOSART (Massachusetts Outcome Study of Assisted Reproductive Technology) database* includes just over 1 million deliveries and covers the years 2004 through 2017.
- The *OMEGA* women's cohort includes women and children conceived by subfertile women who did not conceive by ART.
- The *PEARL (Prolonged Effects of Assisted reproductive technologies on women and children's health: a Record Linkage study for England)* study is designed to assess the impact of successful fertility treatment on the long-term health of women and their children in England.

HEALTH CONDITIONS IN ART OFFSPRINGS

The health conditions that have been studied in ART offsprings are given in the following text.

Malignancies

The findings in most studies are reassuring, showing no elevated risk of overall cancer among children born after ART.[10] However, a higher risk for childhood cancers like acute lymphoid leukemia (ALL), central nervous system tumors, and Wilms' tumors was found among macrosomic children born after FET as also with ART offspring with preterm delivery, respiratory distress, and low APGARS (activity pulse grimace activity respiration score). The possible explanation is genetic and epigenetic changes due to vitrification and adverse perinatal events.[11]

More studies of ART offsprings born due to vitrification rather than the past and outdated slow-freezing method with follow up into adulthood would be relevant.[12]

Asthma

There is an increased risk of childhood asthma in the offspring conceived after ART.

It is not sure whether it is due to ART or related to maternal asthma, paternal subfertility, or adverse perinatal events in ART pregnancies.[13]

Obesity

Assisted reproductive technology conceptions may have an unfavorable lipid profile by way of high cholesterol and triglycerides, low HDL, and high peripheral fat deposition. This predisposes them to cardiovascular and metabolic diseases in later life.[14]

Diabetes

There is an increased risk of type 1 diabetes with FET which is associated with LGA. In general, there is a high risk of impaired glucose tolerance with ART.

However, further prospective studies with follow-up of ART conceptions until late adulthood will throw more light regarding this.[15]

Cardiovascular Disease

Although there is conflicting evidence regarding the risk of suboptimal cardiovascular function, the current data suggests a potential increase in cardiovascular conditions in ART offspring owing to adverse intrauterine and perinatal conditions in ART pregnancies. There is some evidence of more adverse blood pressure and triglyceride (TG) trajectories to young adulthood in those conceived by ART.[7,16]

Only long-term follow-up of the present ART cohort into late adulthood with studies on epigenetics, arterial, and cardiovascular phenotyping will be able to give more accurate results.

Neurodevelopmental Disorders

Based on the CoNARTaS data, the risk of cerebral palsy (CP) diminished over time among ART children due to the lowering of multiple birth rates.[17] Studies have shown association of autism spectrum disease and attention-deficit hyperactivity disorder with preterm birth, advanced paternal age, paternal infertility, hyperandrogenemic polycystic ovary syndrome (PCOS), and very high estradiol levels during stimulation.[18-20]

Cerebral palsy and cognitive development in ART children are reassuring if multiple birth rates are kept low.[7]

Reproductive Function

Male conceptions after ICSI show low sperm count and motility in their young adulthood. It would have been due to genetic etiology behind male infertility which warranted ICSI.[21]

Epilepsy

Severe parental infertility requiring ART and clomiphene-based ovulation induction are associated with raised risk of epilepsy.[22,23]

Thyroid Disorders

Hypothyroidism is seen in FET offspring whose maternal estradiol levels were high. Hence, follow-up of ART conceptions in childhood for thyroid disorders irrespective of the results of neonatal screening is necessary.[24]

SPECIAL SITUATIONS

Postpreimplantation Genetic Test-Aneuploidy Conceptions

Few studies in this aspect showed no difference in perinatal outcomes and birth defects in ART conceptions with preimplantation genetic test-aneuploidy (PGT-A) and without PGT-A.[25]

Third-party Reproduction

No added risks with donor sperm were seen. However, the risk of preeclampsia is seen in artificial FET cycles in case of donor oocyte IVF.[26,27]

Measures to Prevent Long-term Adverse Outcomes

- ART should be done only if medically indicated to increase reproductive outcomes
- ICSI, elective freezing, artificial FET endometrial preparation protocols, and PGT-A should be done only if indicated.
- Fresh transfer should be avoided in the presence of high maternal estradiol levels.
- Single embryo transfer should be adopted whenever possible.
- Optimization of laboratory and culture medium should be done.
- Avoid excessive weight gain in ART pregnancies.
- Encourage exclusive breast feeding up to 6 months to prevent early weight gain in newborns.
- Prenatal supplements like vitamin D and folic acid can mitigate the risk of asthma and structural abnormalities.

CONCLUSION

Although ART is a boon for millions of infertile women, it is imperative for fertility specialists and beneficiaries to understands the risks that come with it. Long-term follow-up studies of ART conceptions into late adulthood might give us more useful and valid inputs regarding long-term health outcomes and their association with infertility or its treatment. Indicated and safe practices in ART will bring meaningful hope to millions of people worldwide.

REFERENCES

1. Wyns C, De Geyter C, Calhaz-Jorge C, Kupka MS, Motrenko T, Smeenk J, et al. ART in Europe, 2018: results generated from European registries by ESHRE. Hum Reprod Open. 2022;2022(2):hoac022.
2. Sullivan-Pyke CS, Senapati S, Mainigi MA, Barnhart KT. In vitro fertilization and adverse obstetric and perinatal outcomes. Semin Perinatol. 2017;41(6):345-53.
3. Manna C, Lacconi V, Rizzo G, De Lorenzo A, Massimiani M. Placental dysfunction in assisted reproductive pregnancies: perinatal, neonatal and adult life outcomes. Int J Mol Sci. 2022;23(2):659.
4. Berntsen S, Soderstrom-Anttila V, Wennerholm UB, Laivuori H, Loft A, Oldereid NB, et al. The health of children conceived by ART: 'the chicken or the egg?'. Hum Reprod Update. 2019;25(2):137-58.
5. Wadhwa PD, Buss C, Entringer S, Swanson JM. Developmental origins of health and disease: brief history of the approach and current focus on epigenetic mechanisms. Semin Reprod Med. 2009;27(5):358-68.
6. Mani S, Ghosh J, Coutifaris C, Sapienza C, Mainigi M. Epigenetic changes and assisted reproductive technologies. Epigenetics. 2020;15(1-2):12-25.
7. Zhang S, Luo Q, Meng R, Yan J, Wu Y, Huang H. Long-term health risk of offspring born from assisted reproductive technologies. J Assist Reprod Genet. 2024;41(3):527-50.
8. Lei X, Zhao D, Huang L, Luo Z, Zhang J, Yu X, et al. Childhood health outcomes in term, large-for-gestational-age babies with different postnatal growth patterns. Am J Epidemiol. 2018;187(3):507-14.

9. Chen W, Peng Y, Ma X, Kong S, Tan S, Wei Y, et al. Integrated multi-omics reveal epigenomic disturbance of assisted reproductive technologies in human offspring. EBio Medicine. 2020;61:103076.
10. Pinborg A, Wennerholm UB, Bergh C. Long-term outcomes for children conceived by assisted reproductive technology. Fertil Steril. 2023;120(3 Pt 1):449-56.
11. Bjorge T, Sorensen HT, Grotmol T, Engeland A, Stephansson O, Gissler M, et al. Fetal growth and childhood cancer: a population-based study. Pediatrics. 2013;132(5):e1265-75.
12. Pomeroy KO, Comizzoli P, Rushing JS, Lersten IL, Nel-Themaat L. The ART of cryopreservation and its changing landscape. Fertil Steril. 2022;117(3):469-76.
13. Wijs LA, Fusco MR, Doherty DA, Keelan JA, Hart RJ. Asthma and allergies in offspring conceived by ART: a systematic review and meta-analysis. Hum Reprod Update. 2021;28(1):132-48.
14. Narapareddy L, Rhon-Calderon EA, Vrooman LA, Baeza J, Nguyen DK, Mesaros C, et al. Sex-specific effects of in vitro fertilization on adult metabolic outcomes and hepatic transcriptome and proteome in mouse. FASEB J. 2021;35(4):e21523.
15. Magnusson A, Laivuori H, Loft A, Oldereid NB, Pinborg A, Petzold M, et al. The association between high birth weight and long-term outcomes—implications for assisted reproductive technologies: a systematic review and meta-analysis. Front Pediatr. 2021;9:675775.
16. Elhakeem A, Taylor AE, Inskip HM, Huang JY, Mansell T, Rodrigues C, et al. Long-term cardiometabolic health in people born after assisted reproductive technology: a multicohort analysis. Eur Heart J. 2023;44(16):1464-73.
17. Spangmose AL, Christensen LH, Henningsen AA, Forman J, Opdahl S, Romundstad LB, et al. Cerebral palsy in ART children has declined substantially over time: a Nordic study from the CoNARTaS group. Hum Reprod. 2021;36(8):2358-70.
18. Idring S, Magnusson C, Lundberg M, Ek M, Rai D, Svensson AC, et al. Parental age and the risk of autism spectrum disorders: findings from a Swedish population-based cohort. Int J Epidemiol. 2014;43(1):107-15.
19. Sandin S, Nygren KG, Iliadou A, Hultman CM, Reichenberg A. Autism and mental retardation among offspring born after in vitro fertilization. JAMA. 2013;310(1):75-84.
20. Djuwantono T, Aviani JK, Permadi W, Achmad TH, Halim D. Risk of neurodevelopmental disorders in children born from different ART treatments: a systematic review and meta-analysis. J Neurodev Disord. 2020;12(1):33.
21. Belva F, Bonduelle M, Roelants M, Michielsen D, Van Steirteghem A, Verheyen G, et al. Semen quality of young adult ICSI offspring: the first results. Hum Reprod. 2016;31(12):2811-20.
22. Kettner LO, Ramlau-Hansen CH, Kesmodel US, Bay B, Matthiesen NB, Henriksen TB. Parental infertility, fertility treatment, and childhood epilepsy: a population-based cohort study. Paediatr Perinat Epidemiol. 2016;30(5):488-95.
23. Kettner LO, Matthiesen NB, Ramlau-Hansen CH, Kesmodel US, Henriksen TB. Fertility treatment with clomiphene citrate and childhood epilepsy: a nationwide cohort study. Hum Reprod. 2021;36(9):2567-75. doi:10.1093/humrep/deab110.
24. Onal H, Ercan O, Adal E, Ersen A, Onal Z. Subclinical hypothyroidism in in vitro fertilization babies. Acta Paediatr. 2012;101(6):e248-52.
25. Ginstrom Ernstad E, Hanson C, Wanggren K, Thurin-Kjellberg A, Hulthe Soderberg C, Syk Lundberg E, et al. Preimplantation genetic testing and child health: a national register-based study. Hum Reprod. 2023;38(4):739-50.
26. Pohjonen EM, Soderstrom-Anttila V, Bergh C, Loft A, Magnusson A, Pinborg A, et al. Obstetric and perinatal risks after the use of donor sperm: a systematic review and meta-analysis. Eur J Obstet Gynecol Reprod Biol. 2022;274:210-28.
27. von Versen-Hoynck F, Griesinger G. What is the true preeclampsia risk in oocyte donation pregnancies?—lack of deconfounding may lead to risk overestimation. Hum Reprod. 2022;37(8):1692-3.

CHAPTER 27

Endometriosis and Assisted Reproductive Technology

Rekha Rajendra Kumar

INTRODUCTION

"He who knows Endometriosis knows gynecology."

-William Osler

Endometriosis is a benign, estrogen dependent, and progressive gynecological disease in women of reproductive age which is extremely common. Yet, there is much that is still not understood and involves a lot of controversies.

HOW ENDOMETRIOSIS LEADS TO INFERTILITY: PATHOPHYSIOLOGY

Possible Mechanisms

Mechanical Causes

- Altered tubo-ovarian relationships because of distorted anatomy resulting impaired oocyte pickup
- Tubal damage—hydrosalpinx and hematosalpinx—altered tubal motility prevents egg capture.

Molecular Mechanisms: Alterations in Peritoneal Fluid

- Local hostile environment and peritoneal fluid abnormal macrophages and cytokines affect sperm motility, sperm oocyte interaction, and implantation failure.
- Prostanoids, cytokines, growth factors, interleukins, etc., cause chronic inflammation—impairing ovarian, tubal, and endometrial function.[1]

Alteration of Systemic Immune Response

- ↑Antiendometrial antibody (autoimmune reaction)[2]
- Increased polyclonal B cell activity, T cell, natural killer (NK) cell, and monocyte activation
- ↑Cell-mediated gametocyte injury.

Reactive Oxidative Species (ROS) and Free Radicals

Iron is sequestrated by macrophages as ferritin and, thus, macrophages are overloaded with iron. During its attempt to destroy iron, it produces large amount of ROS which leads to many adverse fertility-related issues.

IMPACT OF ENDOMETRIOSIS ON IN VITRO FERTILIZATION OUTCOME

Defective ovarian steroidogenesis and folliculogenesis affect oocyte quality, oocyte fertilization, embryogenesis, and implantation, resulting in fertilization and implantation failure due to:

- Poor ovarian reserve (POR)

- Abnormal and slow follicular and oocyte development
- Lower cytoplasmic mitochondrial content and oocyte defects; alteration in structure and function of oocyte mitochondria
- Spindle abnormalities
- Increased apoptosis of granulosa cells
- Low ovarian response
- Increased gonadotropin requirement
- Atretic follicles and ovulation failure—lesser number of follicles and low oocyte yield
- Number of fertilized oocytes and high-quality embryos are less
- Decreased estrogen production
- Dysregulated endometrial function
- Lower implantation rates
- Lower clinical pregnancy rate (CPR) and increased miscarriage rates luteinized unruptured follicle (LUF) (4–35%)
- Attenuated luteinizing hormone (LH) surge
- Luteinized unruptured follicle
- Luteal phase defect (LPD)
- Deep dyspareunia affects sexual performance.

Assisted reproductive technology (ART) is the first choice for infertility associated with endometriosis. Many studies demonstrated that endometriosis has adverse effects on all aspects of the reproductive process and consequently on in vitro fertilization (IVF)/intracytoplasmic sperm injection (ICSI) success rates.[3]

Cycle cancellation rate is three times higher in women with endometriosis. Monthly fecundity rate is lower in women with mild disease (5–11% vs. 25%). Endometriosis reduces per cycle conception by half.[4] The study by Basheer Alkudmani[5] supports the same reporting clinical and ongoing pregnancy rates (PRs) per cycle to be lower than the control group by 1.8 and 2.2% in patients, respectively, with mild endometriosis, and 17 and 22% in patients with severe endometriosis irrespective of the protocol.[5]

STATISTICS

- Prevalence of endometriosis—1 in 10 women suffer from endometriosis.
- 25–50% of infertile women have endometriosis.
- 30–50% of women with endometriosis are infertile.
- Infertile women are 6–8 times more likely to have endometriosis than fertile women.
- The frequency of endometriosis among women with infertility subjected to diagnostic hysterolaparoscopy was found to be 48%.
- The result of IVF in advanced endometriosis is 36% reduced.
- About 25% conceive after surgery.

TREATMENT

It depends on:
- Woman's age
- Symptoms
- Obstetric status
- Stage of the disease
- Ovarian reserve
- Previous ovarian surgery
- Effects of medical therapy
- Other infertility factors like tubal factor and male factor.

No Single Optional Treatment for Endometriosis

Medical management of endometriosis indicated in:
- Young women with shorter duration of infertility
- Early endometriosis and without much anatomical distortion should be offered

controlled ovarian hyperstimulation (COH) with intrauterine insemination (IUI) without surgery
- Endometrioma <3–4 cm in size
- Those which do not come in the way of ovum pick up (OPU)
- Infertile women with POR, elderly, or advanced disease
- Recurrent endometrioma.

MEDICAL MANAGEMENT

Medical management for pain by suppression of ovulation with oral contraceptive pills (OCP), dienogest, and progesterone are of no benefit for fertility treatment.

Medical management for infertility includes:[4]
- Controlled ovarian hyperstimulation and intrauterine insemination
- In vitro fertilization
- Aromatase inhibitors (AI)
- Gonadotropin-releasing hormone analog (GnRHa)—before and after surgical treatment.

INTRAUTERINE INSEMINATION EUROPEAN SOCIETY FOR HUMAN REPRODUCTION AND ENDOCRINOLOGY) GUIDELINES 2014

- Women with endometriosis must be referred to ART earlier.
- Endometriosis has decreased per cycle conception rate in comparison with male factor and unexplained infertility.[6]
- Controlled ovarian hyperstimulation with IUI should be considered within 6 months following surgery in the treatment of subfertile women with American Fertility Society (AFS)/American Society for Reproductive Medicine (ASRM) stage I/II endometriosis, when at least one tube is patent instead of expectant management, as it increases live birth rates (LBRs).
- In minimal and mild endometriosis, success rate per cycle with superovulation with IUI for consecutive 3–4 cycles is 10–15%. They have a plateau effect after 3–6 cycles. However, pregnancy rate is lower than with unexplained infertility.[7]

CONTROLLED OVARIAN HYPERSTIMULATION AND INTRAUTERINE INSEMINATION

There is no exact method to distinguish which stimulation protocol is the best for such patients.
- Clomifene citrate (CC) and IUI triples mean fertility rate from 3.3 to 9.5%
- Clomifene citrate and IUI versus letrozole and IUI gave similar results
- Follicle-stimulating hormone (FSH)/ human menopausal gonadotropin (HMG) and IUI—stages I and II (15%) and stages III and IV (8%).

INDICATIONS FOR IN VITRO FERTILIZATION—INTRACYTOPLASMIC SPERM INJECTION IN ENDOMETRIOSIS

- Diminished ovarian reserve
- Failed COH-IUI three cycles
- Presence of adenomyosis
- Female age >35 years
- Recurrent endometrioma
- Presence of other factors like male or tubal factor
- Bilateral endometrioma
- Infertility duration >5 years
- Stage III/IV disease

In Vitro Fertilization or Intracytoplasmic Sperm Injection—Which is Better?

Intracytoplasmic sperm injection is always better than IVF. In endometriosis, it is "ICSI for all" instead of IVF. Barnhart et al.[8] reported less fertilization in IVF in patients with endometriosis.

IVF protocols in women with endometriosis: The debate about the best protocol is ongoing.

- Extended GnRH analog treatment
- Ultralong protocol
- Gonadotropin-releasing hormone analog long protocol
- Antagonist protocol
- Prolonged OCP or danazol before IVF
- Short protocol
- Clomiphene plus gonadotropins
- Aromatase inhibitors plus gonadotropins
- Natural cycle IVF.

Extended Gonadotropin-releasing Hormone Agonist Protocol

There is evidence to suggest that the use of prolonged downregulation (extinguishes the disease) with GnRH agonist (11.25 mg, 3 months) prior to ovarian stimulation for IVF increases CPR by fourfold.[4]

The administration of extended GnRHa to patients with diminished ovarian reserve (DOR) may further diminish ovarian response to subsequent gonadotropin treatment. Hence, stimulation prior to GnRHa, vitrification of all those embryos, and transferring in a thaw cycle following extended GnRHa treatment may be more appropriate.

Ultralong Protocol

The ultralong protocol extends the usual 3–4 weeks of GnRHa administration with a 3.75 mg depot dose. Despite mixed findings, with one study showing no enhancement in reproductive outcomes, several retrospective studies and a Cochrane review involving three randomized controlled trials (RCTs) suggest that this protocol could indeed improve the likelihood of conception, particularly in women with stages III–IV endometriosis. This review specifically noted higher CPR and LBR in women following the ultralong protocol compared to shorter ones.[9]

Gonadotropin-releasing Hormone Agonist Long Protocols

Gonadotropin-releasing hormone analogs used in the long protocol for COH are the gold standard in fertility treatments, especially recommended for women with a good ovarian reserve. However, its efficacy decreases in women with a low ovarian reserve, who require higher doses of gonadotropins and longer stimulation periods (supported by significant statistical findings: $p < 0.001$ for dosages and $p < 0.05$ for duration).[10]

A review of six RCTs involving 286 patients showed that using GnRH agonists for 3–6 cycles before IVF-ICSI significantly increased the CPR by fourfold and reduced miscarriage rates. This efficacy is attributed to the modulation of uterine NK cells and the normalization of endometrial aromatase expression by GnRH agonists. NK cell modulation suggests an improved immune environment for embryo implantation and aromatase is crucial for estrogen synthesis, essential for a pregnancy-supportive environment.[11]

Higher number of embryos were available for cryopreservation in agonist group.[12]

The Cochrane database reviews from 2006 and 2007 collectively highlight the effectiveness of GnRHa in fertility treatments. The 2006 review, analyzing three trials with 165 women, showed that GnRHa significantly increased LBR and CPR emphasizing its potency in improving fertility outcomes (OR: 9.19; 95% CI: 1.08–78.22). The CPR per woman was also significantly higher (three studies: OR: 4.28; 95% CI: 2.00–9.15).

The 2007 review compared depot and daily GnRHa in 552 women in six studies and found no difference in CPR between the two, suggesting equal effectiveness (OR: 0.94; 95% CI: 0.65–1.37). However, it noted that depot GnRHa required more gonadotropin ampules and longer ovarian stimulation, highlighting practical differences in administration.

In a retrospective analysis comparing three groups of patients with endometriosis undergoing assisted procreation procedures, distinct approaches were evaluated:

1. The use of GnRHa (buserelin) for 3 months, followed by COH with HMG
2. The administration of GnRHa for 3 weeks, then continuing with ovarian stimulation using HMG
3. Treatment with clomiphene citrate in combination with HMG.

The results indicated that the use of GnRHa significantly increased the number of oocytes retrieved. Notably, the group treated with GnRHa for 3 months exhibited the highest fertilization rate. Comparatively, treatment with GnRHa for either 3 months or 3 weeks was found to be more effective than the combination of clomiphene citrate and HMG. This suggests that for patients with endometriosis, GnRHa based treatments, particularly the longer duration of 3 months, are more efficient in enhancing the outcomes of assisted reproduction.

The use of GnRHa in fertility treatments for endometriosis patients yields mixed effectiveness. GnRHa administration before IVF is associated with improved fertilization rates, but not necessarily higher implantation rates. While cleavage, pregnancy, and delivery rates are generally higher with GnRHa, not all studies show statistical significance. A key retrospective study by Liu et al.[13] found that the long agonist protocol in IVF significantly increased cumulative conception rates (50.3%) compared to short or ultrashort protocols (8.3%). This highlights the long agonist protocol's superior efficacy in enhancing fertility outcomes in endometriosis patients.

In evaluating the effectiveness of different approaches to enhancing pregnancy rates, two specific approaches were compared. The use of GnRH agonists (GnRHa) showed an odds ratio (OR) of 1.68 for achieving pregnancy while surgical intervention had the OR of 1.63 for the same outcome. Both these approaches resulted in pregnancy rates within the range of 25–35%. This data suggests that both GnRH agonists and surgical methods are comparably effective in increasing the likelihood of pregnancy.

Gonadotropin-releasing Hormone Antagonist Protocol

Gonadotropin-releasing hormone antagonists (cetrorelix and ganirelix) help to avoid prolonged pituitary suppression. Antagonist protocols reduce the cost and time of gonadotropin treatment compared to long and ultralong ones.

Agonist and Antagonist Protocol—Comparison

A GnRH agonist protocol appears to result in higher PR and LBR after fresh ET in women with endometriosis associated infertility suggesting that antagonist protocol might negatively impact endometrial receptivity.[14]

No significant difference was observed between the groups with freeze—thaw embryo transfer. In frozen embryo transfer (FET) cycles, the antagonist protocol has comparable clinical pregnancy outcome with long or prolonged agonist protocol, especially in those with DOR.[15]

Studies by Canis et al.[16] and Pabuccu R[12] highlight the effectiveness of COH using

TABLE 1: CPR in fresh embryo transfers of agonist versus antagonist cycles.

	Agonist cycle	*Antagonist cycle*
CPR per ET (embryo transfer) (fresh)	25%	13%
LBR per ET (fresh)	22%	10%

(CPR: clinical pregnancy rate; ET: embryo transfer; LBR: live birth rate)

both GnRH agonist and antagonist protocols. These treatments are equally effective in terms of IR and CPR in FET cycles, as evidenced in randomized trials.[14,17]

The findings, therefore, show that GnRH agonist protocol leads to higher PR and LBR after fresh embryo transfer in women with endometriosis-associated infertility, as mentioned in **Table 1** whereas the antagonist protocol might have encouraging response in FET cycles.

Anti-Müllerian Hormone and Protocol Selection

Although the mean number of oocytes retrieved was higher in the agonist group compared to the antagonist group, there was a trend for higher number of embryos and pregnancy rates in the antagonist group compared to the agonist group in low AMH population.

In a recent study, Hosseini et al.[3] showed that the expression levels of some genes involved in the cytoplasmic maturity, antiapoptotic process, and ATP production were higher in human oocytes of the women in the GnRH antagonist protocol versus those in the GnRHa protocol. For these reasons, antagonist protocol may have a positive influence on both oocyte and embryo quality; consequently, on the PR.

However, in the normal range of AMH (1.1–2.8), long agonist protocol is the best choice for these patients. Therefore, individualized IVF protocols, according to various ranges of AMH, may improve clinical outcomes of IVF/ICSI in patients with endometriosis.

Letrozole

Letrozole is an interesting drug resulting in improved endometrial receptivity. Those with poor prognosis for IVF might be improved with letrozole cotreatment. The administration of letrozole 5 mg daily for days 2–6 of gonadotropin stimulation. Letrozole gives better IVF-ET result of CPR 61 versus 14% and LBR 50 versus 7% by improving endometrial receptivity.[18]

A study of 84 patients with 121 cycles with letrozole—GnRH antagonist protocol was associated with significantly better implantation rate (IR), CPR, and LBR per embryo transfer concordant with the theory that letrozole may correct endometrial receptivity defects.

Other Protocols

Short protocol with GnRH analog should be avoided in these women because it results in lower number of oocytes yield when compared with the long protocol.

With *natural cycle IVF* protocol, possible problems such as disease progression and poor responsiveness to hyperstimulation can be avoided.

The use of combined oral contraceptive pills (COCPs) prior to ART may increase IVF success and should be considered like longer GnRH agonist downregulation. Pretreatment with OCP for 6–8 weeks before IVF-ET improves outcome.[19]

Surgery is indicated in:

- Pain attributable to endometrioma or other related symptoms

- Potential for rupture
- Size >4 cm (>3 cm as added by Donnez et al.[20]), because it may give compression effect on follicles and interfere with ovarian responsiveness during COH
- Inability to access follicles during OPU and, thus, avoid technical difficulties and follicular fluid contamination
- Concern of occult malignancy/for histological diagnosis
- Associated with infection or ovarian abscess
- Deep infiltrating endometriosis (DIE).

Presence of large endometriomas at the time of OPU significantly reduces the number of oocytes retrieved compared to the healthy ovary in contrast to normal ovaries: 31 versus 69%.[21] Cumulative pregnancy rate is 43–60% following laparoscopic surgery.

Counseling

The woman should be counseled thoroughly regarding the risks of recurrence, reduced ovarian function after surgery and sometimes, even loss of the ovarian function. ART can be offered as first-line treatment or after surgery. The decision to proceed with surgery should be considered carefully if the woman has had previous ovarian surgery.

Advantages of Laparoscopy

- Prevents endometriosis progression
- Decreased toxicity to the embryos and gamete
- Enhances uterine receptivity.

What are the Limitations of the Surgery?

- Surgery has risk of incomplete surgery and recurrence. High risk of recurrence: 25% at the end of 2 years and 40–50% at 5 years.
- Postoperative medication is required to reduce the recurrence.
- Excision/cystectomy is preferable because of less recurrence (6 vs. 20%), but excision results in more reduction of ovarian reserve as mentioned in **Table 2**.
- Unable to reverse the inflammatory and biomolecular changes.

Negative Impact of Surgery on Ovarian Reserve

Surgical intervention, particularly the excision and ablation of endometriotic lesions **(Figs. 1 and B)**, raises concerns about the balance between benefits and potential harm, such as the loss of ovarian reserve. Studies highlight the cautious approach of "less is more," with evidence showing healthy ovarian tissue (found in 97% of the cyst specimen) often removed during cyst wall stripping, as mentioned in **Table 2**. Stripped cyst wall consisted of primordial, primary, and secondary follicles in 69% cases leading to the loss of primordial follicles, especially in larger cysts.[20]

TABLE 2: Pros and cons: Laparoscopic ablation versus cystectomy.

Ablation	*Cystectomy*
• Cyst wall is ablated, not excised • Diathermy is more used • Less bleeding • A proportion of follicles may be destroyed because of thermal injury • Lesser loss of primordial follicles • Higher risk of recurrence because cyst wall is not removed	• Internal cyst wall is excised by stripping from underlying stroma–traction and countertraction • Diathermy less used, more bleeding • A proportion of follicles may get lost along with the stripped cyst wall • More loss of primordial follicles • Lower risk of recurrence as cyst wall is removed

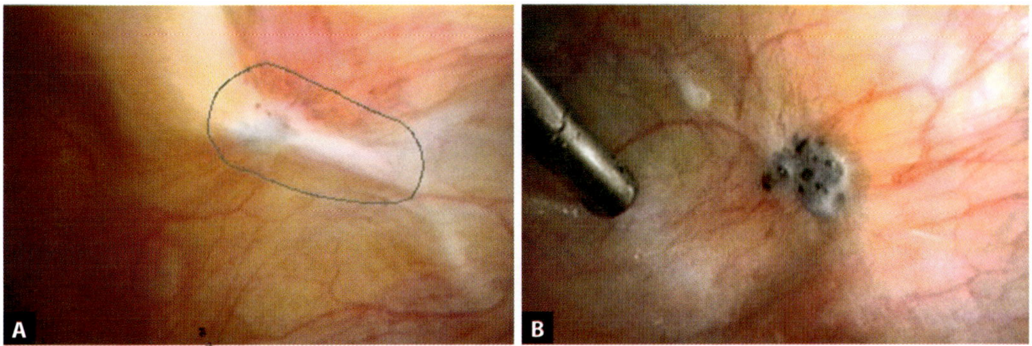

Figs. 1A and B: Endometriotic spots on the peritoneal surface.

Extensive coagulation and surgery close to the ovarian hilum are best avoided to preserve ovarian blood supply. Also, there is a negative correlation between the stage of endometriosis and the pregnancy rate postsurgery, indicating that more advanced stages of the disease can lead to lower chances of conception following surgical intervention.[22]

Proper operative laparoscopy increases pregnancy rates than just diagnostic.

Excision of the endometriotic capsule increases spontaneous PR compared to drainage and electrocoagulation of the cyst wall.

Patients with complete removal of endometriotic lesion had spontaneous PR of 25% and LBR of 19%. After surgical ablation and fulguration in stages I and II with superovulation with gonadotropins and IUI, there was 2–3 times higher LBR compared to just medical treatment. It gave shorter time to pregnancy and LBR with IVF. In patients who had IVF-ICSI after laparoscopic surgery, 48.9% conceived in stage I/II and 28.3% conceived in III/IV.[23,24] Conception rates were maximum in first 6 months and dropped after 1 year of surgery.

For small endometriomas (<3 cm), initial medical management with ovarian stimulation and IUI is advised for 3–4 cycles before considering laparoscopy, as cystectomy prior to ART does not significantly improve pregnancy rates. However, for larger endometriomas (over 3 cm), laparoscopic cystectomy before ART is recommended, improving follicle accessibility, (as mentioned in **Table 3**) and reducing pain, followed by GnRHa treatment and IVF-ICSI[25] and, thus, higher fertility rates.

TABLE 3: Advantages and disadvantages of surgery for endometrioma.

Advantages of surgery	*Disadvantages of surgery*
• Better IVF success rate • Prevents rupture • Facilitates oocyte retrieval • Avoids contamination of follicular fluid with contents • Occult malignancy can be detected • Prevents progression	• Cystectomy prior to IVF does not improve PR • Surgery and anesthesia risks • Potential risk of reduction of ovarian reserve • Aspiration prior to IVF does not increase PR

(IVF: in vitro fertilization; PR: pregnancy rate)

Challenges with endometriomas >4 cm **(Figs. 2A to D)** include difficulties in oocyte retrieval, the risk of cyst puncture, follicular-fluid contamination, and potential infection.[21]

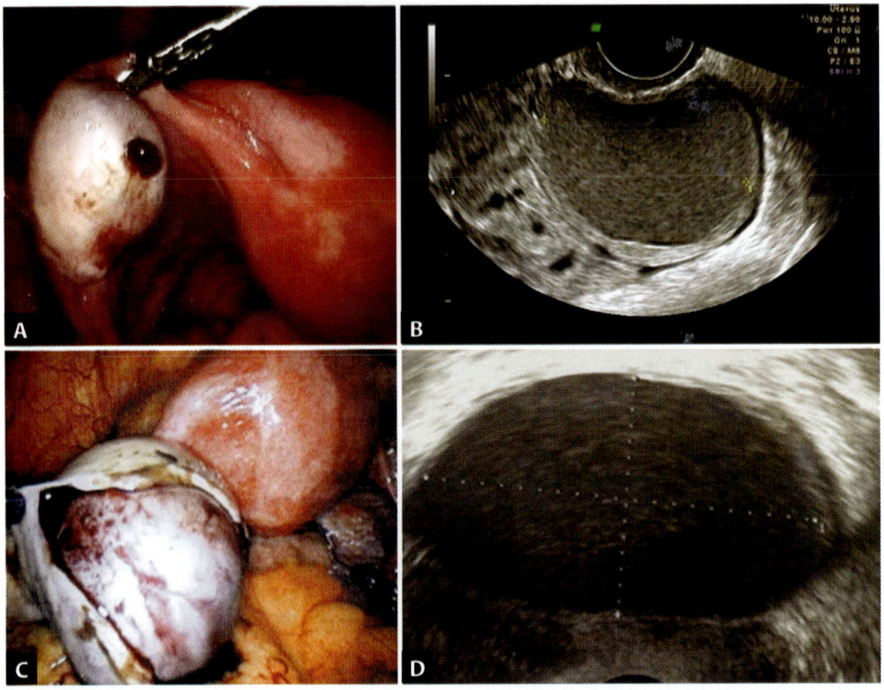

Figs. 2A to D: Endometrioma presentation. (A and C) Laparoscopic and (B and D) Sonography.

TABLE 4: Comparison of benefits and risks of expectant management versus surgical management.

	Expectant management	*Surgical management*
Potential benefits	• Avoids surgery and its complications • No further compromise on ovarian reserve • Avoids delay in commencing ART	• Alleviates symptoms • Histological confirmation and excludes malignancy • Decreased risk of cyst complication • Facilitates ovarian access during OPU
Potential risks	• Pain of various presentation persists • Cyst rupture • Difficult ovarian access during OPU • Infection of endometrioma • No histological diagnosis • May accelerate	• Surgical and anesthetic risks • Decreased ovarian reserve • Postoperative adhesions • Potential delay of ART

(ART: assisted reproductive technology; OPU: ovum pick up)

Surgery is generally avoided in older patients, those with low ovarian reserve, asymptomatic cases, bilateral or recurrent endometrioma due to risks such as reduced ovarian response, decreased oocyte yield, and a higher likelihood of recurrence (as mentioned in **Table 4**).

In vitro fertilization or intracytoplasmic sperm injection cycles postendometrioma excision can face these difficulties:

- Reduced ovarian volume and antral follicle count (AFC)
- Reduced ovarian response on stimulation and oocyte yield

- So, COH needs more gonadotropins and longer stimulation days
- Reduced E2 (estradiol) level.

Advantages of Preoperative Gonadotropin-releasing Hormone Agonist

- Reduction in cyst size
- Reduction of hypervascularization and inflammation
- Reduction in cyst wall thickness
- Reduction of adhesions.

Endometriotic Cyst Aspiration

No statistically different response is seen, with or without cyst aspiration. So, it is not recommended to make ultrasound-guided aspiration with or without sclerotherapy. It is reserved in cases of recurrent endometrioma that may hinder oocyte retrieval like ones >4 cm or in symptomatic infertile women with low-ovarian reserve.

Sclerotherapy

Ethanol sclerotherapy decreases the recurrence rate of endometrioma without altering the results of IVF, where a second surgery would have a deleterious effect. CPR was same in both cystectomy and sclerotherapy, in some clinical trials.[26]

Precautions to be Taken During Ovum Pick Up in the Presence of Endometrioma

- Antibiotic prophylaxis
- 2% betadine vaginal wash followed by thorough saline wash before OPU
- Strict asepsis to be maintained during OPU
- Avoid repeatedly exposing needle tip to vagina and outside
- Avoid puncture and aspiration of the endometrioma.

Fertility Preservation in Women with Endometriosis

Vitrification of the embryos, cryopreservation of the oocytes, or of ovarian tissue is a good practical option in women with bilateral endometriomas or POR.[27]

To summarize, the management of endometriosis-related infertility requires a comprehensive and nuanced approach without delay, prioritizing both fertility restoration and symptom relief. Laparoscopy is the gold standard for diagnosis, offering precision with minimal invasiveness and respectful handling of ovaries. In treating endometriosis, particularly large endometriomas, cystectomy is often the preferred surgical option. For early-stage endometriosis (I/II), combining COH with IUI has proven more effective than expectant management. In advanced stages (III/IV), operative laparoscopy increases pregnancy rates compared to a nonintervention approach.

In IVF treatments for endometriosis, downregulation for 3–6 months prior to ART improves the success, although overall ART success rates are low. Ovulation stimulation, regardless of the protocol chosen, does not appear to exacerbate endometriosis.

Gonadotropin-releasing hormone agonist protocol is associated with improved fertilization rates and a higher yield of mature oocytes and embryos for cryopreservation, thereby increasing the cumulative fecundity rate. Conversely, the antagonist protocol with FET is particularly advantageous for patients with low AMH.

Objectives of the treatment should be not only on restoring fertility at the earliest but also on alleviating pain and other symptoms to improve the patient's quality of life. Controlling the underlying disease to prevent recurrence and regular monitoring are critical.

CONCLUSION

Endometriosis reduces the fertility potential because of many mechanisms, right from egg, embryo, and endometrial quality to take-home baby rates. Once diagnosed, women should initiate her fertility treatment as early as possible rather than wait -and -watch policy. Surgery improving the fertility is not necessary in all the cases. ICSI is always better than IVF for these oocytes. Though there are many treatment protocols, success rates of all appear almost same. The reproductive physician's previous experience has a great impact in deciding the protocols and the ART success.

REFERENCES

1. Garcia Garcia JM, Vannuzzi V, Donati C, Bernacchioni C, Bruni P, Petraglia F. Endometriosis: cellular and molecular mechanisms leading to fibrosis. Reprod Sci. 2023;30(5):1453-61.
2. Gajbhiye R, Suryawanshi A, Khan S, Meherji P, Warty N, Raut V, et al. Multiple endometrial antigens are targeted in autoimmune endometriosis. Reprod Biomed Online. 2008;16(6):817-24.
3. Hosseini E, Mehraein F, Shahhoseini M, Karimian L, Nikmard F, Ashrafi M, et al. Epigenetic alterations of CYP19A1 gene in Cumulus cells and its relevance to infertility in endometriosis. J Assist Reprod Genet. 2016;33(8):1105-13.
4. Dunselman GA, Vermeulen N, Becker C, Calhaz-Jorge C, D'Hooghe T, De Bie B, et al. ESHRE guideline: management of women with endometriosis. Hum Reprod Oxf Engl. 2014;29(3):400-12.
5. AlKudmani B, Gat I, Buell D, Salman J, Zohni K, Librach C, et al. In vitro fertilization success rates after surgically treated endometriosis and effect of time interval between surgery and in vitro fertilization. J Minim Invasive Gynecol. 2018;25(1):99-104.
6. Filip L, Duică F, Prădatu A, Crețoiu D, Suciu N, Crețoiu SM, et al. Endometriosis associated infertility: a critical review and analysis on etiopathogenesis and therapeutic approaches. Medicina (Mex). 2020;56(9):460.
7. Kennedy S, Bergqvist A, Chapron C, D'Hooghe T, Dunselman G, Greb R, et al. ESHRE guideline for the diagnosis and treatment of endometriosis. Hum Reprod. 2005;20(10):2698-704.
8. Barnhart K, Dunsmoor-Su R, Coutifaris C. Effect of endometriosis on in vitro fertilization. Fertil Steril. 2002;77(6):1148-55.
9. Cao X, Chang HY, Xu JY, Zheng Y, Xiang YG, Xiao B, et al. The effectiveness of different down-regulating protocols on in vitro fertilization-embryo transfer in endometriosis: a meta-analysis. Reprod Biol Endocrinol. 2020;18(1):16.
10. Georgiou EX, Melo P, Baker PE, Sallam HN, Arici A, Garcia-Velasco JA, et al. Long-term GnRH agonist therapy before in vitro fertilisation (IVF) for improving fertility outcomes in women with endometriosis. Cochrane Database Syst Rev. 2019;2019(11):CD013240.
11. Sallam HN, Garcia-Velasco JA, Dias S, Arici A, Abou-Setta AM, Jaafar SH. Long-term pituitary down-regulation before in vitro fertilization (IVF) for women with endometriosis. Cochrane Database Syst Rev. 2006;2006(1):CD004635.
12. Pabuccu R, Onalan G, Kaya C. GnRH agonist and antagonist protocols for stage I-II endometriosis and endometrioma in in vitro fertilization/intracytoplasmic sperm injection cycles. Fertil Steril. 2007;88(4):832-9.
13. Liu S, Xie Y, Li F, Jin L. Effectiveness of ultra-long protocol on in vitro fertilization/intracytoplasmic sperm injection-embryo transfer outcome in infertile women with

endometriosis: a systematic review and meta-analysis of randomized controlled trials. J Obstet Gynaecol Res. 2021;47(4):1232-42.

14. Kolanska K, Cohen J, Bendifallah S, Selleret L, Antoine JM, Chabbert-Buffet N, et al. Pregnancy outcomes after controlled ovarian hyperstimulation in women with endometriosis-associated infertility: GnRH-agonist versus GnRH-antagonist. J Gynecol Obstet Hum Reprod. 2017;46(9):681-6.
15. Yu Y, Wei K, Yao Q, Tian S, Liang K, Zhou L, et al. Controlled ovarian stimulation protocols in endometriosis patients: with antagonist or agonist? Zhejiang Da Xue Xue Bao Yi Xue Ban. 2019;48(2):165-73.
16. Canis M, Pouly JL, Tamburro S, Mage G, Wattiez A, Bruhat MA. Ovarian response during IVF–embryo transfer cycles after laparoscopic ovarian cystectomy for endometriotic cysts of >3 cm in diameter. Hum Reprod. 2001;16(12):2583-6.
17. Bastu E, Yasa C, Dural O, Mutlu MF, Celik C, Ugurlucan FG, et al. Comparison of ovulation induction protocols after endometrioma resection. JSLS. 2014;18(3):e2014.00128.
18. Miller PB, Parnell BA, Bushnell G, Tallman N, Forstein DA, Higdon HL 3rd, et al. Endometrial receptivity defects during IVF cycles with and without letrozole. Hum Reprod. 2012;27(3):881-8.
19. Xu L, Ding L, Jiang J, Liu P, Wei D, Qin Y. Effects of oral contraceptive pretreatment on IVF outcomes in women following a GnRH agonist protocol. Reprod Biomed Online. 2019;39(6):924-30.
20. Donnez J, Nisolle M, Smoes P, Gillet N, Beguin S, Casanas-Roux F. Peritoneal endometriosis and "endometriotic" nodules of the rectovaginal septum are two different entities. Fertil Steril. 1996;66(3):362-8.
21. Benaglia L, Somigliana E, Vercellini P, Abbiati A, Ragni G, Fedele L. Endometriotic ovarian cysts negatively affect the rate of spontaneous ovulation. Hum Reprod. 2009; 24(9):2183-6.
22. Adamson GD, Pasta DJ. Surgical treatment of endometriosis-associated infertility: meta-analysis compared with survival analysis. Am J Obstet Gynecol. 1994;171(6):1488-505.
23. Kuivasaari P, Hippeläinen M, Anttila M, Heinonen S. Effect of endometriosis on IVF/ICSI outcome: stage III/IV endometriosis worsens cumulative pregnancy and live-born rates. Hum Reprod. 2005;20(11):3130-5.
24. The ESHRE Capri Workshop. ESHRE: Guidelines to the prevalence, diagnosis, treatment and management of infertility, 1996. Hum Reprod. 1996;11(8):1775.
25. RCOG. (2023). Endometriosis, Investigation and Management (Green-top Guideline No. 24). [online] Available from https://www.rcog.org.uk/guidance/browse-all-guidance/green-top-guidelines/endometriosis-investigation-and-management-green-top-guideline-no-24/ [Last accessed Feb., 2026].
26. Chauffour C, Pouly JL, Gremeau AS. Prise en charge en FIV en cas d'endométriose, RPC Endométriose CNGOF-HAS. Gynécologie Obstétrique Fertil Sénologie. 2018;46(3): 338-48.
27. Llarena NC, Falcone T, Flyckt RL. Fertility preservation in women with endometriosis. Clin Med Insights Reprod Health. 2019; 13:1179558119873386.

Index

Page numbers followed by *b* refer to box, *f* refer to figure, *fc* refer to flowchart, and *t* refer to table.

A

Aberrant oocyte maturation 114
Actinomycin D 139
Acute lymphoid leukemia 216
Adenomyosis 50
Adenosine triphosphate 159
Adiponectin 116
Adipose tissue 117
Adnexal lesions 50
Adnexal torsion, recurrent 68
Adrenoleukodystrophy 100
Adriamycin 139
Agglutination 37
Aggregation 37
Air pollution 17
Alcohol 175
Alkylating agents 73
Allelic dropout 94
Allergic reactions 48
Amenorrhea 26
American Society for Reproductive Medicine 25, 72, 125, 181, 184
Amniocentesis 102
Androgen
  aromatization of 117
  excess 114
  peripheral conversion of 117
Androgenic acne 114
Androstenedione 111
Anesthesia 134
Aneuploidy 100
  conceptions 218
  risk of 72
Angiogenesis 166*f*
Anovulation 113, 117
Anti-Müllerian hormone 27, 42, 43, 44*f*, 125, 167, 225
  levels 42
Antioxidants 130, 157, 158*t*, 159, 171*f*
  role of 156, 171*f*
  supplementation 40
  therapy 160, 171*f*
Anti-sperm antibodies, presence of 37
Antral follicle 45
  count 44*f*, 45, 125, 228
    drops 121
Aphrodite criteria 132
Apoptotic cells 92
Appendix 109
Aromatase 111
  inhibitor 71, 143, 149, 150, 222
Array comparative genomic hybridization 91
Artificial gametes 213
Artificial intelligence 52, 71*f*, 78, 79, 81, 82, 181, 192, 206
  assisted noninvasive embryo assessment 96
  diagnostics 135
  models, continuous improvement of 86
Artificial reproductive 65
Asherman's syndrome 164, 166
Aspermia 33
Assisted reproductive technology 17, 59, 60, 100, 125, 130, 149, 170, 171*f*, 197-201, 201*fc*, 203-205, 205*t*, 209-211, 211*t*, 212, 215, 220, 228
  Act 201
  advances in 188
  and surrogacy
    Acts, key provisions of 212*b*
    landmark case laws in 211*b*, 212*b*
  applications in 52
  conceptions 217
  counseling for 206
  encompasses 198
  ethical principles in 209*b*
  evolution of 197
  guidelines 204*t*
  legal
    considerations in 211
    pathways 212*fc*
  long-term health of 215
  lower 10
  Massachusetts outcome study of 216
  medications 149
  overview of 198
  planning 50
  possible long-term adverse outcomes of 215
  procedure 70
    types of 198, 198*fc*
Asthenoteratozoospermia 34
Asthenozoospermia 33
Asthma 217
Atretic follicles 221
Attenuated luteinizing hormone 221
Autism spectrum disease 217
Autoimmune
  diseases 68
  disorders 73
Autonomy 209
Azathioprine 139
Azoospermia 5, 33
  functional 5
  nonobstructive 132, 171*f*

B

Balloon-tipped devices 48
Basal serum follicle-stimulating hormone levels 42
Beta-thalassemia 100
Bevacizumab 139
Biochemical tests 42
Bioinformatics 95
Bisphenol A 16
Blastocoel fluid 89, 92
  aspiration
    advantages of 92*t*
    disadvantages of 92*t*
  deoxyribonucleic acid 92

Blastocyst 89
  transfer 100
Bleomycin 139
Blood cells 35
Body
  mass index 4, 16, 18
  weight 170
Breast cancer 68, 139
Bromocriptine 149
Busulfan 139

C

Cabergoline 149
Caffeine 19, 175
Cancer 140
  breast 68, 139
  gynecological 140
  hematological 140
  therapy 138
  treatment, impact of 138
Carbohydrates 172, 173
Carbon monoxide 17
Carboplatin 139
Cardiovascular disease 217
Carmustine 139
Carnitine esters 160
Cell
  count 35
  types, variety of 71
Cellular components 37
Central nervous system tumors 216
Cerebral palsy 217
Cervical factors 182
Cetuximab 139
Chemotherapy 67
  incorporating alkylating agents 140
Chlorambucil 139
Chlormethine 139
Chorionic villus sampling 102
Chromosomal structural rearrangements 89, 100
Circadian rhythms 175
Cisplatin 139
Cleavage-stage 89
  embryo transfer 102
Clinical pregnancy rate 221, 225
Clomiphene 134, 154
  citrate 149, 150, 222, 224
    challenge test 42, 43
Coelomic metaplasia 109
Coenzyme Q10 157, 171*f*
Combined oral contraceptive pills, use of 225
Committee of Nordic ART and safety 216
Comparative genomic hybridization 100
Computer-assisted semen analysis 129
Controlled delivery systems 168
Controlled ovarian
  hyperstimulation 121, 222
  stimulation 125, 149
Conventional testicular sperm extraction 75
Cortical ovarian biopsy 73
Counseling
  couple 202
  family 202
  importance of 200
  informative 200
  role of 200
  supportive 200
Cryopreservation 71, 74, 210
  methods 76
  technique of 71
Cryptozoospermia 33
Culture strategy 95
Cyclophosphamide 139
Cyst 68
  ovarian 50
Cystectomy 226*t*
Cytarabine 139
Cytokines 220
Cytological stains 131
Cytosine 94

D

Dacarbazine 139
Dactinomycin 139
Daunorubicin 139
Decision-making counseling 200
Deep learning models 96
Deep neural networks 80
Defective ovarian steroidogenesis 220
Dehydroepiandrosterone 125, 126, 159
  sulfate 28
Deoxyribonucleic acid 38, 89, 159, 182
  embryonic 95*fc*
  extraction 95
  fragmentation 39, 156
Diabetes 217
Dietary interventions 19, 171
Digital
  counseling platforms, integration of 206
  solutions 191
  subtraction hysterosalpingogram 48
Dilated epididymal tubules 135
Diminished ovarian reserve 43, 223
Donor
  anonymity 201
  rights 205
  selection 197
  transparency 201
Dopamine agonist 149, 153
Down syndrome 100
Doxorubicin 139
Dual stimulation 71, 142

E

Ejaculation
  retrograde 5
  volume 33
Elective fertility preservation, ethics of 126
Electro-ejaculation 32
Elevated follicle-stimulating hormone levels 138
Embryo 71, 110
  assessment modalities 78
  creation 210
  cryopreservation 69, 72
  development 59, 181
  disposal 213
  early 58
  selection 192
    integrating multiple modalities for 80
    techniques 78, 82*t*
  status of 209
  storage 213
  transfer 50, 225
    cleavage-stage 102
    guidance 52
Embryogenesis 220
Embryonic fraction 92
Emotional distress 11, 201
Endocrine
  disrupting chemicals 16, 171*f*
  factors 182
  treatments 140

Endometrial
 assessment 50
 development 111
 function 220
 methylation patterns 59
 morphology, assessment of 50
 quality 230
 receptivity 181
  analysis 181
  assays 183
  defects 181
 response 150
Endometrioma 68, 110, 227*t*, 228*f*, 229
Endometriosis 68, 109, 171*f*, 220-222, 229
 associated infertility 109, 110
 etiology of 110
 impact of 220
 medical management of 221
 pathogenesis of 109
Endometriotic
 capsule 227
 cyst aspiration 229
 spots 227*f*
Endometrium 111, 166*f*
 ectopic 112
 eutopic 112
 thin 166
Epidermal growth factor 164
Epididymal sperm retrieval techniques 74*f*
Epididymal tubule 74*f*
Epididymis 74*f*
Epigenetic 18, 58
 aberrations 215
 changes 122
 findings 61
 mechanisms 57
 regulation 58
 role of 59*t*
Epilepsy 217
Epithelial cells 37
Epithelial proliferation 166*f*
Estradiol 111
Estrogen-dependent benign inflammatory disease 109
Estrone 111
European Society for Human Reproduction and Endocrinology guidelines 222
European Society of Human Reproduction and Embryology 25, 81, 184
Exogenous human chorionic gonadotropin 151
Extracellular matrix 164, 166*f*

F

Fallopian tube 48*f*, 109, 110
Fats 172, 173
Fatty acids, polyunsaturated 173
Female fertility 121, 171*f*, 176*f*
 effects on 17
 preservation 70*fc*
Female infertility 157
 stigma instrument 11
Female reproductive
 health 172*t*
 tract 60
Ferriman-Gallway score, modified 114
Fertility 58*b*, 138
 decline, age-related 121, 125, 125*fc*
 female 121, 171*f*, 176*f*
 male 171*f*, 176*f*
 outcomes 61
 preservation 67, 70, 76, 138, 141, 229
  current strategies for 141
  indicator 67
  interventions 141
  technique 67, 69
 problem inventory 10
 quality 10
Fertilization 59, 60, 72, 181
Fibers 172, 174
Fibroids 50
Flavonoids 171*f*
Fludarabine 139
Fluorescence in situ hybridization technique 100
Fluorouracil 139
Folate 57, 58*b*, 58*f*, 61, 172
 pathway variants 57
 supplementation 62
Folic acid 159, 218
 periconceptional 61
Follicles, activated primary 114
Follicle-stimulating hormone 19, 149, 222
 cells 117
 measurement of 27, 42
 secretion 10
Follicular development 150
Folliculogenesis 220
 impaired 113
Fragile X premutation 69
Free radicals 220
Freezing 210
Fresh embryo transfers 225*t*
Frozen embryo transfer conceptions 215
Functional ovarian reserve 43, 44*f*

G

Gamete 110
 development 59
 donation 209
 dysfunction 181
 formation 60
 in vitro maturation of 76
 intrafallopian transfer 198
 quality defects 181
 transport 110
Gametogenesis 57, 58
Gemcitabine 139
Genetics 110
 counseling 103, 202
 data 52
 testing 131
Germ cells 58, 75*f*
 immature 37
Germinal vesicle 72
Gestational age, large for 215
Glucocorticoids 61, 153
Glucose transporter 174
Glycoprotein hormone 43
Gonadotoxic treatments 67, 138
Gonadotropin-releasing hormone 10, 19, 125, 126, 152*f*
 agonist 70*fc*, 152, 229
  protocol 223
 analogs 73, 152, 222
 antagonists 71, 224
  protocol 142, 224
 therapy 149
Gonadotropins 149, 151, 154
 ampules 224
Granulocyte colony-stimulating factor 168
Granulosa cell 43, 44*f*
 luteinization, premature 114
Green fluorescent protein 111

Growing follicles, granulosa cells of 43
Growth factor 164, 165, 220
release of 166*f*, 168
Guanine 94
Gut microbial folate production 61

H

Head defects 38
Health and diseases paradigm, developmental origins of 215
Hematopoietic stem cell 100
transplantation 73
Hematopoietic system 100
Hematosalpinx 220
Hematospermia 34
Heterosexual couples 199
Higher-resolution copy number variations 94
Hirsutism 114
Hodgkin's lymphoma 140
Homeobox A10 dysregulation 181
Homocysteine 61, 62
Hormonal balance 176*f*
Human chorionic gonadotropin 84, 152*f*
Human Fertilization and Embryology Authority register 216
Human leukocyte antigen 89
Human menopausal gonadotropin 149
Human reproduction 59*t*, 60*t*
Hydrogels 168
Hydrosalpinx 48*f*, 220
Hyperandrogenism 113, 216
Hyperestrogenism, maternal 216
Hyperhomocysteinemia, persistent 61
Hyperinsulinemia 113-115
Hyperspermia 33
Hypogonadism 134
Hypospermia 33
Hypothalamic-pituitary
adrenal axis 10, 18, 19
gonadal axis 18, 19, 170
Hypothesis, developmental 114
Hysterolaparoscopy 183
Hysterosalpingo-contrast sonography 28, 51
Hysterosalpingography 28, 47, 48, 48*f*, 182, 183

I

Ifosfamide 139
Immotile sperm 36
Immune
dysregulation 57, 60*t*
epigenetics 60
factors 61
regulation 59
therapies 62
Immunity, altered 109
Immunology 181
Implantation 58-60, 220
failure 166
In vitro fertilization 4, 9, 18, 31, 52, 59, 74, 151, 159, 171*f*, 174, 181-184, 188, 189, 197, 198, 209, 211, 221, 222, 227, 228
challenging aspects of 78
failures 166
incidence of 4
indications for 222
outcome 220
In vitro maturation 69, 70*fc*, 72, 76
In vivo environment, lack of 72
Infections 40, 48, 171*f*
Infertility 3, 9, 13, 16, 17*t*, 18*t*, 31, 47, 113, 156, 171*f*, 175, 199, 220
assessment 26
pivotal tools in 47
basic diagnostic workup of 25*fc*
burden of 188
causes of 149, 170*f*
diagnosis, substantial proportion of 57
disorders 59
epidemiology of 3, 188
female 157
history of 3
idiopathic 181, 183*t*
male 129, 160, 189
management 171*f*, 222
parental 216
prevalence of 188
primary 188
psychological impact of 202*t*
relational dimensions of 11
secondary 188
sociocultural dimensions of 189
stigma scale 11
unexplained 5, 52, 57, 61, 171*f*, 181, 183*t*
Inflammation 61, 220
Informed consent 103, 204
Inner cell mass 78
Inositol 157
Insulin
like growth factor 1 159, 164
resistance 113
sensitizing drug 153
Interleukins 220
receptor 174
International Committee for Monitoring Assisted Reproductive Technologies 188
International Evidence-based Guideline Criteria 113
International Legal Perspectives 211
Intracytoplasmic sperm injection 74, 130, 151, 171*f*, 182-184, 197, 198, 209, 215, 221, 222
cycles postendometrioma excision 228
Intratesticular testosterone 134
Intrauterine
growth restriction 60
infusion technique 167
insemination 31, 171*f*, 181-183, 222
pathology 51
detection of 47
Invasive pre-natal genetic tests 102
Irinotecan 139
Iron 172

L

Laboratory sperm handling 74*f*, 75*f*
Laparoscopic ovarian drilling 153
Laparoscopy, advantages of 226
L-carnitine 161, 171*f*
Leptin 116
Letrozole 143, 149, 150, 154, 225
Leukemia 68

Leukocyte 168
Leukocytospermia 34
Leverage digital technologies 192
Ligaments 109
Live birth rate 125, 225
Longer stimulation period 150
Low ovarian reserve 143
Low-cost in vitro fertilization models 190
Low-density lipoprotein receptor 174
Low-osmolar iodinated contrast agents 48
Luteal phase defect 221
Luteinizing hormone 10, 19, 27, 114, 117, 125, 126, 149
  surge 71
Lymphoma 68

M

Major artificial intelligence-based embryo assessment systems 84*t*
Makler's chamber 35
Male fertility 171*f*, 176*f*
  effects on 17
Male infertility 129, 160, 189
Male reproductive tract 60
Malignancies 216
  hematological 68
Masturbation 31
Maternal-fetal immune balance 59
Mechlorethamine 139
Media portrayals 199
Medicine, regenerative 164
Mediterranean diet 173
Melatonin 159
Melphalan 139
Menstrual cycle 27, 47
  irregular 26, 113
Menstruation, retrograde 109
Mercaptopurine 139
Metabolic diseases 100
Metabolic syndrome 114, 115
Metformin 153
Methotrexate 139
Methylation 60, 96
Methylenetetrahydrofolate reductase 57
Microbiome 61, 114
  dysbiosis 181
  profiling 183
Microfluidics 131
Micronutrient 174
  status 156
Microorganisms 35
Microscopic examination
  primary 35
  secondary 37
Microsurgical epididymal sperm aspiration 32, 74*f*, 75, 135
Microsurgical testicular sperm extraction 75, 75*f*, 134
Minerals 172
Minimally invasive
  blastocoel fluid aspiration 95*fc*
  preimplantation genetic testing 89, 92
Miscarriage, recurrent 171*f*
Mitochondrial deoxyribonucleic acid deletions 181
Mitochondrial dysfunction 122
Mitomycin 139
Monoclonal antibodies 139
Monogenic gene defects 100
Mood change 10
Morphology 33, 37
Mosaicism 90, 94
  low rates of 92
Motility 33, 35
Müllerian ducts, regression of 43
Multidisciplinary teams, role of 205, 205*t*
Multidose antagonist protocol 153*f*
Multimodal embryo selection 83
Multiple pregnancy, chances of 150
Multivitamins 172
Myoinositol 157, 161
Myometrial lesions 50
Myotonic dystrophy 100

N

N-acetylcysteine 159, 171*f*
National Institute for Health and Care Excellence 181, 184
Neck defects 38
Necrozoospermia 33
Neural tube defect 61
Neurodevelopmental disorders 217
Neuroendocrine 116
Next-generation sequencing 89, 91, 94, 96
Nitrogen dioxide 17
Nongenetic factors influence fertility 16
Nongrowing follicles 121*f*
Noninvasive preimplantation genetic testing 92
Nonphysiologic steroid hormone environment 216
Nonsteroidal anti-inflammatory drugs 49
Normozoospermia 33
Nutrigenomics, role of 173*t*
Nutrition 18, 170
  impact of 176*f*

O

Obesity 113, 217
Oligoasthenoteratozoospermia 34, 216
Oligoasthenozoospermia 34
Oligomenorrhea 26
Oligoteratozoospermia 34
Oligozoospermia 33
Omega-3 fatty acids 160
Oncofertility, pivotal advancement for 71
One-carbon metabolism 57, 58*b*, 58*f*
Oocyte 71
  cryopreservation 69, 71
  fertilization 220
  immature 69
  multiple 70
  quality 72, 220
Oral contraceptive pills 114, 222
Ovarian
  applications 164
  cortex strips 73
  decline 121
  disorders 167, 167*t*
  factors 182
  failure, premature 125
  function, endocrinology of 42
  hyperstimulation syndrome, complication of 70
  injection technique 167
  insufficiency 165*f*
    primary 69, 149
  reserve 42, 43, 221, 226
    assessment 42, 45
    tests 127, 141

response 42
stimulation 69, 70, 142, 149
mild 151
protocols 125
suppression 73
tissue
cryopreservation 68, 69, 72, 73, 143
transplantation 143
transposition 69
tumors, benign 68
volume 45
Ovaries
protection of 141
ultrasound imaging of 45
Ovulation
assessment 182
disorders, World Health Organization classification of 149
failure 221
induction 149, 183
protocols 149
monitoring of 150
Ovulatory dysfunction 5
Ovum pick up 228
way of 222
Oxaliplatin 139
Oxidative stress 17, 72, 113, 122, 156, 161, 171*f*, 176*f*
assays 131
impact of 171*f*
mechanism of 157*f*
Oxygen tension 215

P

Paracervical block 49
Paternal genome integrity 216
Patient-oriented strategies encompassing individualized oocyte number 125
Pelvic pathology 5
Penile vibratory stimulation 31
Percutaneous epididymal sperm aspiration 74, 74*f*, 135
Percutaneous sperm retrieval methods 74
Percutaneous testicular sperm aspiration 75*f*
Perfluoroalkyl substances 16
Peritoneal fluid 110, 220
Peritoneal mesothelial cells 109
Peroxisome proliferator-activated receptor gamma 174
Pesticides 17
agricultural 17
pH 35
Placental dysfunction 215, 216
Platelet
biology 165
concentration 164, 168
derived growth factor 164
rich plasma 126, 164-167
administration, methods of 167
biological basis of 165
clinical studies of 166*t*, 167*t*
effect of 166*f*
infusion 166*f*
injection 168*f*
preparation techniques 165
timing of 166*f*
use of 165*f*
Polar body biopsy 89
Polyamines 35
Polycystic ovarian
morphology 113
syndrome 5, 16, 26, 59, 113, 149, 157, 171*f*, 174, 216
prevalence of 189
Polyzoospermia 33
Poor cytoplasmic maturation 72
Poor ovarian reserve 125*fc*, 167, 220
management strategies for 125, 126
Poor ovarian response 121, 122, 126
Posterior cul-de-sac 109
Postpreimplantation genetic test 218
Preeclampsia 215
Pregnancy
loss, recurrent 48, 61, 182
planning 159
rate 183, 184, 183*f*, 227
Preimplantation
development 57
genetic
diagnosis 89
testing 69, 79, 81*f*, 82, 89, 90*f*, 93*t*, 94, 100-102, 210
Pre-in vitro fertilization screening 52
Premature granulosa cell luteinization 114
Premature ovarian
failure 125
insufficiency 167
Preoperative gonadotropin-releasing hormone agonist, advantages of 229
Procarbazine 139
Progesterone
receptors, dysregulation of 112
resistance 112
Progestin-primed ovarian stimulation 71
Progressive motility 36, 37
Prostanoids 220
Proteomic data 52
Provocative tests 42
Psychological counseling 202
Pus cell 37
Pyospermia 34

Q

Quantifies oxidation-reduction potential 131

R

Radiation 171*f*
safety 48
Radiotherapy 68
Randomized controlled trial 125, 173, 174
Random-start stimulation protocols 70, 142
Reactive oxygen species 131, 156, 159, 220
generation 72
Recombinant luteinizing hormone 125
Recurrent implantation failure 52
Reproduction 58, 157*f*
female 156
male 156
third-party 218
Reproductive
care, quality of 87
function 217
health
female 172*t*
worldwide, major component of 188
medicine 101, 200
outcomes 61

problems 116
tract
female 60
infections 189
male 60
Rheumatoid arthritis 68

S

S-adenosylmethionine 57, 60
Saline infusion sonohysterography 28, 47, 51, 183
Sclerotherapy 229
Scrotal skin 74*f*, 75*f*
Scrotum 75*f*
Selective estrogen receptor modulators, co-administration of 143
Selenium 160, 173, 174
Semen 37
analysis 31, 32, 37, 57, 182
computer-assisted 129
appearance 34
collection, methods of 31
handling of 32
microscopic examination of 35
nomenclature of 33*t*
quality 33, 171*f*
poor 40
volume 36
Seminal oxidative stress status 171*f*
Seminal plasma 135
Seminiferous tubules 75*f*, 134
microdissection of 75*f*
Sertoli-cell-only regions 134
Serum estradiol levels 150
Sex hormone-binding globulin 114
Sexual and Reproductive Health and Rights Agenda 3
Sexual intimacy 11
Sexually transmitted infections 40
Sickle cell anemia 100
Sigmoid colon 109
Single antagonist protocol 152*f*
Single cell
signals 96
whole-genome amplification innovations 94
Single embryo transfer 78
Single gene defects 100
Single nucleotide
polymorphism array 100
variants, detection of 96
Skin 117
incision 75*f*
Sleep 175
disruption 10
Social stigma 201
Soft catheters 48
Sonohysterography 47, 51
Spend culture medium 89, 92, 93*t*
advantages of 94*t*
disadvantages of 94*t*
Sperm 35, 37
binding head-to-tail 37
chromatin maturity tests 131
concentration 33
cryopreservation 40, 74
defects in 38*f*
deoxyribonucleic acid 31
integrity 171*f*
deoxyribonucleic acid fragmentation 16, 39*f*, 40, 160, 181
assays 130*t*
index 39, 181
testing 130, 183
freezing 40
indications for 73
gentle sorting of 131
motility 35
parts of 38
selection
devices 131
techniques 40
Spermatogenesis 19, 75*f*, 134
Spermatozoa 75*f*
Standalone decision systems 85
Stem cells 109168
Stimulation protocol 127
mild 151, 153*f*, 190
Stress 19
activates 19
management 154, 170
strategies 175
oxidative 17, 72, 113, 122, 156, 161, 171*f*, 176*f*
psychological 16, 171*f*, 175
reduction 19
Stressor, psychological 9
Submucosal fibroids 48
Substance use 18, 175
Subtle oocyte dysfunction 181
Sugars 172
Sulfur dioxide 17
Supplements 157, 158*t*
Surgery 226
advantages of 227*t*
disadvantages of 227*t*
limitations of 226
negative impact of 226
tubal 48
Surgical sperm retrieval 134
Surrogacy (Regulation) Act 201
Surrogacy
altruistic 210
commercial 210
ethics 210
gestational 210
laws 201, 213
regulations 205
Systemic immune response, alteration of 220
Systemic lupus erythematosus 68, 73

T

Tail defects 38
Telehealth solutions 191
Telemedicine 52
Teratozoospermia 33
monomorphic 33
Testicle 75*f*
Testicular
dysgenesis syndrome 16
fragments 75*f*
homogenates 75*f*
parenchyma 75*f*
specimens 75*f*
sperm
aspiration 74
cryopreservation 73
extraction 32, 73, 74, 75*f*
retrieval techniques 75*f*
use of 130
tissue 75*f*
Testis 75*f*, 134
Testosterone 28, 111
Thalassemia 100
Thiotepa 139
Thrombophilia screening 183
Thyroid
disorders 217
function testing 27
Traditional preimplantation genetic testing 89

Trans-fatty acids 172
Transforming growth factor beta 43, 164
Transgender 69, 200
Triglyceride 217
Trophectoderm 78, 89
  biopsy 102
Tubal
  block 199
  damage 220
  factor 182
    infertility 48*f*
  flushing 49
  patency 51, 57
    assessment 183
    bilateral 48*f*
    primary evaluation of 48
  pathology 5
Tuberculin syringe 74*f*
Tubules
  enlarged 75*f*
  nonenlarged 75*f*
Tunica albuginea 134
Turner syndrome 69, 100
Tyrosine kinase inhibitiors 139

U

Ubiquinone 157
UK Human Fertilisation and Embryology Authority 211
Ultrasound
  contrast-enhanced 51, 52
  three-dimensional 47, 49, 50*f*
  transvaginal 45, 150
Unexplained infertility 5, 52, 57, 61, 171*f*, 181, 183*t*
Urinary chorionic gonadotropin 152*f*
Uterine 164, 165*f*
  anomalies, congenital 50
  cavity 48*f*, 50*f*
    abnormalities, assessment of 48
  disorders 166, 166*t*
  perforation 48
  transplants 213
Uterosacral ligaments 109
Uterus 109

V

Varicocele 40, 171*f*
  repair 40
Varicocelectomy 130, 132
Vascular endothelial growth factor 164, 174
Vasoepididymostomy 133, 134*t*
Vasovasostomy 133, 134*t*
Vinblastine 139
Vinca alkaloids 139
Vincristine 139
Viscosity 35
Vitamin 159, 171*f*, 172
  B 174
  C 160
  D 62, 172, 218
    receptor 174
  E 160
Vitrification 69, 71, 72
  effect of 216
  progress in 76

W

Weight
  loss 153, 154
  management 19
Western diet 18, 173
White blood cells 37
Whole ovary biopsy 73
Whole-genome amplification 89, 95, 96
Wilms' tumors 216
Wingless pathway 111
World Health Organization 149, 182
  semen analysis reference values 36*t*

Y

Y-chromosome
  deletion 216
  microdeletion testing 129, 131

Z

Zinc 160, 172, 174
Zona
  binding, defective 181
  hardening 72